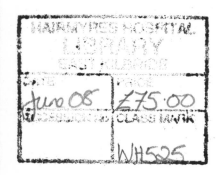

LYMPHOMA

Pathology, Diagnosis and Treatment

Major advances have occurred in almost every aspect of the diagnosis and treatment of lymphoma in recent years. Our understanding of the molecular biology and genetics of the disease has increased exponentially, and significant developments in imaging of this malignancy have resulted in earlier and more accurate diagnosis. At the same time, advances in therapeutic immunology have led to the development of several new treatment options.

This landmark new text describes these advances in a single concise volume, placing them in the context of daily clinical practice. Introductory chapters review epidemiology, prognostic factors, imaging and therapeutic immunology. These are followed by chapters on each lymphoma subtype, dealing comprehensively with all aspects of the diagnosis and treatment of the disorder.

Unique features

- Pathology and cytogenetics information is fully integrated into the discussion of each disease entity, enabling the reader to review all the key diagnostic information for each disorder in one place.
- Treatment algorithms are provided for each lymphoma subtype to guide the reader through the decision-making process for first- and second-line treatment strategies.

Highly illustrated in full color throughout and written and edited by the leading authorities in the field, *Lymphoma: Pathology, Diagnosis and Treatment* provides all the information needed to diagnose and manage these complex disorders.

Robert Marcus is Consultant Haematologist at Addenbrooke's NHS Foundation Trust, and Assistant Lecturer in Pathology, University of Cambridge.

John Sweetenham is Professor of Medicine at the Cleveland Clinic Lerner College of Medicine of Case Western Reserve University, and Director of Clinical Research at the Cleveland Clinic Taussig Cancer Center.

Michael Williams is the Byrd S. Leavell Professor of Medicine and Professor of Pathology, and Director of the Hematologic Malignancy Program, Hematology/Oncology Division and Cancer Center of the University of Virginia School of Medicine.

LYMPHOMA

Pathology, Diagnosis and Treatment

Edited by

Robert Marcus MB FRCP FRCPath
Addenbrooke's NHS Foundation Trust, Cambridge

John W. Sweetenham DM FRCP
Cleveland Clinic Lerner College of Medicine, Case Western
Reserve University

Michael E. Williams MD FACP
University of Virginia School of Medicine, Charlottesville

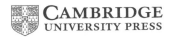
CAMBRIDGE
UNIVERSITY PRESS

CAMBRIDGE UNIVERSITY PRESS
Cambridge, New York, Melbourne, Madrid, Cape Town, Singapore, São Paulo

Cambridge University Press
The Edinburgh Building, Cambridge CB2 8RU, UK

Published in the United States of America by Cambridge University Press, New York

www.cambridge.org
Information on this title: www.cambridge.org/9780521865449

First published 2007
Reprinted 2007

Printed in the United Kingdom at the University Press, Cambridge

A catalog record for this publication is available from the British Library

ISBN 978-0-521-86544-9 hardback

Every effort has been made in preparing this book to provide accurate and up-to-date information which is in accord with accepted standards and practice at the time of publication. Although case histories are drawn from actual cases, every effort has been made to disguise the identities of the individuals involved. Nevertheless, the authors, editors and publishers can make no warranties that the information contained herein is totally free from error, not least because clinical standards are constantly changing through research and regulation. The authors, editors and publishers therefore disclaim all liability for direct or consequential damages resulting from the use of material contained in this book. Readers are strongly advised to pay careful attention to information provided by the manufacturer of any drugs or equipment that they plan to use.

CONTENTS

Contents

CONTRIBUTORS

Neil L. Berinstein
Toronto–Sunnybrook Regional Cancer Centre,
2075 Bayview Avenue, Toronto, Ontario M4N 3M5,
Canada

Francesco Bertoni
Functional Genomics Unit, Laboratory of
Experimental Oncology, Oncology Institute of
Southern Switzerland, 6500 Bellinzona, Switzerland

Kristian Bowles
Department of Haematology, Addenbrooke's
NHS Trust, Cambridge CB2 2QQ, UK
Current address: Norfolk & Norwich
NHS Trust, Norwich NR4 7UY, UK

Guillaume Cartron
Equipe EA 3853, Immuno-Pharmaco-Genétique des
Anticorps Thérapeutiques, Université François
Rabelais, 37000 Tours, France

Lisa M. DeAngelis
Department of Neurology, Memorial Sloan-Kettering
Cancer Center, 1275 York Avenue, New York,
NY 10021, USA

Adrian K. Dixon
Department of Radiology, Addenbrooke's NHS Trust,
Cambridge CB2 2QQ, UK

Martin Dreyling
University Hospital Grosshadern, Department of
Internal Medicine III, Ludwig Maximilians
University, 81377 Munich, Germany

Andreas Engert
First Department of Internal Medicine, University
Hospital Cologne, 50924 Cologne, Germany

Andrew M. Evens
Division of Hematology/Oncology, Department
of Medicine, Northwestern University Feinberg
School of Medicine, 303 E Superior Street, Chicago,
IL 60611, USA

Andrés J. M. Ferreri
Medical Oncology Unit, Department of Oncology,
San Raffaele H. Scientific Institute, Via Olgettina 60,
20132 Milan, Italy

Susan M. Geyer
Division of Hematology, Mayo Clinic College of
Medicine, Rochester, MN 55901, USA

Thomas M. Habermann
Division of Hematology, Mayo Clinic College of
Medicine, Rochester, MN 55901, USA

Eugenia Haralambieva
Institute of Pathology, University of Würzburg,
Josef-Schneider-Str 2, Würzburg 97080,
Germany

Peter Hillmen
Department of Haematology, Leeds Teaching
Hospitals NHS Trust, Leeds General Infirmary, Great
George Street, Leeds LS1 3EX, UK

Daniel Hodson
Department of Haematology, Addenbrooke's
NHS Trust, Cambridge CB2 2QQ, UK

Robert Marcus
Department of Haematology, Addenbrooke's NHS
Trust, Cambridge CB2 2QQ, UK

Beverly P. Nelson
Section of Hematopathology, Department of
Pathology, Northwestern University Feinberg School
of Medicine, 303 E Superior Street, Chicago,
IL 60611, USA

German Ott
Institute of Pathology, University of Würzburg,
Josef-Schneider-Str 2, Würzburg 97080, Germany

Mujahid A. Rizvi
Division of Hematology/Oncology, Department of
Medicine, Northwestern University Feinberg School
of Medicine, 303 E Superior Street, Chicago,
IL 60611, USA

Eve Roman
Epidemiology and Genetics Unit, Department
of Health Sciences, University of York,
York YO10 5DD, UK

Steven T. Rosen
Robert H. Lurie Comprehensive Cancer Center,
Northwestern University Feinberg School of
Medicine, 303 E Superior Street, Chicago,
IL 60611, USA

Andreas Rosenwald
Institute of Pathology, University of Würzburg, Josef-
Schneider-Str 2, Würzburg 97080, Germany

Stephanie Sasse
First Department of Internal Medicine, University
Hospital Cologne, 50924 Cologne, Germany

Julia Scarisbrick
St John's Institute of Dermatology, Guy's and
St Thomas' Hospital, Lambeth Palace Road,
London SE1 7EH, UK

Ashley S. Shaw
Department of Radiology, Addenbrooke's NHS Trust,
Cambridge CB2 2QQ, UK

Philippe Solal-Céligny
Centre Jean Bernard, 9 rue Beauverger, 72000 Le
Mans, France

Michele Spina
Division of Medical Oncology A, National Cancer
Institute, Via Pedemontana occidentale 12, 33081
Aviano (PN), Italy

John W. Sweetenham
Cleveland Clinic Foundation, Hematology and
Oncology/R35, 9500 Euclid Avenue, Cleveland,
OH 44195, USA

Umberto Tirelli
Division of Medical Oncology A, National Cancer
Institute, Via Pedemontana occidentale 12, 33081
Aviano (PN), Italy

Alan S. Wayne
Pediatric Oncology Branch, Center for Cancer
Research, National Cancer Institute, 9000 Rockville
Pike, Bethesda, MD 20892, USA

Sean Whittaker
St John's Institute of Dermatology, Guy's and St
Thomas' Hospital, Lambeth Palace Road, London SE1
7EH, UK

Eleanor V. Willett
Epidemiology and Genetics Unit, Department
of Health Sciences, University of York,
York YO10 5DD, UK

Michael E. Williams
Hematology/Oncology Division, University of
Virginia Health System, Jefferson Park Avenue,
Charlottesville, VA 22908, USA

Wyndham H. Wilson
Lymphoma Therapeutics Section, Metabolism
Branch, Center for Cancer Research, National
Cancer Institute, 9000 Rockville Pike, Bethesda,
MD 20892, USA

Andrew Wotherspoon
Department of Histopathology, Royal Marsden
Hospital, Fulham Road, London SW3 6JJ, UK

Emanuele Zucca
Lymphoma Unit, Oncology Institute of Southern
Switzerland, Ospedale San Giovanni, 6500 Bellinzona,
Switzerland

PREFACE

Why publish a book on lymphoma in 2007? Surely there are sufficient reviews, meetings and published educational symposia to make such a work redundant. Furthermore, doesn't instant access to online information make any work in print out of date before it appears?

The editors and authors of this work think not. We firmly believe that there is still a place for a clear summary of the diagnosis, staging and therapy of lymphoma in a single volume that reflects the advances in these areas which have taken place over the past five years. The problem with the plethora of information now available is that it is rarely set in a framework of understanding of the major challenges which still face those involved with the diagnosis and therapy of non-Hodgkin's and Hodgkin's lymphomas. We, and our patients, are confronted with many facts but little judgment. This work is our modest attempt to rectify this.

Accordingly the layout of the book should enable the reader to gain an understanding of patterns of disease, methods of staging, principles of new approaches to therapy, and interpretation of clinical trials and prognostic markers by reading the first part of the book. In the second part the reader will find separate succinct yet comprehensive reviews of the individual disease entities which make up the spectrum of diseases comprising the lymphomas. Here we have integrated pathology, molecular biology and therapy for each subtype into a single chapter; the reader will not need to flick backwards and forwards to gain a comprehensive understanding of, say, follicular or diffuse large B-cell lymphoma. Such an integration has posed significant editorial challenges, and has been made possible by a willingness on the part of Dr Wotherspoon, Dr Rosenwald and co-workers to accept that their contributions on histopathology and molecular cytogenetics would be divided and distributed among the relevant chapters. The editors are most grateful for their support.

Each chapter is followed by a select bibliography rather than an exhaustive list of references. We feel that these date very quickly, take up disproportionate amounts of space and are better found by internet searches or perusal of current journals.

This book is intended for senior trainees and fellows in hematology and oncology, together with more experienced practitioners who regularly treat these disorders. It is not intended for those who may feel they could have written the chapters themselves. It is also not a book where the reader will find detailed descriptions of rarities seen once in a professional lifetime.

The appearance of this volume comes at an opportune time: we have seen over the past five years a profound understanding of the pathology of lymphoma, the use of increasingly sophisticated imaging techniques, and the integration of monoclonal antibodies into standard therapy for NHL. Our hope is that these radical changes in the way we diagnose and treat lymphoma have been reflected in the book and will stand the reader in good stead even when newer data become available.

The editors express their sincere and heartfelt thanks to all the authors, who have, in the main, responded promptly to our comments and recommendations, and to all those at Cambridge University Press who have helped with this project: Richard Barling, who set the wheels of this vehicle in motion, and especially Betty Fulford and Deborah Russell, who kept it moving to its final destination whenever it threatened to stall.

Part I

LYMPHOMA OVERVIEW

1 EPIDEMIOLOGY

Eleanor V. Willett and Eve Roman

INTRODUCTION

Lymphomas, a heterogeneous group of malignancies arising in the lymphoid tissue, account for over 3% of cancers occurring worldwide. Most lymphomas are B-cell in origin, with a minority being T-cell. These cancers are primarily divided into Hodgkin's (HL) and non-Hodgkin's lymphomas (NHL), where HLs are B-cell malignancies distinguishable by the presence of Reed–Sternberg cells, and NHLs are of either B- or T-cell origin. A few inherited disorders, immunosuppressive drug therapies and certain viruses are known to be associated with specific types of lymphoma. However, for the most part, little is currently known about the etiology of lymphomas. The heterogeneous nature and inconsistent definitions of the specific lymphomas has hindered the identification of potential risk factors, but with the introduction of the Revised European–American Lymphoma (REAL) classification in 1994 and its 2001 successor, the World Health Organization Classification of Tumours of the Haematopoietic and Lymphoid Tissues, lymphomas are more consistently segregated on the basis of morphology, immunophenotype, and genetic and clinical features.

DESCRIPTIVE EPIDEMIOLOGY

With a view to elucidating potential causes of disease, descriptive epidemiological studies are routinely concerned with measures of disease incidence, prevalence, mortality and survival in well-defined populations and/or subgroups. For cancer, disease occurrence is commonly estimated from national, or specialist, cancer registries and the "population at risk" of disease from national, or local, census data.

Incidence estimates for NHL vary ten- to twelve-fold across countries, ranging from 1.6 to 17.1 cases per 100 000 persons per year among men and 0.7 to 11.7 cases per 100 000 persons per year among women. Among men, rates of NHL are highest in the United States, Canada and Australia and lowest in El Salvador, Mongolia and Fiji; for women, the highest NHL rates are observed in Israel, the United States and Canada and the lowest in El Salvador, Fiji and Bangladesh – although few reliable data are available from Africa (Fig. 1.1). In the UK, where the estimated incidence is relatively high compared to other parts of the world, NHL is diagnosed in 11.4 and 8.2 of 100 000 men and women respectively each year. Across all nations, more men than women are diagnosed with NHL, incidence increases with age, and data from the USA suggest that the incidence is greater among whites than blacks.

Hodgkin's lymphoma accounts for one-sixth of all lymphomas, with worldwide annual incidence estimates ranging from 0.2 to 5.7 and 0.1 to 4.9 per 100 000 men and women respectively. For both males and females, incidence is highest in the Middle East and eastern Europe, relatively high in other areas of Europe, North America and Australia, and lowest in East and South-East Asia (Fig. 1.2). Rates in the UK are 2.7 per 100 000 amongst men and 1.9 per 100 000 amongst women. Like NHL, HL tends to occur more often in men than women, and in whites more than blacks. The incidence of HL, however, has a bimodal pattern with age in developed countries, peaking at ages 15 to 34 and again at ages over 60, while in developing nations the higher rates are observed in the elderly (Fig. 1.3).

The estimated incidence of NHL has increased over time, whereas rates for HL have remained relatively constant. A rise in NHL occurrence has been reported

Lymphoma: Pathology, Diagnosis and Treatment, ed. Robert Marcus, John W. Sweetenham and Michael E. Williams. Published by Cambridge University Press. © Cambridge University Press 2007.

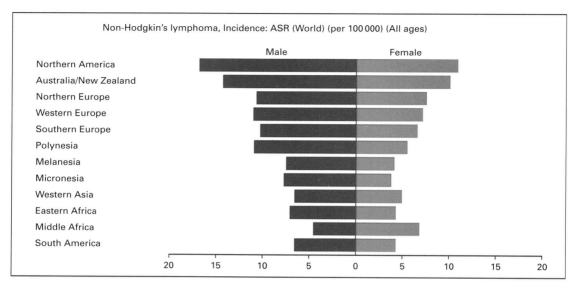

Figure 1.1. Incidence of non-Hodgkin's lymphoma by sex and region. (From *GLOBOCAN 2002.*)

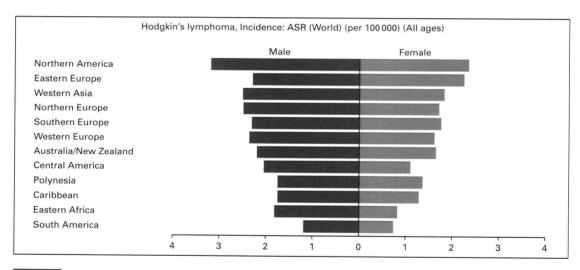

Figure 1.2. Incidence of Hodgkin's lymphoma by sex and region. (From *GLOBOCAN 2002.*)

for several countries, both sexes, all adult ages and ethnic groups, although the greatest increases have been observed among young white males and the elderly. Recent data suggest, however, that the rate of increase has begun to slow down. The increasing rates in the 1980s and 1990s have been attributed, at least in part, to improvements in diagnostic techniques, changes in the disease classification and completeness of cancer registration – as well as to the AIDS epidemic.

Current data suggest that the relative proportions of NHL subtypes vary worldwide. In the West, diffuse large B-cell lymphoma (DLBCL) and follicular lymphoma account for over 50% of NHL while other sub-entities, such as mantle cell lymphoma and peripheral T-cell lymphoma, are comparatively rare. The distribution in Eastern nations differs, with relative proportions of T-cell lymphomas being higher, and of follicular lymphoma and chronic lymphocytic

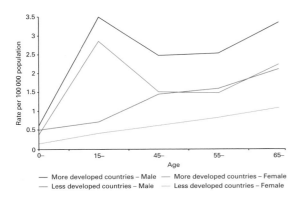

Figure 1.3. Incidence of Hodgkin's lymphoma in more and less developed countries by age and sex. (From *GLOBOCAN 2002.*)

leukemia being lower, than observed in the West. These disparities may reflect the under-presentation or detection of indolent lymphomas in the East, where access to diagnostic tools such as sensitive flow-cytometric methods for use on peripheral blood samples may be more limited. Among HL subtypes, nodular sclerosing HL is the most common, with mixed-cellularity/lymphocyte-depleted less common, and nodular lymphocyte-predominant HL being rare. Most NHL and HL subtypes are more common in men than women except for follicular lymphoma, marginal zone lymphoma and nodular sclerosing HL, where a slight female predominance is observed.

ETIOLOGY

The few known risk factors, such as particular inherited disorders, immunosuppressive drug therapies and certain viruses, are generally accepted to cause lymphoma through severe immunodeficiency. Mild immunosuppression and other alterations to immune function as a consequence of viruses, allergies, autoimmune disorders and ultraviolet light, for example – mediated by genes that influence immune response, such as interleukins and other cytokines – may lead to the development of lymphoma.

Genetics

A family history of lymphoma increases the risk of the disease, with the development of NHL or HL more likely if the relative affected is a sibling. These findings

may imply a genetic component in lymphoma pathogenesis, and there is evidence that the human leukocyte antigens (HLA) are involved in HL. Other variants in genes involved in DNA repair, immune response, xenobiotic metabolism and folate metabolism have generally produced, at best, modest associations with little consistency. Probably the most robust associations – with narrow confidence intervals and evidence of heterogeneity between the two most common diagnostic subgroups – have arisen from a large pooled analysis of 3600 cases and 4000 controls from eight European and North American case–control studies of NHL (Rothman *et al.* 2006). The investigation of 12 single nucleotide polymorphisms (SNPs) in nine cytokine genes suggested that persons homozygous for the A allele at TNF-α-308G >A SNP in the tumor necrosis factor-α (TNF-α) gene were at a 60% increased risk of DLBCL compared to those who were homozygous for the G allele; an association was also suggested between DLBCL and interleukin-10-3575T >A polymorphism. However, the function of these two SNPs remains unknown and the possibility that either SNP is in linkage disequilibrium with other SNPs in the same or neighboring genes cannot be ruled out.

Some interesting findings have been observed in familial studies for chronic lymphocytic leukemia (CLL), now classified as an NHL. Similar risks of CLL among subjects with affected siblings, parents and offspring were reported in one registry linkage study. Further to these observations, unaffected members of families with multiple CLL cases had a monoclonal B-lymphocyte expansion, described as a "CLL-like" phenotype, more often than a randomly selected group of adults. The comparatively high prevalence of this "CLL-like" phenotype in comparison to the occurrence of CLL suggests that a relatively common event initiates the phenotype, but a much rarer one is required for the occult disease to progress to CLL.

Primary/acquired immunosuppression

Rare inherited disorders of the immune system, such as ataxia telangiectasia, Wiskott–Aldrich syndrome and common variable hypogammaglobulinemia, are known in some instances to lead to lymphoma. Since relatives carrying the specific gene (e.g. the *ataxia-telangiectasia mutated* [*ATM*] gene) but without immunodeficiency symptoms are not at risk of

Table 1.1. Human viruses associated with lymphoma.

Virus	Lymphoma	Consistency of association
Human T-cell leukemia virus 1	Adult T-cell leukemia/lymphoma	100%
Epstein–Barr virus	Burkitt's lymphoma	Endemic 98%
		Sporadic < 30%
		Human immunodeficiency virus (HIV) 40%
	Hodgkin's lymphoma	Developed countries 40%
		Developing countries and HIV > 90%
	Post-transplant lymphoproliferative disorder early polymorphic monomorphic	Highest frequency in early onset (<1 year)
Human herpesvirus 8	Plasmablastic non-Hodgkin's lymphoma	Higher frequency in HIV patients
	Primary effusion lymphoma	100%

Sources: M. K. Gandhi and R. Khanna, *Pathology* **37** (2005), 420–433; R. F. Jarrett, *J. Pathol.* **208** (2006), 176–186.

lymphoma, the associated severe immunodepression, rather than the underlying genetic trait, may cause the lymphoma.

The autoimmune conditions rheumatoid arthritis, Sjögren's syndrome, systemic lupus erythematosus (SLE), celiac disease, dermatitis herpetiformis, psoriasis, Crohn's disease and ulcerative colitis are associated with lymphoma. The suspected causal agents include the immunosuppressive therapies azathioprine and methotrexate and the tumor necrosis factor-α blockers infliximab and etanercept, but although an additional effect of these drugs on lymphoma risk cannot be excluded, the severity of the autoimmune disease could also be responsible. Little data are available by lymphoma subtype, but more diffuse large B-cell lymphomas than expected develop among patients with rheumatoid arthritis or SLE, while more T-cell lymphomas are diagnosed among those with celiac disease. Like some autoimmune diseases, atopic conditions stimulate the immune system and impair T-cell function, but little association between lymphoma and atopic dermatitis, hayfever or asthma has been reported.

Infections

Viruses have been implicated in the etiology of several cancers, including lymphoma. A minority of specific lymphoma subtypes are linked with human T-cell leukemia/lymphotropic virus 1 (HTLV-1), Epstein–Barr virus (EBV) and human herpesvirus 8 (HHV-8) (Table 1.1). Human immunodeficiency virus (HIV) and hepatitis C virus (HCV) may be involved in lymphoma pathogenesis although it is likely that, for the most part, the roles of these viruses are indirect. Other suspected viral agents include simian virus 40 (SV40) but evidence is currently inconsistent.

HTLV-1, a deltaretrovirus, causes adult T-cell leukemia/lymphoma (ATLL). The geographical distribution of ATLL follows the regions where the virus is endemic, namely Japan, parts of South America, the Caribbean, central Africa, Melanesia, Papua New Guinea and the Solomon Islands. In other areas of the world, persons at risk of ATLL are immigrants from endemic areas and intravenous drug users positive for HTLV-1. It is suggested from Japanese data that 7% of male and 2% of female HTLV-1 carriers will develop ATLL, with the highest risks amongst those infected at a young age.

The ubiquitous herpesvirus EBV is involved in several types of lymphoma, particularly Burkitt's lymphoma (BL), HL and lymphomas in immunosuppressed individuals. EBV genomes are found in almost all cases of endemic BL, a childhood tumor prevalent in equatorial Africa and Papua New Guinea in areas with high exposure to malaria, in <30% of sporadic BL which occur elsewhere, and in 40% of

HIV-associated BL. EBV-positive HLs comprise 30–50% of HL tumors in developed, and 50–95% in developing, countries. In developing regions, primary exposure to EBV occurs in childhood, where the virus is usually asymptomatic, while in developed nations, first infection is often delayed until adolescence, resulting in infectious mononucleosis. However, EBV-positive HLs do not explain the young adult peak in HL incidence in industrialized nations but are diagnosed more often at younger and older ages. EBV infection is controlled by cytotoxic T-lymphocyte (CTL) responses and so, among persons with primary, acquired or iatrogenic immunosuppression where the CTL response is compromised, EBV-associated lymphomas can occur. Probably the most investigated of these are the post-transplant lymphoproliferative disorders (PTLD), a heterogeneous group of conditions that arise as a consequence of the associated or drug-induced immunosuppression following organ transplantation. EBV is found in the majority of PTLDs, with the greatest likelihood of EBV-positive disease within a year or two of transplantation. Other rarer lymphomas that are EBV-associated include primary effusion lymphoma (PEL) and T/NK-cell lymphoma, particularly of the nasal type. Within all EBV-associated lymphomas EBV is clonal, suggesting viral infection occurs prior to the proliferation of the malignant clone. A causal role for EBV is not necessarily implied, however, and given that the vast majority of adults have been exposed to EBV infection, the EBV-positive lymphomas, at least at older ages, may arise from some host : virus imbalance.

HHV-8 (also known as Kaposi's sarcoma herpesvirus) is associated with several benign and malignant lymphoproliferative disorders. It is detected in a plasmablastic variant of multicentric Castleman's disease, a benign condition which in some cases can transform into HHV-8-positive plasmablastic lymphoma. HHV-8 is also found in all cases of the rare lymphoma PEL. Many PEL tumor cells are co-infected with EBV, but HHV-8 is thought to be the main transforming virus. For the majority of NHLs, however, HHV-8 does not appear to be a major etiological factor, and while this virus and other human herpesviruses, type 6 (HHV-6) and type 7 (HHV-7), are present in HL biopsies, their low prevalence in HL tumors probably reflects impaired immunosurveillance rather than a role in pathogenesis.

The immunosuppressive retrovirus HIV substantially increases the risk of lymphoma. Monoclonal HIV is seldom integrated into lymphoma tumor cells and so, in most instances, HIV leads to lymphoma through immunosuppression or B-cell activation. Other viruses are observed in HIV-associated lymphomas, with EBV being present in more than 50% of cases and HHV-8 more rarely. HIV-associated NHLs are predominantly aggressive lymphomas such as BL with plasmacytoid differentiation, DLBCL, PEL and plasmablastic lymphoma of the oral cavity. HL also develops in some HIV patients, with almost all cases being EBV-positive and from the poorer prognostic subtypes of mixed-cellularity and lymphocyte-depleted. Since the introduction of highly active antiretroviral therapy, the risk of HIV-associated lymphomas, particularly those of the central nervous system, has declined.

An association between HCV and lymphoma was first suspected when some patients with essential mixed cryoglobulinemia, an autoimmune condition with 90% HCV seropositivity, developed lymphoplasmacytoid NHL. HCV prevalence is much lower in the general population but varies widely geographically, ranging from around 12% in Italy and Japan to 1% in other Western countries. Recent epidemiological studies conducted in areas of both high and low prevalence suggest HCV is associated with B-cell NHL. Since HCV is an RNA virus incapable of integrating into host-cell DNA, the virus is not directly oncogenic and its involvement in lymphoma is probably related to chronic antigenic stimulation.

Poliovirus vaccines administered to millions of people across the USA and Europe from 1955 to 1962 were contaminated with SV40, a primate polyomavirus. Involvement of SV40 in lymphoma etiology has been suspected since lymphomas, as well as other malignancies, can develop in rodents exposed to SV40. In humans, the virus has been detected in some series of NHL DNA, but not in others. These inconsistent observations could be explained by, for instance, differences in polymerase chain reaction (PCR) testing methods, and since the virus was detected with low copy number, PCR contamination or other laboratory artifact. Epidemiological studies have been more consistent in suggesting that SV40 is not a risk factor for lymphoma. Investigations of birth cohorts likely to have received the contaminated poliovirus vaccine reported similar lymphoma incidence to other birth cohorts where SV40 exposure from the vaccine was unlikely. While a high proportion of individuals born during the 1955–62 period received the contaminated vaccine, specific antibody responses against SV40 were detectable after the injected formaldehyde inactivated (IPV) poliovirus vaccine but not with the oral attenuated live (OPV) vaccine; moreover, SV40 antibodies are present in persons born after this period, suggesting human-to-human SV40 transmission. Serological measurement of SV40 antibodies provides a direct measurement of SV40 exposure and two case–control studies found no difference in the SV40 seroprevalence among lymphoma cases and unaffected controls.

Bacterial, as well as viral, infections have been suspected in the etiology of lymphoma, particularly of extranodal marginal zone lymphomas that occur in mucosa-associated lymphoid tissue (MALT). Chronic inflammation caused by persistent bacterial infection is thought to encourage development of MALT, and so possibly lymphoma, in organs such as the gastrointestinal tract, ocular adnexa and skin which are normally devoid of native lymphoid tissue. The most established association is between gastric MALT lymphoma and *Helicobacter pylori*. Infection with *H. pylori* can persist for decades in the stomach, where the organism can cause lymphoid follicles and so MALT to develop. The link with these lymphomas was first made in 1991, when the majority of gastric MALT lymphomas in one case series were found to be infected with *H. pylori*. Although this study could not confirm that the infection preceded the lymphoma, it has subsequently been shown that lymphoma B-cell clones are present in biopsy specimens of chronic gastritis taken before the onset of lymphoma, and that lymphoma growth can be stimulated in cultured *H. pylori* strain-specific T cells when crude lymphoma cells were exposed to the organism in vitro. Case–control studies have also reported increased risks of gastric lymphoma following prior *H. pylori* infection. Furthermore, treating the organism with antibiotics has caused, in 75% of cases, the gastric lymphoma to regress, with many patients sustaining remission after several years of follow-up.

Immunoproliferative small intestinal disease (IPSID), a MALT lymphoma arising in the small intestine, can also be successfully treated in the early stages with antibiotics. This suggests that, like the majority of gastric MALT lymphomas, IPSID is bacterial in origin. Following identification of *Campylobacter*

jejuni in intestinal tissue from an IPSID patient, Lecuit *et al.* found evidence of the infection in a further four of six cases. Unlike *H. pylori*, however, *C. jejuni* does not appear to persist in the host and future work is required to determine whether infection by this organism occurs as a consequence of altered immunity or whether it is truly a precursor for this rare lymphoma.

Borrelia burgdorferi has been suspected of causing primary cutaneous marginal zone lymphomas. Evidence of *B. burgdorferi* infection in lymphoma tissue has been reported in several European cases. *B. burgdorferi*, which is transmitted by tick bites, has some parallels with *H. pylori* in its potential to induce lymphoma. The organism is capable of persisting in the host despite immune response and it can induce the development of acquired lymphoid tissue in organs where lymphoid tissue is not normally present. Moreover, treatment of the *B. burgdorferi* infection with antibiotics has led to the regression of early-stage primary cutaneous marginal zone lymphomas. However, some US series of these lymphomas have not found *B. burgdorferi* DNA in lesional skin. The geographical difference between Europe and the USA may be explained by the epidemiology of the organism's genospecies as *B. burgdoferi sensu stricto*, *B. garinii* and *B. afzelli* have been isolated in Europe while only the first has been detected in the USA.

Another bacterial infection suspected of involvement in MALT lymphomas is *Chlamydophila psittaci* (formerly *Chlamydia psittaci*), although published data are preliminary. Ferreri *et al.* first detected this microorganism in 80% of ocular adnexal lymphomas in an Italian case series and reported evidence of lymphoma regression among a small sample of cases treated with antibiotics. Subsequent case series of ocular adnexal lymphomas from other parts of the world had lower proportions, and often no cases, with *C. psittaci* DNA.

Delayed exposure to infections has been proposed as a possible explanation of the young-adult peak in HL incidence. Recent studies show little association between HL and low number of childhood infections, low birth order, small sibship size and other surrogate markers for late exposure to infections, although few report risks among young adults. Without exposure to infections, T helper type 1 (Th1) lymphocyte reactions are not developed, and the human body instead mounts a Th2 immune response. The hypothesis of delayed infection has now been considered for NHL, with a few preliminary reports examining similar proxy variables. Whether early exposure to a specific infection protects against lymphoma remains unanswered, but perhaps the most consistent decreased risks exist for measles, a virus which is present in some lymphoma tumors.

Other medical conditions and therapies

Hodgkin's and non-Hodgkin's lymphomas occur in patients diagnosed with a previous cancer, and both lymphomas can precede other malignancies. Although chemo- and radiotherapies are possible causes, some cancers were treated with neither, and genetic alterations or immunodepression from lymphoma or surgery may be responsible.

While long-term immunosuppressive drug therapy is an accepted risk factor for lymphoma, evidence for other medications remains inconclusive. Antibiotics and sulphonamides have been positively associated with lymphoma, although underlying infection could explain the increased risks with these drugs. Nonsteroidal anti-inflammatory drugs (NSAIDs) are anticipated to protect against lymphoma since NSAIDs inhibit cyclooxygenase-catalysed synthesis of proinflammatory prostaglandins, and further, aspirin can block nuclear factor κB, a transcription factor essential for immune function and survival of lymphoma cells. The direction of risk estimates with aspirin and other NSAIDs have however been mixed. There has been little consistency too in published findings for steroids, drugs with both immuno-suppressive and anti-inflammatory properties. Treatments for hypertension and high cholesterol have been linked with decreased risks while anti-depressants, psychotropics and histamine-2 blockers have generally shown no association with lymphoma.

Since the greatest sex difference in HL incidence occurs between the ages of 25 and 44, with women having lower rates than men, high levels of estrogen exposure may protect young women from this lymphoma. Studies of reproductive histories have provided some support for this hypothesis, but the evidence is inconclusive. Incidence of NHL is also lower among women than men, but contraceptive use, hormone replacement therapy, parity and other reproductive factors have largely shown little association with NHL or its subtypes.

Several case reports have been published describing the occurrence of diffuse large B-cell lymphoma following replacement of hip and knee joints, although epidemiological studies have yet to support this association. The metallic implants are suspected of being carcinogenic, but it is also possible that inflammation or infection could be involved. It has also been suggested that hemophiliacs, and those who have undergone blood transfusions, may be at increased risk due to the transmission of viruses such as HCV.

Radiation

Lymphoma appears not to be associated with low-dose ionizing radiation, radiofrequency electromagnetic fields or power-frequency electromagnetic fields. Recently, the potential role of ultraviolet radiation in lymphomagenesis has received some attention since UV rays, particularly UVB, can cause immunosuppression. Contrary to the hypothesized positive association, protective effects have been reported with various proxy variables for UV exposure, including latitude, outdoor work, recreational exposure, number of vacations, use of sunlamps and sunbathing. Vitamin D is suggested to protect against other cancers, but this fails to explain the occasional occurrence of lymphoma among skin cancer patients, and vice versa.

Occupation

Certain occupations and related exposures have been extensively studied for NHL, but less so for HL. Farmers and agricultural workers may be at increased risk of NHL, possibly due to exposure to pesticides or animals. Several groups of pesticides, such as organophos-phates, organochlorines, phenoxy herbicides, carbamates and atrazines, have been linked with NHL, but identification of a specific compound is difficult given the frequent use of multiple products. Positive associations with animal exposures are more consistent for cattle than for other livestock, perhaps suggesting a bovine viral agent, but butchers, meat processors and packers do not appear to be at risk of NHL.

Exposure to solvents may increase the risk of lymphoma. Benzene, a known leukemogen, is however probably not a risk factor for lymphoma. Recent studies of workers exposed to styrene, ethylene oxide, butadiene and tetrachloroethylene, as well as those employed in the synthetic rubber, chemical, printing,

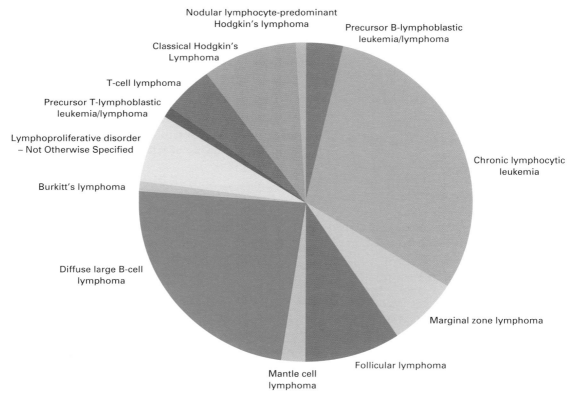

Figure 1.4. Distribution of WHO lymphoma subtypes, based on incidence data in the Yorkshire and Humberside Strategic Health Authority, 2004–5 (www.hmrn.org).

painting, leather and dry-cleaning industries could not definitely confirm associations between solvents and either NHL or HL.

HL may be associated with exposure to wood dust. Cotton dust may also increase the risk of HL as excesses of this lymphoma have been reported among textile workers, tailors, sewers and dress-makers. Organic dusts seem less likely to cause NHL.

Lifestyle

Tobacco smoke shows little consistent association with NHL, most NHL subtypes and HL. An increased risk of follicular lymphoma is suggested, although convincing dose–response trends have rarely been reported. Emerging epidemiological evidence sup-ports a smoking relationship specific to EBV-positive, as opposed to EBV-negative, HL, possibly caused by CD95/CD95L (Fas/FasL)-mediated apoptosis of

Hodgkin/Reed–Sternberg cells being inhibited by both EBV and tobacco smoke.

Alcohol, particularly wine, may decrease the risk of NHL and its subtypes, although evidence is inconsist-ent; studies of HL are fewer and inconclusive. Similarly, investigations of diet lack consistency, but some general patterns have been observed. Consumption of vegeta-bles, fruit and grains may decrease the risk of lym-phoma while dairy products, fat, animal protein and total food intake may elevate the risk; no associations were observed with intake of coffee, tea, folate or vita-min B12. Use of hair dyes has previously been asso-ciated with NHL, but more recent data suggest no effect for NHL, its subtypes or HL.

Several studies report positive associations between NHL and obesity, while others have not. Risks of dif-fuse large B-cell lymphoma generally rise with increas-ing body mass index, patterns for follicular lymphoma are less consistent, and little data are available for rarer

NHL subtypes. Findings for HL are inconsistent, although positive associations have been observed among men. Polymorphisms in genes involved in energy homeostasis which can also modulate immune response, such as leptin, leptin receptor, adiponectin and ghrelin, have been related to NHL but these polymorphisms do not modulate the risk of NHL associated with body mass index.

SUMMARY

While many agents have been proposed, there are few that have been accepted as risk factors for lymphoma. Most potential risk factors cause modulation to the immune system, either through immunodeficiency or chronic inflammation. Probably the largest area of interest for lymphoma etiology is infections, and, while several viral and bacterial agents have been proposed, further work is required to confirm observed associations. Few of the investigated environmental exposures appear to be involved in lymphoma, with perhaps the exception of pesticides. One of the major problems in identifying risk factors for lymphoma has been the heterogeneity of this group of malignancies. More consistent diagnostic techniques, which continue to be improved and modified, have identified more homogeneous subtypes of lymphoma (Fig. 1.4). Availability of these better-quality pathological diagnostic data has enabled the most recent epidemiological studies to explore risks by the distinct disease subtypes. The frequency of the rarer subtypes within some individual studies has been low and so sufficient power to detect risks may only be achieved through collaborative study.

FURTHER READING

Clarke, C. A. and Glaser, S. L. Changing incidence of non-Hodgkin lymphomas in the United States. *Cancer* **94** (2002), 2015–2023.

Farinha, P. and Gascoyne, R. D. *Helicobacter pylori* and MALT lymphoma. *Gastroenterology* **128** (2005), 1579–1605.

Ferreri, A. J., Guidoboni, M., Ponzoni, M. *et al.* Evidence for an association between *Chlamydia psittaci* and ocular adnexal lymphomas. *J. Natl. Cancer Inst.* **96** (2004), 586–594.

Gandhi, M. K. and Khanna, R. Viruses and lymphoma. *Pathology* **37** (2005), 420–433.

Harris, N. L. Hodgkin's disease: classification and differential diagnosis. *Mod. Pathol.* **12** (1999), 159–176.

Harris, N. L., Jaffe, E. S., Stein, H. *et al.* A revised European–American classification of lymphoid neoplasms: a proposal from the International Lymphoma Study Group. *Blood* **84** (1994), 1361–1392.

Harris, N. L., Jaffe, E. S., Diebold, J., Flandrin, G., Muller-Hermelink, H. K. and Vardiman, J. Lymphoma classification: from controversy to consensus. The R.E.A.L. and WHO Classification of lymphoid neoplasms. *Ann. Oncol.* **11** Suppl 1 (2000), 3–10.

IARC CancerBase. *GLOBOCAN 2002: Cancer Incidence, Mortality and Prevalence Worldwide* (Lyon: IARC Press, 2004).

Jaffe, E. S., Harris, N. L., Stein, H. and Vardiman, J. W. *World Health Organization Classification of Tumours: Pathology and Genetics of Tumours of Haematopoietic and Lymphoid Tissues* (Lyon: IARC Press, 2001).

Jarrett, R. F. Viruses and lymphoma/leukaemia. *J. Pathol.* **208** (2006), 176–186.

Lecuit, M., Abachin, E., Martin, A. *et al.* Immunoproliferative small intestinal disease associated with *Campylobacter jejuni*. *N. Engl. J. Med.* **350** (2004), 239–248.

Morton, L. M., Hartge, P., Holford, T. R. *et al.* Cigarette smoking and risk of non-Hodgkin lymphoma: a pooled analysis from the International Lymphoma Epidemiology Consortium (InterLymph). *Cancer Epidemiol. Biomarkers Prev.* **14** (2005), 925–933.

Morton, L. M., Zheng, T., Holford, T. R. *et al.* Alcohol consumption and risk of non-Hodgkin lymphoma: a pooled analysis. *Lancet Oncol.* **6** (2005), 469–476.

Rawstron, A. C., Green, M. J., Kuzmicki, A. *et al.* Monoclonal B lymphocytes with the characteristics of "indolent" chronic lymphocytic leukemia are present in 3.5% of adults with normal blood counts. *Blood* **100** (2002), 635–639.

Rothman, N., Skibola, C. F., Wang, S. S. *et al.* Genetic variation in TNF and IL10 and risk of non-Hodgkin lymphoma: a report from the InterLymph Consortium. *Lancet Oncol.* **7** (2006), 27–38.

Willett, E. V., O'Connor, S., Smith, A. G. and Roman, E. Does smoking or alcohol modify the risk of Epstein–Barr virus genome-positive or -negative Hodgkin lymphoma? *Epidemiology* **18** (2007), 130–136.

Willett, E. V., Skibola, C. F., Adamson, P. *et al.* Non-Hodgkin's lymphoma, obesity and energy homeostasis polymorphisms. *Br. J. Cancer* **93** (2005), 811–816.

2 PATHOLOGY AND CYTOGENETICS

Andrew Wotherspoon, German Ott, Eugenia Haralambieva and Andreas Rosenwald

PREPARATION OF SPECIMENS FOR HISTOLOGY AND CYTOLOGY

The diagnosis of hematolymphoid tumors requires a combination of morphological, immunophenotypic, molecular genetic and clinical data. Successful morphological analysis is easiest to achieve by examination of intact lymph nodes that have been excised whole with the capsule intact. Fragmentation, while difficult to avoid in some areas (such as the mediastinum), inhibits analysis. Core biopsies are increasingly used for the diagnosis of lymphoid-related conditions, but these should be restricted to cases in which nodal excision is difficult or impossible, due either to access-related problems (intra-abdominal location) or to patient-related factors. Core biopsies, by their very nature, represent a small percentage of the lesional tissue and may fail to demonstrate focal variations in the tumor such as a diffuse component in follicular lymphoma. Fine needle aspiration (FNA) cytology has a role to play in the diagnosis of lymphoid pathology, but is best performed where there is access to high-quality flow cytometry that allows immunophenotyping of the lymphoid cells. FNA is particularly useful in the head and neck region for the exclusion of metastatic tumour.

Choice of the lymph node for sampling is of great importance. Where there is choice of areas the inguinal region is best avoided, as these nodes frequently show distortion of the normal architecture by fibrosis. Cervical lymph nodes are most easily interpreted. Clearly the lymph node sampled should be one that is most likely to show the pathological changes, and in cases where transformation needs to be excluded, a node showing rapid enlargement should be chosen.

Ideally tissue should be rapidly transported to the pathology department in a fresh state. This allows preparation of imprint sections that can be used for cytological examination and fluorescence *in-situ* hybridization (FISH) studies, collection of fresh material for conventional cytogenetic studies and microbiologic studies (if appropriate), and preparation of frozen material for DNA and RNA analysis if required. The lymph node should be thinly sliced and allowed to fix in adequate amounts of fixative for an appropriate time. In the UK fixation is usually in buffered formalin for 12–24 hours. Longer fixation may inhibit antigen reactivity (although this may be compensated for by antigen retrieval processes), while under-fixation may irretrievably interfere with morphological preservation. Core biopsies provide limited tissue but this can be maximized by embedding separate cores in different blocks.

Histological sections should be cut at 3–5 μm and stained with hematoxylin and eosin. Staining with giemsa, periodic acid Schiff and reticulin may give valuable additional information. Immunophenotypic staining of lymphoid infiltrates is an essential part of the diagnosis of lymphoma. There is now a wide panel of immunological markers that are reactive in fixed paraffin embedded material and the need for frozen-section immunophenotyping has diminished, although some antigens remain undetectable in fixed tissue. Flow cytometry of solid tissues can be of use for antigens unreactive in fixed material and can be helpful in the detection of light chain expression and membrane immunoglobulin. Flow cytometry can also demonstrate co-expression of different antigens on the same cell, which can be difficult even on serial sections of embedded material.

Immunocytochemical staining is currently frequently performed using automated staining machines that allow a high throughput of cases and provide a constant and controlled environment. Retrieval of antigens that are masked by fixation is achieved using a mixture of heat (pressure cooker, microwave or both) and enzyme pre-treatment in an appropriate buffer. The exact pre-treatment required varies between antigens, laboratories and automated stainer. In all laboratories the staining runs should be performed with the inclusion of appropriate positive and negative control sections. All laboratories involved with hematolymphoid tumor diagnosis should participate in appropriate external quality-assurance schemes.

Immunocytochemical analysis should only be undertaken by individuals who are familiar with the patterns of reactivity of the antigens (cytoplasmic vs. membrane vs. nuclear) and the expected profiles seen in the various lymphoma types. Ideally immunological panels should be employed for analysis. Care must be taken to avoid the diagnostic pitfalls that are associated with aberrant antigen expressions and the antigen losses that are frequently associated with neoplastic lymphoid infiltrates, and the immunocytochemical stains must be interpreted in the context of the histological features of the infiltrate.

MOLECULAR AND CYTOGENETIC TECHNOLOGIES

Genotypic studies are of pivotal importance in the diagnosis of malignant lymphomas. The identification of clonally expanded lymphoid cells is possible, because lymphoid cells, in the process of maturation, rearrange their immunoglobulin heavy chain (IgH) and light chain (IgL) genes or their T-cell receptor genes. Other gene rearrangements, e.g. in chromosomal translocations, are also accessible to DNA rearrangement studies. The sensitivity of the Southern blot technique is estimated to be in the range of detecting 1–5% clonal cells in a given population. Since T and B cells rearrange their specific receptor genes, these analyses also distinguish T- and B-lineage neoplasms.

The sensitivity of the Southern blot technique can be greatly enhanced by use of the polymerase chain reaction (PCR) approach. The PCR represents a technique in which small amounts of DNA can be amplified in vitro by use of primers with DNA sequences flanking regions of interest. Because of the requirement for only minimal amounts of short-sequence DNA, the PCR technique can be used for the detection of clonal cell populations or DNA rearrangements also in paraffin-embedded formalin-fixed material (in which the DNA normally is largely degraded). Because of its high sensitivity, the PCR can also be employed in the monitoring of minimal residual disease (MRD), especially if clonotypic primers are used.

By DNA sequence analysis of Ig-receptor genes, non-mutated (naive) prefollicular and mutated (memory) postfollicular B cells can be distinguished. In follicular cell populations so-called "ongoing" somatic mutations are the reflection of the germinal-center-associated process called affinity maturation. The detailed analysis of Ig-receptor genes, therefore, allows us to reach conclusions about the status of antigen-dependent selection and mutation as well as the immunoglobulin heavy chain variable (IgV$_H$) gene repertoire.

CYTOGENETIC ANALYSES

Malignant lymphomas are well-characterized neoplasms from the cytogenetic perspective. Apart from proving the neoplastic nature of a lymphoid cell proliferation, the description of characteristic cytogenetic aberrations in certain types of malignant lymphomas has greatly added to our understanding of the biology of lymphoid neoplasms (Fig. 2.1), and

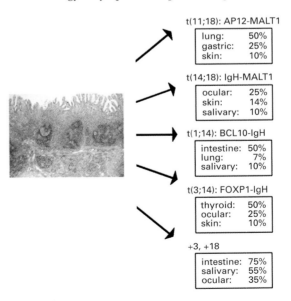

t(11;18): AP12-MALT1

lung:	50%
gastric:	25%
skin:	10%

t(14;18): IgH-MALT1

ocular:	25%
skin:	14%
salivary:	10%

t(1;14): BCL10-IgH

intestine:	50%
lung:	7%
salivary:	10%

t(3;14): FOXP1-IgH

thyroid:	50%
ocular:	25%
skin:	10%

+3, +18

intestine:	75%
salivary:	55%
ocular:	35%

Figure 2.1. Genetic alterations in MALT-type lymphomas. (From Streubel *et al.* 2004.)

Table 2.1. Overview of the most common and characteristic chromosome aberrations in malignant lymphoma.

Diagnosis	Chromosome aberration	Genes involved
Precursor B-lymphoblastic lymphoma/ leukemia	t(12;21)(p13;q22)	TEL/AML1
	t(1;19)(q23;p13)	E2A/PBX1
	t(4;11)(q21;q23)	AF4/MLL
	del(6q)	
	t(9;22)(q34;q11)	BCR/ABL
B-cell chronic lymphocytic leukemia / small lymphocytic lymphoma	del(13)(q14)	
	Trisomy 12	
	del(11)(q22–23)	ATM
	del(17)(p13)	TP53
Mantle cell lymphoma	t(11;14)(q13;q32)	Cyclin D1
Follicular lymphoma	t(14;18)(q32;q21)	BCL-2
Extranodal marginal zone B-cell lymphoma of MALT type	t(11;18)(q21;q21)	API2–MALT1
	t(1;14)(p22;q32)	BCL-10
	t(14;18)(q32;q21)	MALT1
	t(3;14)(p13;q32)	FOXP1
Splenic marginal zone B-cell lymphoma	t/del(7)(q22–32)	
	del(10)(q22–24)	
Diffuse large B-cell lymphoma	t(3;14)(q27;q32) and variants	BCL-6
	t(14;18)(q32;q21)	BCL-2
	t(8;14)(q24;q32)	MYC
Burkitt's lymphoma	t(8;14)(q24;q32)	MYC
	t(2;8)(p12;q24)	MYC
	t(8;22)(q24;q11)	MYC
Plasmacytoma	t(4;14)(p16;q32)	FGFR3/MMSET
	t(6;14)(p25;q32)	MUM1/IRF 4
	others	
	t(14;16)(q32;q23)	C-MAF
	t(11;14)(q13;q32)	Cyclin D1
Precursor T-lymphoblastic lymphoma/ leukemia	14q11	TCR genes
	7p15 or 7q34–35	TCR genes
T-cell prolymphocytic leukemia	inv(14)(q11q32)	TCL1
Angioimmunoblastic T-cell lymphoma	+3, +5, +X	
Anaplastic large cell lymphoma	t(2;5)(p23;q35) and variants	NPM/ALK and variants
Hepatosplenic γδ T-cell lymphoma	i(7)(q10)	
Enteropathy-type T-cell lymphoma	+9q33–34	

has also aided in the universal acceptance of specific separate entities. This principle, for example, is exemplified by the close association of mantle cell lymphoma with the translocation t(11;14)(q13;q32), the recognition of which ultimately led to the general acceptance of mantle cell lymphoma as an entity in its own right. Some of the most important and characteristic chromosomal aberrations in this and other malignant lymphomas are listed in Table 2.1, while Tables 2.2, 2.3 and 2.4 show typical immunophenotypes of B-cell non-Hodgkin's lymphomas, T-cell non-Hodgkin's lymphomas and Hodgkin's lymphoma.

Notwithstanding their importance in the definition of lymphoma entities, primary genetic alterations cannot be used as the sole criteria for the

Table 2.2. Typical immunophenotype of B-cell non-Hodgkin's lymphomas.

	CD20	CD79a	CD10	bcl-6	CD5	CD23	Cyclin D1	bcl-2	Others
Follicular lymphoma	+	+	+/−	+	−	−/+	−	+/−	MUM1−
Small lymphocytic lymphoma/chronic lymphocytic lymphoma	+	+	−	−	+	+	−	+	
Lymphoplasmacytic lymphoma	+	+	−	−	−	−	−	+	CD25−/+, CD11c−
B-cell prolymphocytic leukemia	+	+	−/+	−/+	−/+	−	−	+	
Hairy cell leukemia	+	+	−	−	−	−	−/+	+/−	DBA44+, TRAP+, CD25+, CD11c+
Nodal marginal zone lymphoma	+	+	−	−	−	−	−	+	CD11c−/+
Extranodal marginal zone lymphoma	+	+	−	−	−	−	−	+	CD11c−/+
Splenic marginal zone lymphoma	+	+	−	−	−	−	−	+	DBA44−/+, CD25−/+
Mantle cell lymphoma	+	+	−	−	+	−	+	+	MUM1−, CD11c−
Myeloma/plasmacytoma	−/+	+/−	−	−	−	−	−/+	−	MUM1+, CD138+, CD38+
Diffuse large B-cell lymphoma, germinal center type	+	+	+	+	−/+	−/+	−	+/−	MUM1−
Diffuse large B-cell lymphoma, non-germinal center type	+	+	−	−/+	−/+	−/+	−	+/−	MUM1+
Mediastinal large B-cell lymphoma	+	+	−/+	+	−	+/−	−	+	
Burkitt's lymphoma	+	+	+	+	−	−	−	−	MUM1−

classification of these tumors, because some lack well-defined aberrations, and because the same chromosomal translocation may be detected in different lymphoma entities. For example, the t(14;18) (q32;q21) is present in up to 85–90% of follicular lymphomas, but also in roughly 20% of diffuse large B-cell lymphomas (Fig. 2.2). In addition, characteristic cytogenetic alterations are present only in a fraction of a given lymphoma entity: 10–15% of typical follicular lymphomas, for example, are t(14;18)-negative.

More recently, the use of fluorescent dye-conjugated DNA probes in *in-situ* hybridization has overcome the fundamental shortcoming of conventional banding analyses, that is the need for viable dividing cells. The FISH technique can be performed on interphase cells also in paraffin-embedded material, thus allowing for the recognition of numerical or structural chromosome alterations without the need to cultivate cells. This technique is sometimes also referred to as "molecular cytogenetics."

The comparative genomic hybridization (CGH) technique provides an overview of genetic imbalances (over-representations and deletions) in malignant tumors derived from paraffin-embedded material and may be used to estimate overall genomic instability, which appears to constitute a new and important prognostic feature.

Table 2.3. Typical immunophenotype of T-cell non-Hodgkin's lymphomas.

	CD2	CD3	CD5	CD7	CD4	CD8	TIA-1	Granzyme	CD56	Others
T-cell prolymphocytic lymphoma	+	+	+	+	+	−/+	−	−	−	TCR-beta+
T large granular lymphocyte leukemia	+	+	+/−	+/−	−	+	+	+	−/+	TCR-beta+
Adult T-cell leukemia/ lymphoma	+	+/−	+	−	+	−	−	−	−	TCR-beta+, CD25 +, CD30+/−, EMA−, ALK-1−
Angioimmunoblastic T-cell lymphoma	+	+	+	+	+	−	−	−	−	CXCL13+
Peripheral T-cell lymphoma, unspecified	+	+	+	+	+	−	−/+	−	−	CD30+/−, perforin−, CXCL13−
Anaplastic large-cell lymphoma	+/−	−/+	−/+	+/−	+/−	−	+	+	−	CD25+, CD30+, ALK-1+/−, perforin+
Mycosis fungoides	+	+	+	+	+	−	−	−	−	TCR-beta+, CD30−/+,
Subcutaneous panniculitis-like T-cell lymphoma	+	+	+	+	−	+	+	+	−/+	TCR-beta+, perforin+
Enteropathy-type T-cell lymphoma	+	+	−	+	−	−/+	+	+	−/+	TCR-beta+, CD30+/−, perforin+
Hepatosplenic T-cell lymphoma	+	+	−	+	−	−	+	−	+/−	TCR-beta−, CD30−, perforin−
Extranodal NK-cell lymphoma, nasal type	+/−	−	−	+/−	−	−	+	+	+	TCR-beta−, CD30−/+, perforin+, CD3ε+

Table 2.4. Typical immunophenotype of Hodgkin's lymphoma.

	CD45	CD20	CD79a	CD10	bcl-6	CD30	CD15	EMA	J chain	Oct-2	Bob-1	MUM1	PAX5	Fascin
Nodular lymphocyte-predominant Hodgkin's lymphoma	+	+	+	−	+	−	−	+/−	+/−	+	+	−	+	−
Classical Hodgkin's lymphoma	−	−/+	−/+	−	−	+	+/−	−	−	−/+	−/+	+	+	+

In recent years, the development of high-throughput technologies and especially of DNA microarrays has allowed for the characterization of global transcriptional profiles in human tumors. In lymphomas, gene expression profiling using this technology has led to a more precise molecular classification of various lymphoma subtypes (Fig. 2.3), and in several lymphoma subgroups important gene expression-based survival predictors have been created that may help guide future treatment decisions (Fig. 2.4).

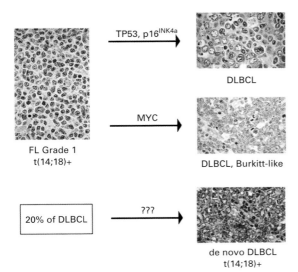

Figure 2.2. Transformational pathways of follicular lymphoma.

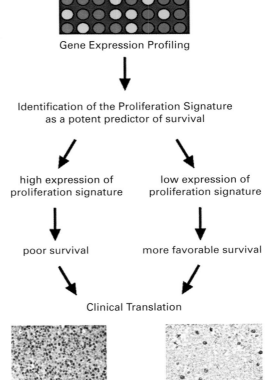

Ki-67 immunostaining

Figure 2.4. Proliferation signature in mantle cell lymphoma.

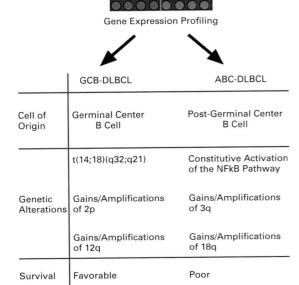

Figure 2.3. Molecular subgroups of diffuse large B-cell lymphoma (DLBCL).

FURTHER READING

Damle, R. N., Wasil, T., Fais, F. *et al.* Ig V gene mutation status and CD38 expression as novel prognostic indicators in chronic lymphocytic leukemia. *Blood* **94** (1999), 1840–1847.

Dave, S. S., Wright, G., Tan, B. *et al.* Prediction of survival in follicular lymphoma based on molecular features of tumor-infiltrating immune cells. *N. Engl. J. Med.* **351** (2004), 2159–2169.

Dohner, H., Stilgenbauer, S., Benner, A. *et al.* Genomic aberrations and survival in chronic lymphocytic leukemia. *N. Engl. J. Med.* **343** (2000), 1910–1916.

Farinha, P. and Gascoyne, R. D. Molecular pathogenesis of mucosa-associated lymphoid tissue lymphoma. *J. Clin. Oncol.* **23** (2005), 6370–6378.

Fernandez, V., Hartmann, E., Ott, G., Campo, E. and Rosenwald, A. Pathogenesis of mantle-cell lymphoma: all oncogenic roads lead to dysregulation of cell cycle and DNA damage response pathways. *J. Clin. Oncol.* **23** (2005), 6364–6369.

Hamblin, T. J., Davis, Z., Gardiner, A., Oscier, D. G. and Stevenson, F. K. Unmutated Ig V (H) genes are associated with a more aggressive form of chronic lymphocytic leukemia. *Blood* **94** (1999), 1848–1854.

Jaffe, E. S. Anaplastic large cell lymphoma: the shifting sands of diagnostic hematopathology. *Mod. Pathol.* **14** (2001), 219–228.

Jaffe, E. S., Harris, N. L., Stein, H. and Vardiman, J. W. *World Health Organization Classification of Tumours: Pathology and Genetics of Tumours of Haematopoietic and Lymphoid tissues* (Lyon: IARC Press, 2001).

Klein, U., Tu, Y., Stolovitzky, G. A. *et al.* Gene expression profiling of B cell chronic lymphocytic leukemia reveals a homogeneous phenotype related to memory B cells. *J. Exp. Med.* **194** (2001), 1625–1638.

Lossos, I. S. Molecular pathogenesis of diffuse large B-cell lymphoma. *J. Clin. Oncol.* **23** (2005), 6351–6357.

Re, D., Kuppers, R., Diehl, V. Molecular pathogenesis of Hodgkin's lymphoma. *J. Clin. Oncol.* **23** (2005), 6379–6386.

Rosenwald, A., Alizadeh, A. A., Widhopf, G. *et al.* Relation of gene expression phenotype to immunoglobulin mutation genotype in B cell chronic lymphocytic leukemia. *J. Exp. Med.* **194** (2001), 1639–1647.

Rosenwald, A., Wright, G., Chan, W. C. *et al.* The use of molecular profiling to predict survival after chemotherapy for diffuse large-B-cell lymphoma. *N. Engl. J. Med.* **346** (2002), 1937–1947.

Rosenwald, A., Wright, G., Wiestner, A. *et al.* The proliferation gene expression signature is a quantitative integrator of oncogenic events that predicts survival in mantle cell lymphoma. *Cancer Cell* **3** (2003), 185–197.

Streubel, B., Simonitsch-Klupp, I., Mullauer, L. *et al.* Variable frequencies of MALT lymphoma-associated genetic aberrations in lymphomas of different sites. *Leukemia* **18** (2004), 1722–1726.

3 IMAGING

Ashley S. Shaw and Adrian K. Dixon

INTRODUCTION

The radiologist plays a key role in the management of patients with lymphoma at several stages, from initial diagnosis through to the evaluation of response to treatment. The possible diagnosis of lymphoma is often raised first by the imaging department. The alert radiologist who identifies an abnormal mediastinum on a chest radiograph may consider lymphoma in the diagnosis, and this may prompt further investigations. With the increasing advent of computed tomography (CT) for all thoracic and abdominal problems, the imaging findings may again point to a very strong likelihood of lymphoma being the responsible cause. A primary-care referral of a patient with a neck lump may lead to an ultrasound examination. Frequently, tissue for histopathological examination is obtained by the radiologist using image-guided techniques, either at ultrasound or at CT. It is important when performing these procedures that the radiologist endeavors to obtain good core biopsies with sufficient tissue for full histopathological evaluation. Fine needle aspiration is often inadequate for accurate diagnosis and should be avoided.

Accurate delineation of the extent of disease is essential both at initial presentation and at follow-up, as this is used to guide management decisions. As lymphoma may involve almost any tissue in the body, a variety of imaging techniques may be required to demonstrate it, both anatomically and functionally, depending upon the tumor biology and location. Moreover, as treatment regimens develop, it is important that the radiologist is able to recognize complications of therapy.

STAGING TECHNIQUES

CT has been the mainstay of lymphoma staging in the chest, abdomen and pelvis for the past two decades, and continues to form the basis of clinical practice and the majority of clinical trials. Developments in CT technology enable detailed three-dimensional images of the whole body to be obtained within a few seconds. With the addition of intravenous contrast medium we are able to identify lesions within, and adjacent to, the solid organs, and from their enhancement patterns try to discern their nature (Figs. 3.1, 3.2). However, despite these advances, the evaluation of lymph nodes with CT is almost exclusively based on size: lymph nodes measuring 1 cm or greater in their short axis are considered abnormal, whereas those less than 1 cm are deemed normal. There are a few sites in the body where nodes smaller than this may be considered suspicious. These include retrocrural, left gastric and obturator regions. Likewise multiple small nodes coalescing to form a larger complex is suspicious of involvement too.

It has long been recognized that a significant proportion of enlarged lymph nodes are hyperplastic, and conversely that many small nodes are infiltrated with malignant cells. There are, however, several patterns of disease seen on CT which are considered characteristic of lymphoma. A paraspinal mass in direct continuity with enlarged para-aortic lymph nodes will often prove to be lymphoma. So too will the appearance of the aorta "floating" away from the vertebral body within a mass of para-aortic nodes (Fig. 3.3). Marked mesenteric nodal enlargement, in the form of a "hamburger" or "sandwich" (Fig. 3.4) encompassing the superior mesenteric arterial

Lymphoma: Pathology, Diagnosis and Treatment, ed. Robert Marcus, John W. Sweetenham and Michael E. Williams. Published by Cambridge University Press. © Cambridge University Press 2007.

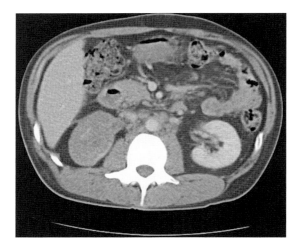

Figure 3.1. Non-enhancing soft tissue mass replacing the right kidney with para-aortic nodes. Renal biopsy confirmed diffuse large B-cell lymphoma (DLBCL).

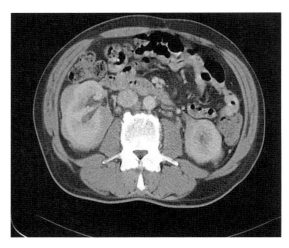

Figure 3.2. A rind of soft tissue is seen in the pararenal fat surrounding the right kidney and invading the cortex, with differential enhancement of the functioning kidney and lymphomatous tissue.

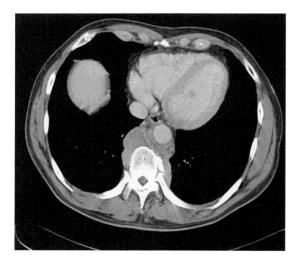

Figure 3.3. Paravertebral soft tissue mass in the lower thorax displacing the aorta anteriorly, the so-called "floating aorta."

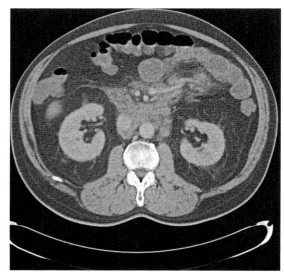

Figure 3.4. Lymph node mass seen around the aorta and IVC, extending into the small bowel mesentery. The nodes surround the vascular arcade to give the "hamburger" or "sandwich" sign.

arcade, is highly likely to be due to non-Hodgkin's lymphoma (NHL). The appearance of lymph nodes in other sites also makes a lymphomatous process highly likely (internal mammary nodal enlargement, splenic hilar enlargement and pericardiacophrenic nodes). Sometimes the root of the mesentery appears somewhat "misty", without a frank mesenteric nodal enlargement (Fig. 3.5). The differential diagnosis is wide, including all possible causes of abnormal fat on CT, but the usual cause is either mesenteric panniculitis

(which some hold to be the harbinger of future malignancy) or non-Hodgkin's lymphoma. Recently PET-CT has been shown to be useful in this situation.

Given the heterogeneity of the lymphomas, the paucity of studies with histopathological correlation at multiple nodal sites, and the variable reporting of results either by individual nodes, disease sites or overall staging, the literature is frequently confusing

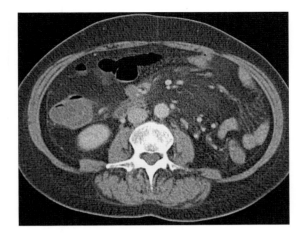

Figure 3.5. Ill-defined increase in opacification of the small bowel mesentery (misty mesentery) in a patient with follicular lymphoma.

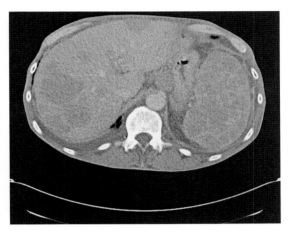

Figure 3.6. Multiple low-attenuation lesions throughout the liver and spleen were demonstrated by CT with small bilateral pleural effusions. Biopsy demonstrated this to be due to DLBCL.

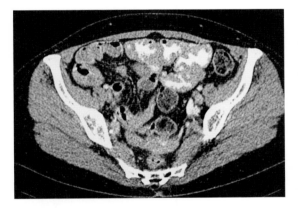

Figure 3.7. Marked thickening of the small bowel loops within the pelvis due to small bowel lymphoma.

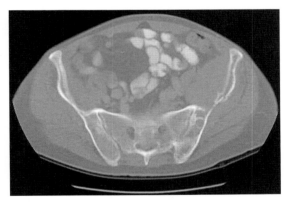

Figure 3.8. Lytic lesions are demonstrated throughout the left ilium, with destruction of the cortex and an associated soft tissue mass, proven to be DLBCL at biopsy.

and contradictory. Using a node-by-node analysis with surgical correlation, one study found CT to have a sensitivity of only 20%, correctly staging only 42% of patients with Hodgkin's lymphoma (HL). Conversely, other workers have reported CT to have 92% sensitivity in staging Hodgkin's lymphoma and 75% sensitivity in staging non-Hodgkin's lymphoma. The majority of published results lie between these findings, suggesting an accuracy of approximately 60–70%.

Splenic involvement may be manifest by either splenomegaly, for which there are many causes, or the presence of focal lesions (Fig. 3.6). Depending on the size and number of lesions, together with the technical parameters relating to intravenous enhancement, these may be easily overlooked and/or difficult to characterize with any confidence.

Extranodal sites of disease can also be difficult to identify with CT. Gastrointestinal wall thickness is difficult to estimate, particularly in the non-distended stomach, and will only be visible when gross (Fig. 3.7). In the stomach, an interrupted rugal pattern and focal thinning may provide the only clue. Bone-marrow disease will only be evident when a lytic or sclerotic lesion has developed or when there is extension into the adjacent soft tissues (Fig. 3.8). Conversely, pulmonary disease is usually readily apparent, but can be very difficult to differentiate from other causes of

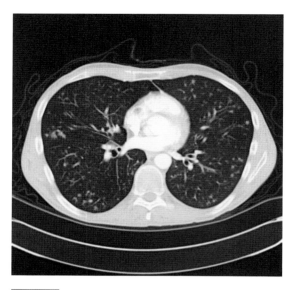

Figure 3.9. Multiple pulmonary nodules bilaterally measuring up to 1 cm in diameter. Biopsy proved these to be DLBCL.

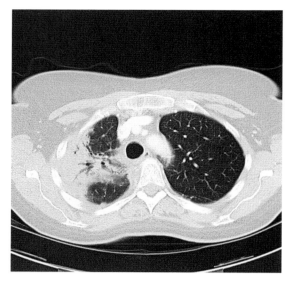

Figure 3.10. Consolidation in the right upper lobe with an air bronchogram demonstrated at CT. Biopsy proved this to be mantle cell lymphoma.

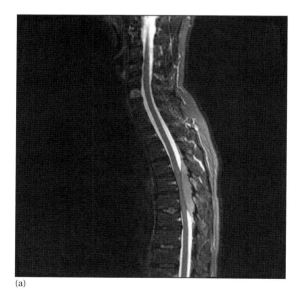

(a)

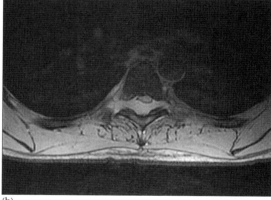

(b)

Figure 3.11. (a) Sagittal T2-weighted MRI of the thoracic spine demonstrating an extradural mass posterior to, and compressing, the spinal cord. (b) Axial images through the lesion demonstrate the extradural mass extending through the neural foramina bilaterally.

nodules and consolidation, particularly infection and drug toxicity (Figs. 3.9, 3.10).

Magnetic resonance imaging (MRI) is primarily used to image the central nervous system (CNS), soft tissue masses and bone marrow. MRI has a greater sensitivity than CT in identifying CNS lesions and provides excellent multiplanar images (Figs. 3.11, 3.12) which may help in radiotherapy planning. Similarly, imaging focal deposits in the limbs with MRI can provide additional information as it offers superior contrast between different soft tissues over CT. MRI of the bone marrow may be useful in identifying patients with focal lymphoma deposits, particularly when bone-marrow biopsy is normal.

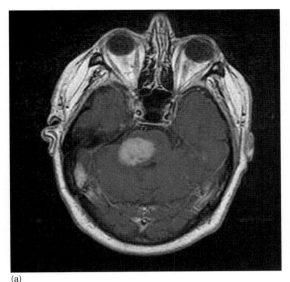 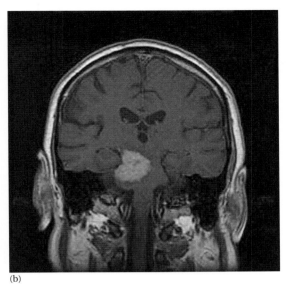

(a)   (b)

Figure 3.12. (a) Axial T1-weighted image following intravenous gadolinium demonstrates a uniformly enhancing mass within the pons extending posteriorly into the right middle cerebellar peduncle. (b) Coronal T1-weighted image demonstrates the lesion extending up into the right midbrain toward the cerebral peduncle. (Images courtesy of Dr. J. Cross.)

Lymphoma deposits are seen as low signal on T1 and high signal on fat-saturated T2-weighted images as the normal fatty marrow is displaced, often with disease spilling out into the extradural or paravertebral spaces. The identification of focal marrow infiltration in patients with normal biopsies is well described, with some investigators having used MRI to guide a further biopsy. The accuracy of MRI in detecting bone-marrow infiltration is thought to be around 80%, but there are clearly difficulties in performing histology-correlated studies. For this reason, MRI is not routinely used to assess the marrow in most centres.

Positron emission tomography (PET) with ^{18}F-fluorodeoxyglucose (FDG), on the other hand, provides functional information about the tissues. FDG mimics the action of glucose in entering the glycolytic pathway, but cannot be metabolized and thus effectively provides a map of glucose utilization. Because of this mode of action, the technique requires the patient to be fasted and have normal blood glucose levels; elevated blood glucose levels stimulate insulin release, which drives glucose, and thus FDG, into the muscles. This is not usually problematic in oncological PET, but may be in cardiac PET. Equally, anxious patients may demonstrate increased uptake within neck muscles, whilst if patients are cold then brown fat uptake may be excessive. Steroid administration usually has little effect in oncological PET studies, although surprisingly low uptake of FDG has been reported in patients with HL and diffuse large B-cell lymphoma (DLBCL) who have received high doses for only 2–3 days prior to imaging. The intensity of FDG uptake within a lesion is expressed as the standardized uptake value (SUV), a semiquantitative measure which broadly represents the ratio of uptake in the tumor compared to that which would be expected if the FDG were evenly distributed throughout the entire body. There have been a number of studies investigating the use of the SUV in lymphoma, which demonstrate that an SUV ≤ 6 often represents indolent histology whereas ≥ 13 usually indicates aggressive histology. However, the significant degree of overlap in the SUV of aggressive and indolent histology, coupled with the known inter-patient variability of the SUV, means that it has limited value in grading NHL.

There have been a large number of studies evaluating the accuracy of FDG-PET in the initial staging of lymphoma, all of which report sensitivity, specificity and accuracy to be considerably superior to that of CT. Indeed, all three of these measures are usually reported to be in the region of 85–98% for both HL and high-grade NHL. This is reported to result in a change of stage in anything up to 59% of patients, although other studies quote 8–40%. In the vast majority of these cases, the additional information from PET results in the disease being upstaged. This stage migration will lead to an apparent improvement in response rates at each clinical stage. Patients with true "early" stage disease will be distinguished from those with occult "advanced" disease, who in turn are likely to have a better prognosis than those with clinically overt disease, thus "improving" response and survival rates in this group too. This new paradigm in lymphoma staging will need to be taken into account when comparing literature from the pre- and post-PET eras. The clinical impact of PET in initial staging is significant, with management changed in many of these cases. Management changes range from modifying radiation treatment volume to changing from local to systemic therapy. Clearly, a degree of caution needs to be exercised when there is a discrepancy between CT and PET findings which will result in treatment modifications, as to over-treat or under-treat could lead to significant morbidity.

The clinical utility of PET imaging in low-grade lymphoma, however, appears to vary with histological subtype and the tissue involved. In patients with follicular lymphoma, PET is again reported to identify 40% more abnormal nodal sites than CT. Conversely, PET identifies less than 60% of the abnormal nodes on CT in chronic lymphocytic leukemia. The limited data available for MALT lymphoma suggest that FDG uptake is poor in the organs but well demonstrated in the lymph nodes. The reason for this is unclear, but it is thought to be possibly due to background tissue uptake.

As with all techniques, FDG-PET is not infallible and may give false-positive studies in a number of conditions, including infection, drug toxicity, radiotherapy, G-CSF therapy, other forms of malignancy and physiological activity in normal tissues. Whereas many of these potential pitfalls are readily identified, others may present diagnostic confusion. In such instances correlation with anatomical imaging is often helpful, and the current generation of PET machines are coupled with CT, to produce PET-CT. This produces two sets of images which may be fused to give a complete structural and functional overview of the whole body. False-negative PET studies are a

reflection of either tumor biology or lesion size, or a combination of the two, and it is therefore difficult to accurately quantify the minimum size of lesion that PET will detect. However, in high-grade disease it is in the order of a few millimetres. In this respect, PET-CT may be particularly useful in evaluating pulmonary disease, as tiny nodules may be beyond the resolution of PET alone. As the evidence base grows and PET-CT technology becomes more widely available, it would seem likely that it will become the standard staging investigation for lymphoma over the next decade.

STAGING CLASSIFICATIONS

The Ann Arbor staging classification with Cotswolds revision (Table 3.1) is used to provide the radiologic staging of Hodgkin's lymphoma and most types of NHL. It is important for the radiologist to understand the impact of staging on management in order that the report is tailored appropriately. For example, in HL, early-stage asymptomatic supradiaphragmatic disease is currently treated by a combination of short-course chemotherapy and involved field radiotherapy, although the use of radiation may alter when results of prospective studies utilizing the results of FDG-PET become available. The presence of disease below the diaphragm will increase the number of planned cycles of chemotherapy. Additionally, the phrase "bulky lymph node mass" in a radiological report should be reserved for those lesions $\geq 10\,\mathrm{cm}$ in diameter, in order to avoid confusion.

However, in indolent follicular lymphoma, a watch-and-wait policy may be adopted for many patients even with advanced-stage disease. There are a number of radiological indications for chemotherapy, including nodal or extranodal mass $\geq 7\,\mathrm{cm}$ in diameter, ≥ 3 nodal sites with a diameter $\geq 3\,\mathrm{cm}$, splenic enlargement, compression syndrome, pleural or pericardial effusion, and the radiologist must be aware of the potential therapeutic implications of the report.

For childhood NHL and adult patients with Burkitt's lymphoma, the St. Jude classification (Table 3.2) is employed. This differs significantly from the Ann Arbor system in the way that extranodal disease is staged, reflecting the different patterns of disease and the prognostic implications for these two groups of patients.

Table 3.1. Ann Arbor staging classification and Cotswolds revision.

Stage	Area of involvement
I	A single lymph-node region or a single localized involvement of an extralymphatic site
I$_E$	Localized involvement of a single extralymphatic organ or site
II	Two or more lymph-node regions on the same side of the diaphragm
II$_E$	Localized involvement of a single extralymphatic organ or site and of one or more lymph-node regions on the same side of the diaphragm
III	Lymph-node regions on both sides of the diaphragm
III$_E$	Lymph-node regions on both sides of the diaphragm accompanied by localized involvement of an extralymphatic organ or site
IV	Diffuse involvement of one or more extranodal organs with or without lymph-node involvement
	Localized involvement of a single extralymphatic organ or site with non-regional lymph-node involvement

Additional qualifiers	
A	Absence of systemic symptoms
B	Presence of systemic symptoms
X	Bulky disease, defined as a nodal mass > 10 cm in maximum diameter or mediastinal mass > one-third of the internal diameter of the thorax on a PA chest radiograph

Table 3.2. St. Jude staging classification.

Stage	Area of involvement
I	Single tumor (extranodal)
	Single anatomic area (nodal)
	Excluding mediastinum or abdomen
II	Single tumor (extranodal) with regional node involvement
	Two single (extranodal) tumors without regional lymph-node involvement on the same side of the diaphragm
	Two or more nodal areas on the same side of the diaphragm
	Primary gastrointestinal tumor with or without involvement of associated mesenteric nodes only, grossly completely resected
III	Two single (extranodal) tumors, one on either side of the diaphragm
	Two or more nodal areas, involving above and below the diaphragm
	Primary intrathoracic tumors (mediastinal, pleural, thymic)
	Extensive primary intra-abdominal disease
	Paraspinal or epidural tumors irrespective of other sites
IV	Any of the above with initial CNS or bone-marrow involvement

RESPONSE ASSESSMENT

The International Workshop Criteria (IWC), published in 1999, have become the widely accepted standard for the assessment of disease response in non-Hodgkin's lymphoma. These have enabled comparability of clinical trials as well as the day-to-day management of patients. Although based primarily on CT findings, the IWC take bone-marrow biopsy, clinical and biochemical information into account (Table 3.3). However, there are a number of drawbacks with the IWC which need to be addressed.

Following treatment for lymphoma, up to 40% of patients with nodal disease will have a residual mass

Table 3.3. International Workshop Criteria (IWC).

Complete response (CR)

Complete disappearance of all detectable disease by imaging, with nodes previously > 1.5 cm regressing to < 1.5 cm and nodes of 1.0–1.5 cm to < 1.0 cm. In addition, resolution of disease-related symptoms, normalization of biochemical abnormalities and normal bone-marrow biopsy.

Complete response unconfirmed (CRu)

As for CR, but with a residual mass > 1.5 cm in diameter that has regressed by $> 75\%$.

Partial response (PR)

At least 50% reduction in the sum of the product of the greatest diameters (SPD) of the six largest nodes. There should be neither increase in the size of other nodes nor any new sites of disease. Hepatic and splenic lesions should also reduce $> 50\%$ in the SPD.

Stable disease (SD)

Where response is less than a PR but there is not progressive disease.

Progressive disease (PD)

More than 50% increase in the product of the diameters in any previously abnormal node or the development of new disease sites either during or at the end of therapy.

Relapsed disease (RD)

The appearance of any new disease or an increase in size of over 50% of residual lesions in patients who had previously achieved CR or CRu.

on CT. Of these, only a small proportion (up to 20%) will be positive for lymphoma on re-biopsy. Moreover, if a patient has been imaged too soon following treatment, there may have been insufficient time for any significant volume reduction. As outlined above, whilst CT provides excellent morphological information, it is impossible to tell whether this tissue represents residual disease, inflammation or fibrosis. Thus, a significant proportion of patients are designated as having either a partial response (PR) or complete response unconfirmed (CRu). Similarly, CT may detect numerous lymph nodes measuring < 1 cm in diameter, which are thus deemed normal and the patient considered to have had a complete response (CR). In the lungs, a number of changes may occur related to chemotherapy, radiotherapy, infection or disease progression. Bony abnormalities resolve slowly, if at all, whilst gastrointestinal lesions may not be visible at all and cannot be reliably measured.

As with initial staging, there is a growing body of evidence regarding the clinical utility of FDG-PET in assessing response to therapy. Rapid decreases in the tumoral uptake of FDG-PET have been demonstrated

within seven days of commencing chemotherapy. Early response assessment has been studied by a number of groups, with results of FDG-PET performed after 1–4 cycles of chemotherapy correlated with clinical follow-up. A recent meta-analysis of these studies calculated that FDG-PET had an overall sensitivity of 79%, a specificity of 92% and an overall accuracy of 85% in predicting response. Similarly, early and mid-treatment PET studies have been shown to be a good predictor of progression-free survival and overall survival. However, no published study has yet clearly shown that PET can be used at an early stage to alter treatment with an improvement in outcome.

The integration of FDG-PET results into IWC has so far received comparatively little attention in the published literature, with just one series reported. In this retrospective analysis of 54 patients, comparison of IWC alone versus IWC including FDG-PET results demonstrated only 61% concordance in response classification. The study highlights that the principal advantage of PET in this situation is in patients with a residual mass who are classified as either CRu or PR

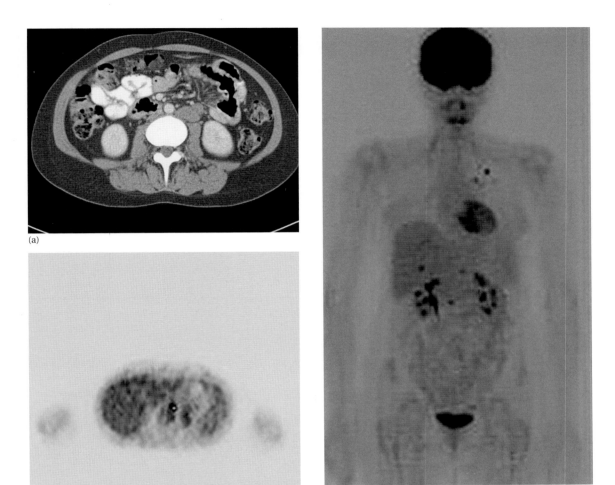

(a)

(b)

(c)

Figure 3.13. (a) CT demonstrates a residual soft tissue mass in the left para-aortic region following chemotherapy. (b) Axial FDG-PET image through the mass demonstrates tracer uptake. (c) Coronal FDG-PET image demonstrates multiple foci of tracer uptake in the left supraclavicular fossa, mediastinum and abdomen. These nodes all measured less than 1 cm on CT.

by CT criteria (Figs. 3.13, 3.14). PET enabled reclassification of CRu to either CR or PR, whilst half of those designated PR were changed to CR. All but one of the ten patients reclassified as CR by this method remained disease-free at a median 32 months follow-up. The overall progression-free survival in the groups designated CR by IWC and IWC+PET were 88% vs. 91% at 2 years and 74% vs. 80% at 3 years. Crucially, this group contained only 17/54 patients using IWC, but 35/54 using IWC+PET. These results need to be validated in the setting of a prospective trial, but it would seem likely that the IWC will need to be modified to include PET along the lines used by the authors of this study (Table 3.4) in the near future. The timing of this post-treatment study should ideally be at least 3–4 weeks following completion of chemotherapy, three months or more following completion of radiotherapy.

The use of PET to evaluate residual lesions in indolent disease is less clear and studies should be interpreted with caution, particularly if PET was not used during initial staging.

Table 3.4. International Workshop Criteria modified to include PET findings.

IWC+PET	Description
CR	CR by IWC with a completely negative PET
	CRu, PR or SD by IWC with a completely negative PET and a negative BMB if positive prior to therapy
	PD by IWC with a completely negative PET and CT abnormalities ≥ 1.5 cm (≥ 1.0 cm in the lungs) and negative BMB if positive prior to therapy
CRu	CRu by IWC with a completely negative PET but with an indeterminate BMB
PR	CR, CRu or PR by IWC with a positive PET at the site of a previously involved node or nodal mass
	CR, CRu, PR or SD by IWC with a positive PET outside the site of a previously involved node or nodal mass
	SD by IWC with a positive PET at the site of a previously involved node or nodal mass that regressed to < 1.5 cm if previously > 1.5 cm, or < 1.0 cm if previously 1.1–1.5 cm
SD	SD by IWC with a positive PET at the site of a previously involved node or nodal mass (i.e. residual mass)
PD	PD by IWC with a positive PET finding corresponding to the CT abnormality (new lesion, increasing size of lesion)
	PD by IWC with a negative PET and a CT abnormality (new lesion, increasing size of lesion) of < 1.5 cm (< 1.0 cm in the lungs)

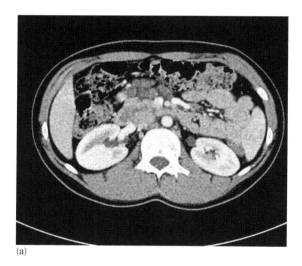

(a)

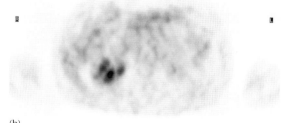

(b)

Figure 3.14. (a) Residual nodal mass measuring 4 cm in diameter in the root of the small bowel mesentery following chemotherapy. (b) FDG-PET images did not demonstrate any tracer uptake at this or any other site. Note normal excretion in the right kidney but less in the left, which had previously been involved with disease. (Image courtesy of Dr. J. Wat.)

COMPLICATIONS OF THERAPY

Patients with lymphoma may be treated with an array of cytotoxic agents and radiation therapy, which can themselves result in significant morbidity and occasionally death. The lungs appear to be particularly sensitive to these insults and this can manifest itself in a number of ways, the more common of which are listed in Table 3.5.

Diffuse alveolar damage (DAD) is the histopathological pattern that results from necrosis of type II pneumocytes and alveolar endothelial cells. The clinical correlate of this is the acute respiratory distress syndrome (ARDS). In the acute phase (first week after insult), there is interstitial and alveolar edema and hyaline membranes. Following this is a reparative phase, with proliferation of type II pneumocytes and interstitial fibrosis (usually at 1–2 weeks). The chest radiograph may demonstrate bilateral focal areas of consolidation, often in the mid and lower zones. At this stage, CT often demonstrates a combination of

Table 3.5. Manifestations of pulmonary drug toxicity in lymphoma.

Presentation	Drugs most commonly involved
Diffuse alveolar damage	Bleomycin, carmustine, cyclophosphamide
Organizing pneumonia	Bleomycin, cyclophosphamide
Pulmonary hemorrhage	Cyclophosphamide, cytarabine, amphotericin B
Non-specific interstitial pneumonia	Chlorambucil, carmustine

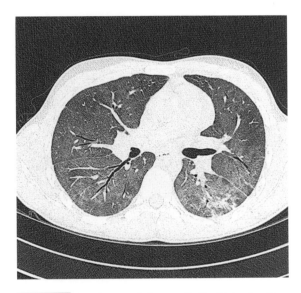

Figure 3.15. Extensive ground-glass opacification bilaterally with areas of consolidation in the left lower lobe. A presumptive diagnosis of bleomycin toxicity was made, with the patient responding to drug withdrawal and a course of corticosteroids.

consolidation, ground-glass opacification and fibrosis (Fig. 3.15). In the chronic phase, fibrosis may improve, remain stable or progress. The fibrotic changes depicted at CT are predominantly peripheral and subpleural. A number of drugs have been implicated, cyclophosphamide, carmustine and bleomycin being the commonest in the context of lymphoma. Cyclophosphamide-related injury is not dose-related and has been reported up to 13 years after administration. Conversely, carmustine has a clear dose-related toxicity, with the overall incidence rising from 20–30% to 50% once a cumulative dose of $1.5\,g/m^2$ has been exceeded. Bleomycin pulmonary toxicity is reported to occur in up to 18% of patients, with a mortality of 4.2%. There appear to be a number of risk factors associated, including age > 40 years,

cumulative dose > 450 units and use of granulocyte colony-stimulating factor. Of note, the same group observed that omitting bleomycin from the therapeutic regimen had no impact on rates of complete remission, progression-free survival and overall survival.

Patients with an organizing pneumonia typically present with progressive dyspnea, fever and a dry cough. The chest radiograph demonstrates bilateral scattered opacities with a peripheral distribution. At CT, ill-defined areas of consolidation, nodules and plugging of the small airways ("tree in bud" appearance) will be evident. Withdrawal of the causative agent, with or without steroid therapy, typically results in a good response. Non-specific interstitial pneumonia (NSIP) and pulmonary hemorrhage are less frequently observed manifestations of pulmonary drug toxicity. NSIP is an inflammatory condition that results in mild interstitial fibrosis with areas of ground-glass opacification on CT. Diagnosis of NSIP may be difficult at both histology and radiology, but the prognosis is good. Diffuse pulmonary hemorrhage results in acute respiratory distress with focal areas of consolidation demonstrated on the plain radiograph. CT will delineate multiple foci of consolidation and/or ground-glass opacification. Diagnosis may be confirmed by demonstrating an increase in the diffusion capacity for carbon monoxide (D_LCO). The outcome is heavily dependent on the underlying cause.

Radiation therapy has evolved significantly over the past decade, with the introduction of three-dimensional conformal radiotherapy and, more recently, intensity-modulated radiotherapy. This has resulted in a significant reduction in the volume of "normal" tissue that is irradiated. As a result, frank radiation pneumonitis is rarely seen, and only minimal paramediastinal fibrosis is seen on CT. However, as more patients are cured of their initial disease, the risk of radiation therapy in the development of a second malignancy is becoming more apparent. In the context of lymphoma, it is particularly important to minimize the dose to the breasts of young female patients with mediastinal disease. To this end, the role of PET-CT in defining active disease for radiotherapy planning requires further investigation.

Severely immunocompromised patients are also susceptible to a variety of infectious agents that carry a high morbidity and mortality. Angioinvasive aspergillosis classically demonstrates variably sized nodules of consolidation with a halo of ground-glass opacification or pleural-based wedge-shaped areas of consolidation, and is elegantly shown on thin-section CT sections (especially with an HRCT algorithm) (Fig. 3.16). This represents infarcted lung with a zone of hemorrhage peripherally. The patient will usually be severely neutropenic, but as the neutrophil count increases, a crescent of air may be seen as the necrotic tissue falls away from the viable tissue. This will eventually resolve to leave either a cavity or parenchymal scarring. Unfortunately, the CT features are non-specific, with candida, cytomegalovirus (CMV) and herpesvirus among the infections that can give similar appearances. However, CMV more typically has bilateral ground-glass opacification with numerous ill-defined small nodules. Patchy consolidation is seen commonly, whilst pleural effusions are seen in approximately 60% of cases.

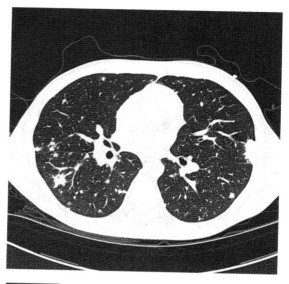

Figure 3.16. Multiple foci of consolidation, some with a rim of ground-glass opacification, typical of angioinvasive aspergillosis.

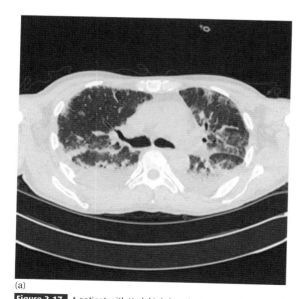

(a)

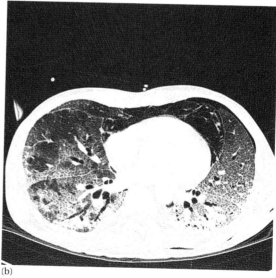

(b)

Figure 3.17. A patient with Hodgkin's lymphoma and HIV presented with acute dyspnea. (a) Initial CT demonstrates multiple foci of ground-glass opacification and bilateral pleural effusions. This was proven to be PCP following bronchoscopy. (b) Eleven days later, the patient deteriorated further and CT demonstrated a pneumomediastinum and left pneumothorax. The ground-glass opacification within the lung parenchyma is now more confluent and the septal thickening is more evident.

Similarly, *Pneumocystis carinii* pneumonia (PCP) presents in severely immunocompromised patients and has a number of radiographic manifestations. Most commonly, there is a combination of fine reticular opacification and ill-defined ground-glass opacification which progresses to consolidation over a period of days. Less commonly, PCP may present as a focal area of consolidation, mimicking pulmonary lymphoma, pleural effusions, mediastinal lymphadenopathy or with military nodules. Approximately one-third of patients go on to develop pneumatoceles (thin-walled cysts), most often in the upper lobes. These usually resolve spontaneously within a year of the acute episode, but may rupture to produce a pneumothorax (Fig. 3.17).

FURTHER READING

Cheson, B. D., Horning, S. J., Coiffier, B. *et al.* Report of an international workshop to standardize response criteria for non-Hodgkin's lymphomas. NCI Sponsored International Working Group. *J. Clin. Oncol.* **17** (1999), 1244.

Grubnic, S., Vinnicombe, S. J., Norman, A. R. and Husband, J. E. MR evaluation of normal retroperitoneal and pelvic lymph nodes. *Clin. Radiol.* **57** (2002), 193–200.

Hoffmann, M., Kletter, K., Diemling, M. *et al.* Positron emission tomography with fluorine-18-2-fluoro-2-deoxy-D-glucose (F18-FDG) does not visualize extranodal B-cell lymphoma of the mucosa-associated lymphoid tissue (MALT)-type. *Ann. Oncol.* **10** (1999), 1185–1189.

Jerusalem, G., Beguin, Y., Najjar, F. *et al.* Positron emission tomography (PET) with 18F-fluorodeoxyglucose (18F-FDG) for the staging of low-grade non-Hodgkin's lymphoma (NHL). *Ann. Oncol.* **12** (2001), 825–830.

Jerusalem, G., Hustinx, R., Beguin, Y. and Fillet, G. Evaluation of therapy for lymphoma. *Semin. Nucl. Med.* **35** (2005), 186–196.

Juweid, M. E. and Cheson, B. D. Role of positron emission tomography in lymphoma. *J. Clin. Oncol.* **21** (2005), 4577–4580.

Juweid, M. E., Wiseman, G. A., Vose, J. M. *et al.* Response assessment of aggressive non-Hodgkin's lymphoma by integrated International Workshop Criteria and fluorine-18-fluorodeoxyglucose positron emission tomography. *J. Clin. Oncol.* **23** (2005), 4652–4661.

Kazama, T., Faria, S. C., Varavithya, V., Phongkitkarun, S., Ito, H. and Macapinlac, H. A. FDG PET in the evaluation of treatment for lymphoma: clinical usefulness and pitfalls. *Radiographics.* **25** (2005), 191–207.

Lister, T. A., Crowther, D., Sutcliffe, S. B. *et al.* Report of a committee convened to discuss the evaluation and staging of patients with Hodgkin's disease: Cotswolds meeting. *J. Clin. Oncol.* **7** (1989), 1630–1636.

Myers, J. L. Pathology of drug-induced lung disease. In *Katzenstein and Askin's Surgical Pathology of Non-Neoplastic Lung Disease*, 3rd edn, ed. A. A. Katzenstein and F. B. Askin (Philadelphia, PA: Saunders, 1997), pp. 81–111.

Moon, J. H., Kim, E. A., Lee, K. S., Kim, T. S., Jung, K.-J. and Song, J.-H. Cytomegalovirus pneumonia: high-resolution CT findings in ten non-AIDS immunocompromised patients. *Korean J. Radiol.* **1** (2000), 73–78.

Rimmer, M. J., Dixon, A. K., Flower, C. D. R. and Sikora, K. Bleomycin lung: computed tomographic observations. *Br. J. Radiol.* **58** (1985), 1041–1045.

Rossi, S. E., Erasmus, J. J., McAdams, H. P., Sporn, T. A. and Goodman, P. C. Pulmonary drug toxicity: radiologic and pathologic manifestations. *Radiographics* **20** (2000), 1245–1259.

Surbone, A., Longo, D. L., DeVita, V. T. Jr. *et al.* Residual abdominal masses in aggressive non-Hodgkin's lymphoma after combination chemotherapy: significance and management. *J. Clin. Oncol.* **6** (1988), 1832–1837.

Zissin, R., Metser, U., Hain, D. and Even-Sapir, E. Mesenteric panniculitis in oncologic patients: PET-CT findings. *Br. J. Radiol.* **79** (2006), 37–43.

PROGNOSTIC FACTORS FOR LYMPHOMAS

Guillaume Cartron and Philippe Solal-Céligny

INTRODUCTION

The prognosis for lymphoma patients has improved markedly with the introduction of cytotoxic chemotherapy. Treatment strategies based upon intensified chemotherapy have also demonstrated improved survival of patients with relapsed lymphoma. It is necessary, however, to define the populations with adverse prognostic factors in order to justify such a strategy. Consequently prognostic indices have been developed from the results of clinical trials to define therapeutic strategies. Such prognostic indices have usually been based on retrospective studies, which have certain methodological problems in the new monoclonal antibody era. The recent development of technologies analyzing gene expression profiling also gives us new tools for a more accurate diagnosis with prognostic implications, using biological prognostic factors based upon lymphoma-specific risk factors. Technologies such as positron emission tomography using ^{18}F-fluorodeoxyglucose (FDG-PET) should also improve assessment of tumor response and introduce new prognostic factors.

METHODOLOGY FOR BUILDING PROGNOSTIC INDICES

The goals of a prognostic index (PI) are multiple:
(1) for a single patient, to help the physician at diagnosis to predict the probable course of the disease and propose a specific treatment, to give the patient and his or her family accurate information;
(2) to compare the results of clinical trials in order to ascertain whether the groups of patients share the same prognosis;

(3) to design clinical trials in homogeneous subgroups of patients.
A good PI must fulfill several qualities.

It must be accurate

(1) It must include patients having the same lymphoma subtype. This is most often achieved in individual entities like Hodgkin's lymphoma (HL). It may be much more difficult for subtypes whose diagnosis requires highly experienced pathologists, such as mantle cell lymphoma. In a retrospective analysis, the best approach would be to organize pathology review. In prospective studies, precise pathological, immunohistochemical and/or cytogenetic diagnosis criteria should be defined, common to all patients within the group.
(2) Patients should ideally represent the whole spectrum of the lymphoma subtype.
(3) In subtypes where treatment has a significant influence on the course of the disease, only patients optimally treated should be included.

It must be simple

(1) Although molecular biology and/or sophisticated cytogenetic studies (FISH) may improve the accuracy of prognostic indices, these tests are cumbersome, costly and available only in large centers. Using such tests will limit the usefulness of an index; widely used prognostic indices in lymphoma should, therefore, rely on routinely performed tests.
(2) Some tests can require a consensus before they are incorporated in a prognostic index, such as the cell grade in follicular lymphomas and bcl-2

Lymphoma: Pathology, Diagnosis and Treatment, ed. Robert Marcus, John W. Sweetenham and Michael E. Williams. Published by Cambridge University Press. © Cambridge University Press 2007.

positivity in large B-cell non-Hodgkin's lymphomas (NHL).

(3) The number of parameters included in an index must be limited (i.e. 3–5) in order to be easily memorized, and to separate the patients into a limited number (3–5) of risk groups. However, the widely expanding use of "pocket computers" will permit the development of more complex indices and/or algorithmic programs.

It must rely on overall survival

Overall survival (OS) is the most convenient endpoint. Prognostic indices have been developed from retrospective analyses of large groups of patients. In these retrospective studies, to rely on the time to progression (TTP) or time to treatment failure (TTF) leads to uncertainties and is a potential source of bias.

However, OS cannot be used in analyses of patients with some lymphoma subtypes such as Hodgkin's lymphoma or indolent lymphomas, where the OS is very good, events are rare and an analysis would require many years of follow-up. It is now widely accepted – although not proved – that significant improvement in progression-free survival (PFS) is a good surrogate for an improvement in OS that can be used in the evaluation of the influence of a new treatment in different prognostic subgroups.

It must be discriminant

In order to be useful to clinicians, a PI must separate patients into risk groups with significantly different OS when compared by log-rank test and hazard-ratio for death.

Furthermore, except in some frequent subtypes such as large-cell NHL or Hodgkin's lymphoma, there must be an even distribution between risk groups in order to allow assessment of a new treatment in a large enough number of patients. In developing the PI it may also be useful, in some frequently occurring subtypes, to identify a small group of patients with either a very good or a very poor prognosis.

It must be validated

The first step in building a prognostic index is to collect the data from a large number of patients spanning the entire spectrum of the disease. Then these patients are randomly separated into a test group used for building the index and a second group for internal validation of the index. This method has been used in creating the International Prognostic Index (IPI) for aggressive non-Hodgkin's lymphomas and the Follicular Lymphoma International Prognostic Index (FLIPI). These indices must then be validated by other groups and/or centers in other patients who may differ by age, distribution and treatment modalities. This external validation is mandatory before widespread adoption of the PI. A univariate analysis is the first step. Parameters here are selected from the literature and will include demographic data as well as clinical and biological markers of tumor burden and of consequences of the lymphoma upon the host. This univariate analysis may, however, generate bias: for example when creating the FLIPI it appeared that including the cell subtype of follicular lymphoma would require a pathology review, since the distribution was obviously center-dependent. Another example is the absence, in all indices, of inclusion of comorbidities, since the presence and the severity of a concomitant disease will influence prognosis and treatment selection. This is especially true in the elderly. New scores for evaluating these comorbidities and their severity have been proposed, and their validation is ongoing.

There is no consensus on the optimal method for including continuous variables in univariate analyses. They may be included as a continuous variable – which is the most accurate but the most complex option – or dichotomized according to a threshold change in prognosis beyond a certain point (for instance, the threshold of 60 years was chosen for the IPI since it was considered a maximal age for autologous bone-marrow transplantation). The expansion of computer software in daily use by physicians in their practice will allow more and more use of continuous variables in prognostic indices. Parameters that significantly influence the OS of patients in the univariate analysis should then be included in the multivariate analysis. However, if the number of patients is very high, a selection of parameters has to be made according to statistical and clinical considerations. Parameters that significantly influence OS in the multivariate analysis are chosen for building the PI. Detailed statistical considerations are beyond the scope of this chapter.

DIFFUSE LARGE B-CELL LYMPHOMA

Prognostic factors at diagnosis

Clinical factors

Until the end of the 1980s, age and staging according to the Ann Arbor classification were the most frequent parameters used to identify "high-risk" and "low-risk" patients with aggressive NHL. The Ann Arbor classification was originally developed for Hodgkin's lymphoma, which commonly spreads via contiguous lymph-node groups. Because the patterns of spread are somewhat different between NHL and HL, it is therefore not surprising that the Ann Arbor classification was less efficient for identifying prognostic subgroups of patients with aggressive NHL. Age at diagnosis was also commonly identified as a prognostic factor in numerous studies. However, most studies that included large numbers of older patients demonstrated a tendency to treat elderly patients with lower doses of chemotherapy, to reduce treatment-related toxicity, while others suggested that older patients could benefit from full-dose therapy. In this context, many investigators attempted to identify pre-treatment prognostic factors from their own series of patients with aggressive NHL. Features independently associated with outcome were often used to develop prognostic-factor models in which the individual patient's risk correlated to the number of adverse factors present at diagnosis. Although the clinical features used in these models differed, they were thought to reflect three basic features:

(1) the tumor's growth and invasive potential: lactate dehydrogenase (LDH), Ann Arbor stage, mass size, bone-marrow (BM) involvement, number of nodal and extranodal sites
(2) the patient's reaction to the tumor: performance status (PS), B symptoms
(3) the patient's likely ability to tolerate intensive therapy: PS, BM involvement, age

Those models were similarly predictive for outcome in large series of patients uniformly treated, suggesting that, although they relied on different parameters, they identified the same patient sub-populations.

In 1993, institutions and cooperative groups from the United States, Canada and Europe participated in the International Non-Hodgkin's Lymphoma Prognostic Factors Project to attempt to develop a

Table 4.1. Prognostic factors for survival in the International Prognostic Index (IPI).

	Relative risk	p-value
Patients of all ages		
Age ($\leq$60 years vs. >60 years)	1.96	<0.001
LDH ($\leq$ normal vs. > normal)	1.85	<0.001
ECOG performance status	1.80	<0.001
(0–1 vs. 2–4)		
Ann Arbor stage (I/II vs. III/IV)	1.47	<0.001
Extranodal involvement	1.48	<0.001
($\leq$ 1 site vs. > 1 site)		
Patients $\leq$ 60 years of age		
Ann Arbor stage (I/II vs. III/IV)	2.17	<0.001
LDH ($\leq$ normal vs. > normal)	1.95	<0.001
ECOG performance status	1.81	<0.001
(0–1 vs. 2–4)		

predictive model (the IPI) based on a large cohort of patients with aggressive NHL. This model had to allow comparisons of published clinical trials and to identify patients at high risk for relapse after anthracycline-based chemotherapy. From a study of 2031 patients who were treated with anthracycline-based chemotherapy between 1982 and 1987, clinical features independently predictive for overall survival (OS) and relapse were age, PS, LDH levels, Ann Arbor stage and the number of extra-nodal sites (Table 4.1). These five factors were incorporated into a model (Table 4.2) and an individual patient's relative risk for death was determined by adding the number of adverse prognostic factors present at diagnosis. It was therefore possible to identify four groups, with significantly different predicted 5-year OS: 73% (low-risk group, with either no or one adverse factor), 51% (low-intermediate-risk group, with two adverse factors), 43% (high-intermediate-risk group, with three adverse factors) and 26% (high-risk group, with four or five adverse factors). Since age was an independent predictive factor for outcome, and patients younger than 60 years were often candidates for intensive treatment, an age-adjusted model was also developed. From 1274 patients aged 60 years or younger, three adverse factors were identified: tumor stage, serum concentration of LDH and PS. By adding the number of adverse prognostic factors, this age-adjusted IPI (aaIPI) identified four risk groups, with

Table 4.2. The International Prognostic Index (IPI) and age-adjusted IPI (aaIPI).

Risk group	Risk factors	Distribution of cases (%)	CR rate (%)	RFS (%)		OS (%)	
				2-year rate	5-year rate	2-year rate	5-year rate
International Index (patients of all ages)							
Low (L)	0–1	35	87	79	70	84	73
Low-intermediate (LI)	2	27	67	66	50	66	51
High-intermediate (HI)	3	22	55	59	49	54	43
High (H)	4–5	16	44	58	40	34	26
Age-adjusted Index (patients ≤ 60 yrs)							
Low (L)	0	22	92	88	86	90	83
Low-intermediate (LI)	1	32	78	74	66	79	69
High-intermediate (HI)	2	32	57	62	53	59	46
High (H)	3	14	46	61	58	37	32
Age-adjusted Index (patients > 60 yrs)							
Low (L)	0	18	91	75	46	80	56
Low-intermediate (LI)	1	31	71	64	45	68	44
High-intermediate (HI)	2	35	56	60	41	48	37
High (H)	3	16	36	47	37	31	21

CR, complete response; RFS, relapse-free survival; OS, overall survival.

predicted 5-year OS of 83% (low-risk group, with no adverse factor), 69% (low-intermediate-risk group, with one adverse factor), 46% (high-intermediate-risk group, with two adverse factors) and 32% (high-risk group, with three adverse factors).

When the clinical characteristics of patients above and below 60 years were compared, it was seen that equal percentages of younger and older patients presented with elevated LDH, advanced stage, non-ambulatory PS (2–4) or multiple extranodal sites, demonstrating that the worse outcome of older patients was not due to more extensive disease. The comparison of complete response (CR) and relapse-free survival (RFS) rates between older and younger patients (Table 4.2) indicated also that they had similar CR rates, but lower RFS rates in the older group translated into significant age-related differences in survival. When survival of patients with different Ann Arbor stages was compared according to risk groups defined by the IPI, it was possible to determine a significantly different outcome in each stage, indicating that the IPI was more predictive than the Ann Arbor classification.

The IPI is now used to design therapeutic trials, and to select and compare treatment strategies. Approximately half of all patients are assigned to the high-intermediate or low-intermediate categories, with survival at 5 years of 51% and 43% respectively. This indicates that in these subgroups the IPI is not sufficiently powerful to separate patients who will be cured by conventional treatment from those who will have refractory or relapsing disease. In addition, the IPI has been built from a cohort of patients with aggressive lymphoma, including T lymphoma and different types of aggressive B lymphoma. Thus, these clinical variables clearly represent surrogates for the intrinsic cellular and molecular heterogeneity within aggressive lymphoma, and highlight the need for patient-specific and biologically based risk factors.

Histological factors

The Revised European–American Lymphoma classification system (REAL), subsequently updated as the World Health Organization (WHO) classification in 2001, defined DLBCL as a proliferation of B lymphocytes which diffusely effaces the normal architecture of

Table 4.3. Immunohistochemical markers having prognostic value in diffuse large B-cell lymphoma.

Immunohistochemical markers	Prognostic value
Lineage-associated and immune antigens	
CD5	Expression associated with extranodal presentation and shorter survival
HLA molecules	Defective expression associated with poor prognosis
CD54	Expression associated with shorter relapse-free survival
CD86	Expression associated with shorter relapse-free survival
Proliferation and apoptosis markers	
Ki67	High expression associated with shorter survival
MIB1	High expression associated with shorter survival
p53/p21	p53+/p21− phenotype associated with poor treatment response
Cycline D3	Expression associated with shorter survival
rb	High expression associated with better survival
bcl-2	High expression associated with shorter survival
survivin	Expression associated with shorter survival
Adhesion molecules	
CD44	Expression associated with shorter survival in localized nodal disease
Stage-specific markers	
CD10/bcl-6	CD10+/bcl-6+ phenotype associated with a better survival

nodes or extranodal sites. Malignant B lymphocytes are large transformed lymphocytes, which have been divided into several morphologic variants: centroblastic, immunoblastic, T-cell/histiocyte-rich, and anaplastic variant. Immunoblast-rich tumors have been found to have a worse prognosis in several studies, and in some studies are associated with frequent involvement of the central nervous system (CNS) and BM. Until recently, T-cell/histiocyte-rich large B-cell lymphomas were also considered to have a worse prognosis. However, most of these studies were retrospective and included small numbers of patients, and these results were not confirmed by others. Futhermore, the reproducibility of histologic subclassification in daily practice is low, and subtyping of DLBCL is therefore considered to have minor clinical significance.

DLBCLs usually express CD45 (leukocyte common antigen) and pan-B-cell antigens such as CD19, CD20 and CD79. They can also express other markers detectable by immunohistochemistry, including lineage-associated and immune markers, cell adhesion molecules, proliferation and apoptosis markers. Some of these markers have been considered to have a prognostic impact and are summarized in Table 4.3. Bcl-2

protein expression is found in 30–60% of cases, and is the consequence of either t(14;18)(q32;q21) or *BCL-2* amplification leading to an increase of bcl-2 production. In contrast to the lack of prognostic significance of the presence of t(14;18)(q32;q21) in DLBCL, numerous studies have demonstrated an association between bcl-2 expression and decreased disease-free survival (DFS) or OS. However, there was considerable variation in the criteria used by authors to classify bcl-2-positive cases (ranging from 10% to more than 50% positive cells). Moreover, in cohorts of patients treated with chemotherapy and rituximab, bcl-2 expression did not correlate with survival, emphasizing the ambiguous prognostic value of bcl-2 expression.

CD5, found primarily in T cells is also expressed by a subset of normal B cells. CD5-positive DLBCL is reported to be associated with an older age, predominantly in women, with frequent involvement of extranodal sites (especially BM and spleen) and inferior survival compared to CD5-negative DLBCL. Using an immunostaining approach, it is also possible to distinguish germinal center-like (GC-like) DLBCL (see Gene expression profiling, below), where neoplastic B cells express CD10, may or may not express bcl-6 and lack MUM1 and CD138, from non-GC-like DLBCL, where neoplastic B cells express MUM1 and CD138. In a large cohort of patients previously evaluated by cDNA microarray technology, it has been confirmed that the GC phenotype evaluated by tissue microarray (TMA) predicted a better survival than the non-GC phenotype.

Genetic abnormalities

Several recurrent chromosomal abnormalities have been described in DLBCL, including those involving *BCL-6* (3q27), *BCL-2* (18q21), *TP53* (17p), *REL* (2p14). None of them is a hallmark of DLBCL. *BCL-6* is located on 3q27 and could be involved in chromosomal translocations or mutations leading to deregulation of bcl-6 expression. The chromosomal translocations involving 3q27 are the most frequent genetic abnormalities, detected in 30–40% of DLBCL. Contrary to the predictive value of increased bcl-6 mRNA and bcl-6 protein expression, the clinical importance of such translocations has been controversial, and most studies have failed to demonstrate a significant effect on survival. The translocation t(14;18)(q32;q21) is found in up to 30% of DLBCL, and most previous studies have not shown a prognostic impact of this translocation in *de novo* DLBCL. Mutations and deletion of *P53* are reported in up to 20% of DLBCL, and have been associated with a more aggressive clinical course. However, p53 protein expression is imperfectly correlated with *P53* mutations, and it has been demonstrated that the analysis of p53, associated with its downstream target p21, may identify a subgroup of DLBCL with a poor outcome (p53+/p21−).

Gene expression profiling

Recent studies using gene expression profiling have identified different patterns of gene expression, allowing the separation of DLBCL subtypes deriving from distinct stages of lymphocyte ontogeny. The first group, named germinal center-like (GC-like) DLBCL, expresses genes characteristic of normal B cells in the germinal center, whereas non-GC-like DLBCL consists of activated B-cell-like (ABC-like) and "type 3" subtypes. The ABC-like tumors express genes found in in-vitro activated peripheral-blood B cells as well as some genes expressed normally by plasma cells, suggesting their post-GC origin, and type 3 is a heterogeneous DLBCL subgroup which does not express high levels of either GC or ABC genes.

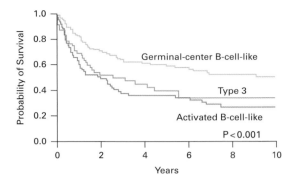

Figure 4.1. Kaplan–Meier estimates of overall survival after chemotherapy in previously untreated DLBCL patients according to gene-expression subgroup (from Rosenwald *et al.* 2002).

This stratification, related to stages of B lymphocyte ontogeny, has been found to be correlated with the OS independently of the IPI. GC-like DLBCL has significantly better OS rates than ABC-like or type 3 DLBCL (Fig. 4.1). However, the microarrays used in these studies were different and there was no overlap between the genes identified in the studies. The clinical utility of such technologies is also limited by high cost and the requirement for fresh or optimally cryopreserved tumor. A simplified six-gene predictive model using quantitative real-time polymerase chain reaction was subsequently developed, demonstrating that the expression of three genes (*LMO2*, *BCL-6*, *FN1*) correlated with prolonged survival whereas the expression of another set of three genes (*BCL-2*, *CCND2*, *SCYA3*) was associated with a shorter survival. The predictive value of the gene expression profile was later confirmed using TMA, suggesting the potential of this technology to replace gene expression profiling in clinical practice. Gene expression profiling has been obtained with tumor samples from patients treated without rituximab, and should be therefore validated with these new treatment modalities including anti-CD20 monoclonal antibodies.

Treatment-related prognostic factors

Although parameters associated directly with response to treatment cannot be used to determine induction therapy, they provide information regarding chemosensitivity of the tumor. The recent introduction of FDG-PET has improved our ability to evaluate the prognostic relevance of response.

Table 4.4. Predictive value of whole-body FDG-PET for treatment evaluation in NHL.

Clinical situation	Sensitivity	Specificity	Positive predictive value	Negative predictive value
Early response	79%	92%	90%	81%
Before transplantation	84%	83%	84%	83%
Post-treatment	67%	100%	100%	83%

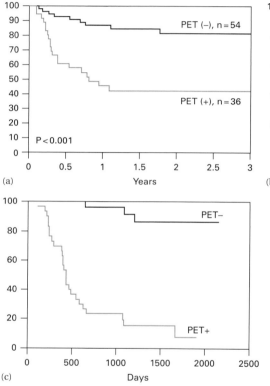

(a)

(b)

(c)

Figure 4.2. Prognostic value of FDG-PET scan in DLBCL. (a) Early prognostic value: Kaplan–Meier estimate of EFS in 54 patients with a negative scan after two cycles of chemotherapy compared to 36 patients with a positive scan after two cycles of chemotherapy (Haioun *et al.* 2005). (b) Prognostic value after completion of treatment: Kaplan–Meier estimate of PFS in 26 patients with a positive scan after therapy compared to 67 patients with a negative scan after therapy (Spaepen *et al.* 2001). (c) Prognostic value before autologous stem-cell transplantation: Kaplan–Meier estimate of PFS in 30 patients with a positive pre-transplant scan compared to 30 patients with a negative pre-transplant scan (Spaepen *et al.* 2003).

Time to complete response

The survival of patients with DLBCL is closely related to achieving CR at the end of treatment, whereas stable and progressive diseases (refractory disease) are both associated with poor survival. The time required to obtain CR has also been identified as an important prognostic factor of OS, patients achieving CR early having the best survival. However, evaluation of response by clinical examination and computer tomography scans is often limited to patients with bulky or disseminated tumors, who frequently (30–60%) have residual abnormalities of uncertain significance.

Positron emission tomography using ^{18}F-fluorodeoxyglucose (FDG-PET)

Gallium-67 (^{67}Ga) scintigraphy was initially used to assess response to treatment. ^{67}Ga scintigraphy suffers from low resolution, lack of specificity, low sensitivity in infradiaphragmatic disease and a large variability of gallium avidity. ^{67}Ga scintigraphy has now been replaced by FDG-PET, which is considered the non-invasive imaging technique of choice for the detection of residual disease after treatment. The positive predictive value of FDG-PET for relapse is close to 100% (Table 4.4), and persistent ^{18}F-FDG uptake after first-line therapy is associated with a high risk of relapse

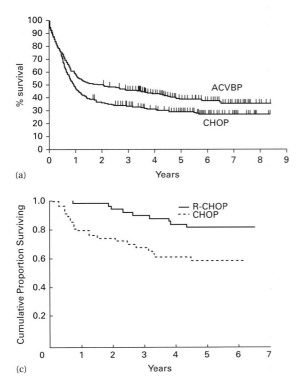

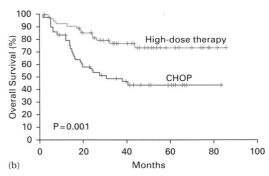

Figure 4.3. Prognostic value of upfront chemotherapy regimen on overall survival. (a) Intensified conventional treatment: ACVBP vs. CHOP in elderly patients (≥ 60 years) with at least one adverse prognostic factor by aaIPI (Tilly *et al.* 2003). (b) High-dose chemotherapy with autologous stem-cell transplantation vs. CHOP in young patients (< 60 years) with HI-risk according to aaIPI (Milpied *et al.* 2004). (c) Addition of rituximab to CHOP: R-CHOP vs. CHOP plus rituximab in elderly patients (≥ 60 years) with L- and LI-risk according to aaIPI (Feugier *et al.* 2005).

(Fig. 4.2b). The follow-up time and the small size of the studies, including often both DLBCL and Hodgkin's lymphoma, are critical factors, and the prognostic impact of FDG-PET needs to be confirmed. It is likely that FDG-PET will be included in response evaluation in the near future.

The prognostic value of FDG uptake has also been evaluated before autologous stem-cell transplantation (ASCT), and a positive FDG-PET scan was again correlated with PFS and OS (Fig. 4.2c). FDG-PET before transplantation should be an even stronger prognostic factor than IPI, and its prognostic significance is higher before than after transplantation. As ASCT is not effective in patients with refractory disease, a positive FDG-PET should influence the choice of salvage regimen before ASCT.

Early prediction of response to therapy could also distinguish those patients who will benefit from standard therapy from those for whom intensive strategies should be developed. A rapid decrease in FDG uptake by tumoral tissue has been observed as early as 7 days after the first administration of chemotherapy in patients with NHL, and it is therefore possible to separate early patients with or without residual

FDG uptake. Nevertheless, the best time to assess response remains unknown, and FDG-PET evaluation after one or a few cycles, or at mid-treatment, can predict response, PFS, and OS. Some authors have found that the predictive value of FDG-PET was independent of IPI, and FDG-PET findings obtained after the first cycle correlated better with PFS than those observed after completion of chemotherapy. Prospective studies evaluating the impact of interim FDG-PET on patient management are expected.

Dose intensity and schedule

Until the advent of rituximab the CHOP regimen (cyclophosphamide, doxorubicin, vincristine and prednisone) was considered as the gold standard for the treatment of DLBCL. Early phase II studies have highlighted the potential role of dose intensity and schedule of treatment on survival rates. These second- and third-generation regimens failed, however, to demonstrate an impact on survival. Several recent randomized trials have focused again on increasing the frequency and intensity of CHOP (Fig. 4.3). They demonstrated that CHOP given every 2 weeks (CHOP-14) or an intensified regimen (ACVBP) could improve OS rates. A more intensive strategy using high-dose chemotherapy followed by ASCT has also been tested in first-line therapy. Results are often conflicting, but could suggest that intensive early therapy might benefit age-adjusted IPI HI-risk patients. The benefit of adding rituximab to CHOP on survival has been demonstrated in both elderly patients with advanced DLBCL and in young low-risk patients (defined by IPI ≤ 1). The impact of adding rituximab to both intensified and high-dose chemotherapy is currently under investigation.

Prognostic factors at relapse

Clinical and treatment-related prognostic factors

Initial therapy of DLBCL with anthracycline-based chemotherapy cures approximately 40–50% of patients, and therefore 50–60% of patients either will have refractory disease to initial therapy or will relapse from a complete response. For them, high-dose chemotherapy followed by ASCT is the most successful approach, obtaining 40–45% 5-year event-free survival in the PARMA trial, which compared a salvage regimen (DHAP) given alone or followed by ASCT. Early studies of high-dose chemotherapy have, however, demonstrated that chemosensitivity to initial second-line therapy was an overwhelming predictor of outcome. Other additional adverse factors identified in many studies include short initial remission duration (lower than 12 months), elevated LDH, bulky disease (greater than 10 cm), three or more chemotherapy regimens before ASCT. The IPI has been evaluated at the initiation of second-line therapy as a predictor of outcome. In a retrospective analysis of the PARMA trial, aaIPI was highly predictive both of response to DHAP and of OS, for the entire cohort of patients and for the standard chemotherapy arm. For chemosensitive patients randomized to autologous stem-cell transplantation, however, aaIPI failed to be predictive of OS. Furthermore, no difference in PFS or OS was found between the two arms for patients with an aaIPI score of 0. The predictive value of aaIPI at relapse has been confirmed more recently.

Gene expression profiling

There are very few studies including gene expression profiling at the time of relapse, and its predictive value is under investigation. The importance of phenotype assessed by TMA in predicting survival in relapse or refractory DLBCL treated with ASCT has been recently reported. No difference in survival was observed for patients with either the GC phenotype or the non-GC phenotype.

FOLLICULAR LYMPHOMAS

Follicular lymphomas (FL) account for 25–30% of all NHLs. Until 20 years ago, treatment of FL was palliative and did not significantly modify the natural history of the disease. Since the development of immunotherapies such as interferon alpha, anti-CD20 monoclonal antibodies and combinations of them with chemotherapy, the overall survival has improved. However, these treatments may have immediate and/or long-term toxicity, may have untoward effects on quality of life and have variable costs. It has thus become essential for clinicians to have information on the potential prognosis of the disease at diagnosis, in order to help select a treatment with optimal efficacy/toxicity/cost ratios.

Prognostic factors at diagnosis

Clinical factors

Until recently, several retrospective analyses have looked for prognostic factors in FLs. The factors that have been reported as having a significant adverse influence on prognosis are listed in Table 4.5. The International Prognostic Index (IPI) proposed for aggressive lymphomas has also been tested in FLs, and almost all these retrospective analyses have shown that the IPI could separate patients into groups with significantly different prognoses. However, there are many caveats for using the IPI in FLs: (1) the statistical methodology is inadequate since some factors which were not significant in aggressive NHLs could influence the prognosis of FLs; (2) the IPI is poorly discriminant, with less than 15% of patients in the high-intermediate-risk and high-risk groups.

This prompted a group of specialists to initiate in 1998 a collection of data from around 5000 patients with FL. After univariate and multivariate analyses, the Follicular Lymphoma International Prognostic Index (FLIPI) has been proposed. The FLIPI relies on five parameters (Table 4.6): age, serum LDH level,

Table 4.5. Adverse prognostic factors in follicular lymphomas (from retrospective analyses of the literature).

Demographic	Advanced age
	Male sex
Pathological	Follicular diffuse architecture
	Cell type grade 3
Cytogenetic	Absence of t(14;18)
	Additional cytogenetic abnormalities
	6q deletion, 17p, 1p abnormalities
	p53 gene mutations
Molecular	Overexpression of macrophage and dendritic cell genes
	Overexpression of p53
Tumor mass	Ann Arbor stage III–IV
	Number of nodal sites involved
	Massive marrow infiltration
	Presence of bulky tumors
	Increased serum LDH level
	Increased serum β_2 microglobulin level
	Increased serum CA125
Consequences upon the host	Poor performance status
	B symptom(s)
	Anemia
	Hypoalbuminemia

Table 4.6. Prognostic factors for survival in the Follicular Lymphoma International Prognostic Index (FLIPI).

	Relative risk	p-value
Age (≤ 60 years vs. > 60 years)	2.38	<0.001
Ann Arbor stage (I–II vs. III–IV)	2.00	<0.001
Hemoglobin level (< 120 g/L vs. ≥ 120 g/L)	1.55	<0.001
LDH ($\leq$ normal vs. $>$ normal)	1.50	<0.001
Number of nodal sites (≤ 4 sites vs. > 4 sites)	1.39	<0.001

Ann Arbor stage, hemoglobin level. From these five parameters, three risk groups have been established. The characteristics of these groups, distribution of patients in the test group, 5-year and 10-year survivals and relative risks of deaths are shown in Table 4.7, and survival curves in Fig. 4.4. The FLIPI has been validated by analysis of other series and other validation tests are ongoing. The FLIPI was based on patients treated with conventional chemotherapy before the era of anti-CD20 monoclonal antibodies (MoAb). Overall survival cannot be used for validation in patients treated with anti-CD20 MoAb because of the scarcity of events. The usefulness of the FLIPI has thus been tested on progression-free survival, and it has been validated on different series of patients treated with CVP followed by rituximab, CVP combined with rituximab, CHOP combined with rituximab or treatment with radiolabeled anti-CD20 MoAb.

Histological factors

In the WHO classification of lymphomas, FLs are separated into three grades according to the cell type: grade 1 or small-cell FL, grade 2 or mixed small and large-cells FL, grade 3 or large-cell FL. Criteria for distinguishing between these three grades have been described by Mann and Berard. However, the concordance between pathologists is poor and patients with grade 1 or grade 2 FL are similarly treated. Grade 3 FLs account for approximately 10% of FLs and represent a separate entity. In addition, they have been separated into grade 3a (neoplastic follicles with more than 15 large cells per high-power field on a background of small cells) and grade 3b (neoplastic follicles in association with sheets of diffuse large-cell infiltration). Grade 3b FLs are also distinguished by cytogenetic characteristics: a lower incidence of t(14;18) than in other cell types, rearrangements in the 3q27 region in cases negative for t(14;18), absence of concomitant rearrangement of *BCL-2* and *BCL-6*. Grade 3b FLs are now considered and treated as DLBCL.

Genetic abnormalities

The t(14;18)(q32;q21) translocation is the hallmark of FLs, leading to overexpression of the *BCL-2* gene. FLs without the t(14;18) as studied by Southern blot may have a worse prognosis, although this remains debatable. Most FL cells carry additional chromosome abnormalities, and cell grade and survival have been demonstrated to be correlated with the number of

Table 4.7. Outcome and relative risk of death according to risk group as defined by the FLIPI.

Risk group	Number of factors	Distribution of patients (%)	5-year OS (%)	10-year OS (%)	Relative risk
Low	0–1	36	90.6	70.7	1.0
Intermediate	2	37	77.6	50.9	2.3
High	≥3	27	52.5	35.5	4.3

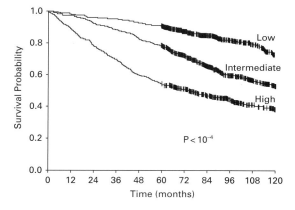

Figure 4.4. Survival of patients with follicular lymphoma according to risk group as defined by the Follicular Lymphoma International Prognostic Index (FLIPI). (Adapted from Solal-Céligny et al. 2004).

abnormalities. Besides, some chromosome abnormalities have per se an influence on prognosis, and may be associated with either a poor (6q deletion, 17p, 1p abnormalities) or a good (trisomy 12, +7, +8) survival. Some abnormalities have been associated with histological transformation of FL into high-grade NHL, such as mutation(s) of *P53*, overexpression of *C-MYC*, inactivation of the *P15* and *P16* cyclin-dependent kinase inhibitors located on chromosome 9 p21. However, these abnormalities are far from constant, and their relative contribution remains unknown.

Gene expression profiling

Recently, studies have been carried out on the gene profile of 191 patients with FL. Two signatures were distinguished, one associated with overexpression of T-lymphocyte genes and the other with macrophage and/or dendritic cell genes. The former signature was associated with a good prognosis while the latter was associated with a poor prognosis, and survival differences were highly significant and independent of clinical factors. The negative influence on prognosis of macrophage infiltration in follicular NHLs has been confirmed recently. Using tissue microarrays, it has been reported that a high macrophage infiltration as demonstrated by CD68 expression (i.e. more than 15 macrophages per high-power field) was associated with a poor prognosis. These studies strongly suggest that the immunologic microenvironment of FL cells plays a major role in the clinical aggressiveness of the disease.

Treatment-related prognostic factors

Several factors may allow the prediction of either response to treatment or duration of response. The significance of the persistence after treatment of t(14;18)-positive cells in the blood and/or bone marrow is controversial. It does not seem to influence the risk of relapse after radiation therapy for localized disease, but it is associated with a short progression-free survival after autologous bone marrow transplantation. Some studies suggest a negative influence for these cells, others an absence of prognostic value. According to a few gene profile analyses, some signatures are associated with an improved response to CHOP or to rituximab.

Prognostic factors at relapse

Histological transformation into DLBCL is by far the most important prognostic factor at relapse, and justifies nodal biopsy whenever possible, but few studies have tested prognostic factors at relapse. The FLIPI was tested and showed different overall survivals according to risk group. Sensitivity to initial chemotherapy, and delay between first and second episodes, also affect prognosis.

In conclusion, the development of new clinical and biological tools for predicting the prognosis of a patient with FL will help in choosing an optimal approach and thus contribute to an improvement in the prognosis of FLs.

MANTLE CELL LYMPHOMAS

Prognostic factors at diagnosis

Clinical factors

Amongst NHL subtypes, mantle cell lymphomas (MCL) have the poorest long-term survival, for several reasons:

(1) the median age is around 65 and few patients can be treated with intensive therapies;

(2) although response rates are high after initial therapy, complete response (CR) rates are low and most patients have residual disease;

(3) even in CR patients, the relapse rate is high after a median duration of response of around 18 months;

(4) after several relapses, most patients have a blastic transformation, which is highly resistant to all treatments.

Because of the low incidence of the disease and its heterogeneity in presentation, there is no consensus on a clinical prognostic index to use in MCL patients. Several retrospective analyses have reported adverse prognostic factors (Table 4.8). The IPI has also been applied to patients with MCL, and has been found to be discriminant in some but not all series. The IPI is poorly discriminant because most patients with MCL have adverse prognostic factors according to the IPI (age > 60, Ann Arbor stage IV disease, more than one extranodal involvement site) and are in the high-intermediate- and high-risk groups.

More recently, the FLIPI, which was designed for patients with follicular lymphoma, has also been applied to patients with MCL. In this study of 93 MCL patients, the 5-year overall survival rates were 65%, 42% and 8% respectively for patients in FLIPI low-, intermediate- and high-risk groups. Confirmative analyses are needed. Elaborating a consensual clinical prognostic index for MCL is one of the ongoing projects of the European Network for Mantle Cell Lymphomas.

Histological factors

MCL initially infiltrates the mantle zone surrounding normal germinal centers, generating a pattern called "nodular" MCL. Progressively, the germinal centers are destroyed by the neoplastic infiltrate, and the MCL becomes the "diffuse" type. In both nodular and diffuse types, the largest neoplastic compartment is made of small to medium-size lymphoid cells, with few large cells. There is no demonstration of a difference in prognosis between the nodular and diffuse types. MCL is sometimes characterized by slightly larger cells with a high mitotic index, and is therefore termed "blastoid" variant. This latter variant is associated with a more aggressive clinical behavior.

Table 4.8. Adverse clinical prognostic factors in mantle cell lymphomas, from retrospective analyses.

Reference	No. of patients	Adverse prognostic factors
R. Oinonen et al.	94	Age > 60 years; Ann Arbor stage III–IV, Leukemic disease; LDH > normal
H. Samaha et al.	121	Age > 70 years; ECOG performance status ≥ 2; Hemoglobin < 120 g/L; Leukemic involvement
D. Weisenburger et al.	68	Age > 60 years; Bone-marrow involvement; Ann Arbor stage III–IV; B symptoms; Performance status ≥ 2; High or intermediate IPI risk group
N. S. Andersen et al.	105	Age > 65 years; Hemoglobin < 120 g/L; Splenomegaly
E. Zucca et al.	65	Performance status ≥ 2; Increased LDH level; Increased β₂ microglobulin; Age > 65 years; High IPI risk group
L. H. Argatoff et al.	80	Performance status ≥ 2
A. J. Norton et al.	66	Age > 70 years; Ann Arbor stage IV; Splenomegaly; Low sodium; Low albumin

Genetic abnormalities

The genetic hallmark of MCL is the chromosomal translocation t(11;14)(q13;q32) that can be detected in virtually all cases of MCL. This translocation leads to overexpression of cyclin D1, which plays a key role in the control of the G1 phase of the cell cycle. An elevated level of cyclin D1 expression in MCL cells accelerates G1/S-phase transition and thus tumor cell proliferation. The level of cyclin D1 expression – as measured by mRNA translation – is directly correlated with tumor cell proliferation rate, as measured by Ki67 expression, and clinical aggressiveness.

Cyclin D1 is a key regulator of the cell cycle, and elevated levels of cyclin D1 in MCL cells promote additional cytogenetic alterations which may contribute to proliferation and prognosis. Other abnormalities of the cell-cycle regulatory pathway which have been reported in MCL are associated with an aggressive behavior and a poor prognosis:

- deletions of the cyclin D kinase (CDK) inhibitor gene (*CDK p16^{INK4a}*) on chromosome 9
- gene amplification of *CDK4*
- decreased expression of *P27KIP1*, which is an inhibitor of cyclin D/CDK complexes
- inactivation of *P53*, mainly observed in blastoid MCL types with a high proliferation index

These genetic alterations share the fact that they all predominantly target cell-cycle regulation and lead to an uncontrolled proliferation of MCL lymphoma cells. This has been confirmed by gene profile studies, which have demonstrated that a "proliferation signature," i.e. an overexpression of proliferation-associated genes, was a strong predictor of a poor survival. This "proliferation signature" probably reflects the combination of the genetic abnormalities mentioned above, and was also found to be associated with overexpression of genes involved in drug resistance. In conclusion, all MCLs have a poor prognosis with conventional treatments. As cell-cycle disturbances are the main factor in the development and clinical course of MCL, abnormalities of genes and proteins of the cell cycle will probably provide the most useful prognostic information. However, this contribution will be improved when new biological tools can be integated with new therapeutic approaches.

PERIPHERAL T-CELL LYMPHOMAS

Prognostic factors at diagnosis

Clinical factors

The importance of the T phenotype has been recognized recently by the REAL and the subsequent updated WHO classification. These classifications have also allowed us to appreciate fully the wide heterogeneity of peripheral T-cell lymphoma (PTCL), which accounts for 10–15% of all NHLs in Western countries. The WHO classification divides them into predominantly leukemic, nodal and extranodal types. Peripheral T-cell lymphoma unspecified (PTCL-u) represents the most common T-cell lymphoma in Western countries, accounting for 60–70% of PTCL. Because of this heterogeneity and the recent histopathological description, retrospective analyses of PTCL prognostic factors have to be treated with caution. For example, earlier reports based on older classifications failed to find a clinical impact of phenotype on outcome, whereas several studies using the REAL classification have indicated that T phenotype has a negative impact on survival (Fig. 4.5). The negative prognostic value of T phenotype is now well recognized, justifying new and innovative therapeutic strategies which differ from those developed for DLBCL.

The prognostic value of the IPI has also been assessed for PTCL. Most of these studies included patients with nodal PTCL, and found that the IPI had predictive value (Fig. 4.6). Another model has been developed in a large study that included some IPI factors (age, LDH, PS) in addition to BM involvement. PTCL-u patients commonly present with unfavorable characteristics including B symptoms, elevated LDH, bulky tumor, poor PS and extranodal disease. The majority of patients (50%) thus fall into the unfavorable IPI category. The IPI has also been evaluated in primary nasal natural killer cell lymphoma, where it was found to be correlated with survival. Application of IPI in the remaining subtypes has not been evaluated because of the scarcity of these subtypes, such as hepatosplenic $\gamma\delta$ T-cell lymphoma (present almost exclusively with high-risk IPI scores) and it is unlikely that the IPI has any clinical utility.

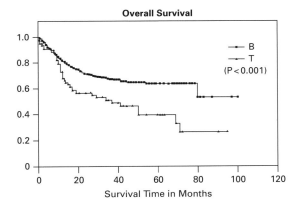

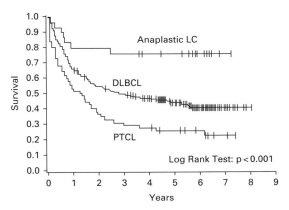

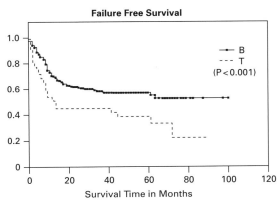

Figure 4.5. Kaplan–Meier estimates of overall survival and failure-free survival in patients with PTCL (T) compared to patients with DLBCL (B) (adapted from Melnyk *et al.* 1997).

Figure 4.7. Prognosis of systemic ALCL compared to other PTCL and DLBCL (adapted from Armitage *et al.* 2004).

Histological factors

Most PTCLs are predominantly nodal NHLs, which include angioimmunoblastic T-cell lymphomas (AITL), peripheral T-cell lymphomas unspecified (PTCL-u) and systemic anaplastic large-cell lymphomas (ALCL). Systemic ALCL has a superior survival compared to other PTCLs (Fig. 4.7), whereas the prognosis of PTCL-u compared to AITL remains controversial, with 5-year overall survival around 30–35%. It has also been demonstrated that systemic ALCL is heterogeneous according to the expression of ALK protein. ALK-negative cases often present in elderly patients, with an advanced stage, elevated serum LDH levels, B symptoms and extranodal involvement and have a prognosis similar to that of other PTCL, whereas ALK-positive cases have a 5-year survival close to 90% (Fig. 4.8). The prognosis for ALK-positive and ALK-negative groups may be further divided based on CD56 positivity, which imparts, independently of IPI, a significantly worse outcome when expressed in either ALCL group. More recent studies have suggested that a high bcl-2 expression or numerous activated (granzyme B+) cytotoxic T lymphocytes were associated with poor outcome in ALK-negative ALCL. For PTCL-u, CXCR3 expression was found to be associated with a better outcome whereas CCR4 expression was associated with a poor outcome and remained significant after adjustment for IPI.

Treatment-related prognostic factors

Because of the low incidence and the wide heterogeneity of PTCL, the evaluation of treatment

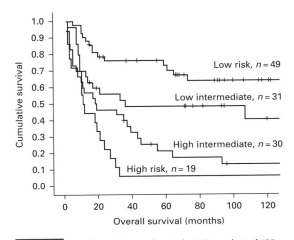

Figure 4.6. Overall survival according to the IPI in a cohort of 125 patients with nodal mature T-cell lymphoma (adapted from Sonnen *et al.* 2005).

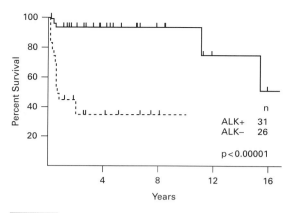

Figure 4.8. Prognostic value of ALK expression in systemic ALCL (adapted from Gascoyne *et al.* 1999).

regimens has been limited to non-randomized and retrospective studies. In addition, most of them have included different subtypes of PTCL known to have different outcomes. As in DLBCL, reaching a CR at the end of treatment probably improves the clinical outcome. However, optimal treatment is not defined and it is therefore difficult to identify prognostic factors related to this treatment.

MARGINAL ZONE LYMPHOMAS

Marginal zone B-cell lymphomas (MZL) encompass three subtypes:
(1) extranodal MZL or mucosa-associated lymphoid tissue (MALT) lymphomas
(2) splenic MZL with or without villous lymphoid cells in the blood and/or bone marrow
(3) nodal MZL with or without "monocytoid" type lymphoid cells in the blood and/or bone marrow
All MZLs have a normal counterpart in B cells of the "marginal zone" of the secondary follicles, which is adjacent to the mantle zone. Because of the rarity of this cell type, data on prognostic factors originate from retrospective analyses of small series with heterogeneous treatments. They therefore have limited value in guiding treatment choices.

MALT lymphomas

The main prognostic factor of MALT lymphomas (or MALTomas) is the demonstration of an infectious agent – *Helicobacter pylori* in gastric, *Chlamydophila psittaci* in adnexal ocular, *Borrelia burgdorferi* in skin

MALT lymphomas – and its eradication by the appropriate antibiotic treatment. Such eradication may result in the cure of the MALT lymphoma. Overall, the prognosis of gastrointestinal MALT lymphomas is better than that of other extranodal MALT lymphomas (median time to progression of 8.9 years vs. 4.9 years, $p < 0.01$). The presence of a large-cell component (so-called MALT lymphoma in transformation) is a rare event but associated with a poorer prognosis. Other clinical factors have been shown to adversely affect the clinical outcome of patients with MALT lymphomas in retrospective analyses: disseminated disease in some series, poor performance status, increased serum LDH levels, bulky tumor, increased serum β_2 microglobulin level, decreased serum albumin level. A t(11;18)(q21;q21) translocation has been described in 30% of gastric MALT lymphomas. It fuses the amino terminal of the *API2* gene to the carboxy terminal of the *MALT1* gene and generates a fusion product that activates nuclear factor kappa B (NF-κB). This translocation is associated with the absence of concomitant *Helicobacter pylori* infection, or with resistance to *Helicobacter pylori* eradication and to therapy with an alkylating agent, but not resistance to rituximab.

Other MZL lymphomas

Studies of prognostic factors in splenic or nodal MZLs are scarce. The International Prognostic Index could not be used in these patients because very few patients are in high-risk groups. A high lymphocyte count, increased serum LDH and/or β_2 microglobulin levels have been described as adverse prognostic factors.

BURKITT'S LYMPHOMA

Prognostic factors at diagnosis

Whereas Burkitt's lymphoma represents 30–50% of pediatric lymphoma, it accounts for only a small percentage of adult lymphomas. The evaluation of treatment regimens in adults is also limited to retrospective and non-randomized studies. Most of our knowledge of prognostic factors for Burkitt's lymphoma, therefore, comes from large prospective randomized pediatric studies, in which very high rates of survival have been obtained (Fig 4.9).

Table 4.9. Burkitt's lymphoma: therapeutic groups according to the Société Française d'Oncologie Pédiatrique (SFOP) and the Berlin–Frankfurt–Münster (BFM) group.

	SFOP	BFM
Low-risk group	Stage I Abdominal stage II	Initial complete resection of lymphoma manifestations

Intermediate-risk group	Unresected stage I
	Non-abdominal stage II
	Any stage III or IV, or
	L3 ALL ($<$ 25% blasts)
		No or incomplete resection of lymphoma manifestations
		  with at least one of the following criteria:
		  only extra-abdominal sites
		  abdominal site and LDH $<$ 500 UI/L

High-risk group	CNS involvement
	L3 ALL ($\geq$ 25% blasts)
		No or incomplete resection of abdominal lymphoma and
		  LDH $\geq$ 500 UI/L
		BM involvement and/or CNS disease and/or multifocal
		  bone involvement

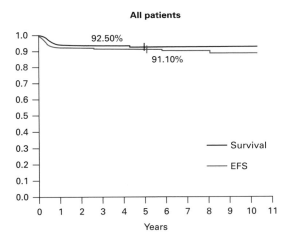

Figure 4.9. Event-free survival and overall survival of 561 children with Burkitt's lymphoma (adapted from Patte *et al.* 2001).

Clinical factors

Age is often considered an adverse prognostic factor for Burkitt's lymphoma. In studies including children and adults treated with the same regimen, this factor was not identified. But in other studies using more intensive chemotherapy, age below 10 years or 15 years has been demonstrated to be associated with favorable outcome. When these chemotherapy regimens have been tested in adult cohorts, researchers have found a decreased overall survival compared to that obtained in a pediatric population, especially for advanced stages. These results could be due in part to an increased toxicity of such intensified conventional chemotherapies, and the exact impact of age on survival remains uncertain.

Burkitt's lymphoma patients more frequently present with extranodal involvement, compared to DLBCL, and the extent of such lymphomas is usually assessed using the Murphy classification. Advanced stages III and IV were initially found to be associated with a decreased survival in both pediatric and adult patients, whereas the use of an adapted and intensified conventional chemotherapy tends toward erasing the influence of stage on survival. Serum LDH level, as a surrogate of cell proliferation, and a tumor mass $\geq$ 10 cm have also been found to impart a poorer prognosis. Central-nervous-system and bone-marrow involvement are recognized to be the most significant adverse prognostic factors, and justify an intensified treatment. Using these prognostic factors, different therapeutic groups have been defined, allowing the development of therapeutic strategies based upon individual risk (Table 4.9).

Treatment-related prognostic factors

Survival of patients with Burkitt's lymphoma requires achieving CR. Stable or progressive diseases (refractory disease) are almost always rapidly fatal. Some other treatment-related prognostic factors have been demonstrated, especially in children. First, the absence of complete response after three multi-agent chemotherapy courses correlated with an adverse outcome, and those patients who achieved a partial response at this time could be salvaged with high-dose chemotherapy with ASCT. Second, patients whose tumors did not respond to the pre-phase (regimen including cyclophosphamide, vin-cristine and prednisone) ultimately failed. More recently, the importance of early intensive treatment has been shown, with significantly lower EFS if the second course of chemotherapy (COPADM2) started after day 21. It is also established that no relapse occurs after one year of CR, and patients without early relapse or progression can be considered to be cured. At relapse, it has been demonstrated that the ability to cure patients with high-dose chemotherapy followed by ASCT is closely related to the chemosen-sitivity of relapse. Burkitt's lymphoma refractory to a second line of chemotherapy has a low probability of cure, whatever the treatment.

PRIMARY CENTRAL NERVOUS SYSTEM LYMPHOMA

Prognostic factors at diagnosis

Clinical factors

Primary central nervous system lymphomas (PCNSL) represent 2% of NHLs, making it difficult to identify robust clinical prognostic factors. A primary brain localization is an adverse prognostic factor compared to localized non-CNSL. Immunodeficiency, whether related to inherited disorders, to HIV or to organ transplantation, increases the risk of PCNSL. Even if these patients are not usually included in prospective trials, they seem also to have a bad prognosis compared with immunocomptent PCNSL. Age and PS are the only two universally accepted prognostic factors for PCNSL. It has been suggested that they are factors influencing therapeutic choice rather than independent survival indicators, but critical review of published data and a more recent large study have confirmed that they are independent variables. The prognostic value of the IPI has been tested in some retrospective studies. The IPI is not accurate for PCNSLs which are localized and fre-quently associated with a poor PS. This explains why

Table 4.10. Prognostic factors for survival in PCNSL.

	Relative risk	p-value
Age ($\leq$ 60 years vs. $>$ 60 years)	1.02	<0.001
LDH ($\leq$ normal vs. $>$ normal)	1.41	0.008
Performance status (0–1 vs. 2–4)	1.64	<0.001
CSF protein level (normal vs. elevated)	1.71	0.003
Deep lesions (no vs. yes)	1.45	<0.001

the IPI was not discriminant in a large retrospective study.

It is also likely that specific prognostic factors influ-ence survival. The influence of lymphoma localiza-tion, number of brain tumors and CSF protein level has therefore been retrospectively evaluated, with conflicting results. More recently, predictors of response and survival were analyzed in an interna-tional multicenter retrospective series of 378 immuno-competent patients with PCNSL in an attempt to propose a prognostic index. More than 90% of patients were treated with radiotherapy alone or with combined radiochemotherapy. In the multivari-ate analysis, five factors have been identified to have a prognostic impact on survival (Table. 4.10): age, PS, LDH serum level, protein CSF concentration and involvement of the deep structures of the brain. Each variable was assigned a value of either 0, if favorable, or 1, if unfavorable, and the overall score was obtained by the addition of the values of these five variables. The number of adverse features was significantly cor-related to survival (Fig. 4.10) and the prognostic value of this index was also found in patients treated with high-dose methotrexate (HD-MTX)-based chemother-apy, with or without radiotherapy.

Histological factors

Over 90% of B-cell PCNSLs are DLBCL, with Burkitt's and low-grade NHL each representing 5%. The T phe-notype is found in fewer than 5% of PCNSL. The phenotype and histological subtypes do not seem to influence survival. Bcl-6 and bcl-2 protein expression have both been found to have a prognostic influence in DLBCL. In a recent study of 83 patients with PCNSL, GC and ABC phenotypes were assessed by TMA; most patients express an ABC phenotype and have survival identical to DLBCL expressing the same phenotype.

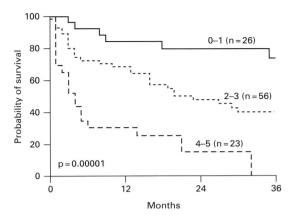

Figure 4.10. Prognostic value of PCNSL prognosis score (adapted form Ferreri *et al.* 2003).

Treatment-related prognostic factors

An important difference from NHL located outside the CNS is that in the case of PCNSL obtaining a CR does not seem to have a prognostic impact. In a retrospective study, patients with CR and PR did not have statistically different 5-year survivals. However, such results highlighted the difficulty of accurate evaluation of these tumors by CT scan and MRI. The impact of FDG-PET in PCNSL evaluation has not yet been examined.

PCNSL treatment influences the outcome of patients. Surgery is not recommended, and radiotherapy and chemotherapy are usually used. Prospective randomized studies have failed to demonstrate an impact of treatment on survival, but retrospective analyses have shown that radiotherapy or chemotherapy alone give lower survival rates compared to combined chemoradiotherapy. HD-MTX-based chemotherapy has been found to have significant impact on survival in several studies using multivariate analysis. Concomitant intrathecal chemotherapy did not have any impact.

HODGKIN'S LYMPHOMA

Prognostic factors at diagnosis

Clinical factors

There are numerous studies analyzing the impact of clinical characteristics at diagnosis on outcome in patients with Hodgkin's lymphoma (HL). However, most of them included few patients, and were heterogeneous and retrospective, and the prognostic factor models developed should be considered carefully before they are used as a basis for deciding on treatment for a patient with HL. Moreover, prognostic factors are closely related to the treatment used, and with the improvement in outcome for patients with limited-stage HL these models are no longer clinically relevant. In advanced-stage HL, prognostic factors can also be helpful in identifying patients at high risk of relapse and in developing new therapeutic strategies. All prognostic factors described are related to tumor spread, tumor burden, patient characteristics or interaction of tumor and host.

Related to tumor spread and tumor burden

The Ann Arbor classification describes the anatomic spread of tumor cells via contiguous lymph-node groups, and has been demonstrated to be of prognostic relevance for disease-free survival (DFS) and OS in many studies testing different therapeutic regimens in HL. It is therefore possible to separate "early disease" (stages I/II), which represents two-thirds of patients, with an estimated 5-year OS close to 90%, and "advanced disease" (stages III/IV), which represents one-third of patients, with 5-year OS lower than 70%. The Ann Arbor classification has been used for more than 30 years to influence therapeutic strategies, but clinical studies have clearly demonstrated differences of survival among patients with the same stage, demonstrating the need for additional prognostic factors to adapt the therapeutic strategy to individual risk.

The amount of tumor cells is an important prognostic factor and the presence of bulky disease, especially in the mediastinum, is associated with a poor prognosis. Bulky disease is defined as either a single mass of tumor tissue exceeding 10 cm in largest diameter or a mediastinal mass with a ratio of largest transverse diameter of the mass to transverse diameter of the thorax at T5–6 of ≥ 0.35 on chest radiograph. This definition has been included in the Ann Arbor classification and is often referred to as the Cotswolds modification. A ratio of more than 0.45 has been found to be independently associated with a poor DFS and OS. Bulky mediastinum, found in 15–20% of patients with early disease, correlated with a reduced DFS after radiotherapy or chemotherapy alone as well as after combined treatment, whereas in advanced-stage HL treated with more aggressive therapies there are less consistent data on the prognostic significance of mediastinal bulk. The prognosis value of bulky disease outside the mediastinum is more uncertain. Some have calculated tumor burden according to both the number and the size of involved nodes. These authors have demonstrated that, in early stages, tumor burden correlates with both DFS and OS. Other specific sites of HL were shown to be of prognostic significance, such as BM, spleen or pleural involvements. Their prognostic value is controversial and seems to have only a little impact on survival. The number of organs involved has been correlated with OS and DFS by some, but this has not been found in larger studies. LDH could be viewed as a surrogate of tumor burden, and an elevated LDH level has been found to have a prognostic value in HL, being associated with involvement of marrow and at least two organs.

Related to patient characteristics

Some patient characteristics including age and sex are important in prognosis. Age is considered as an adverse prognostic factor in many malignant diseases but increased morbidity and mortality in older patients due to other causes has to be considered and results have to be matched to the general population. Secondly, increased comorbidity leads to increased therapy-related mortality. Nevertheless, considering studies matching patients to the general population and including multivariate analysis, age has been shown to have an adverse prognostic impact especially in advanced stages. Gender seems also to influence outcome in HL. This could be due in part to the association of female gender with other favorable parameters including localized stage and lack of B symptoms or nodular sclerosis. In a large cohort of patients, multivariate analysis demonstrated that male gender was independently associated with a reduced OS.

Related to interaction of tumor and host

B symptoms (fever, weight loss and night sweats) have been known to have clinical relevance for many years and have been included in the Ann Arbor classification. They are more frequent in advanced stages compared to early stages and correlate with other biological parameters including increased erythrocyte sedimentation rate (ESR) and

decreased serum albumin or hemoglobin. Despite this, their independent prognostic value has not been confirmed in multivariate analysis, but the presence of B symptoms is used by most cooperative groups to inform therapeutic strategies. An elevated ESR was shown to have independent prognostic significance for DFS and OS for different stages and several regimens especially in early-stage disease. The European Organisation for Research and Treatment of Cancer (EORTC) lymphoma group defined a group of patients with either ESR > 50 without B symptoms or ESR > 30 with B symptoms, who have a worse outcome and an increased rate of relapse. Anemia has also been reported to be associated with decreased survival in both early and advanced stages. In large retrospective analyses, lymphopenia $< 0.6 \times 10^9$/L was independently associated with decreased survival. Many other biological parameters easily available in peripheral blood, such as ferritin, C-reactive protein, β_2 microglobulin, coeruloplasmine or thymidine kinase, have been described as influencing outcome in HL, but their significance falls to insignificant levels when multi-parametric analysis is used.

Prognostic models

From studies conducted during the 1980s prognostic models have been developed (Table 4.11). Most of these studies included few patients with both early and advanced stages, patients were treated with different approaches, and these prognostic models have not been validated on other groups of patients. Furthermore, they failed to identify a subgroup of advanced HL patients with a very high risk of relapse when applied in a cohort of patients treated homogeneously. In 1998, Hasenclever *et al.* used the international database on HL to develop a parametric model for predicting survival. This model was based on data from 5023 patients who were at various stages of the disease and who received various treatments. Seven prognostic factors – sex, age, hemoglobin level, white blood-cell and lymphocyte counts, serum albumin and disease stage – were found to influence freedom from progression (FFP) in a Cox model (Table 4.12). These factors were therefore incorporated into a model and an individual patient's relative risk for relapse and death was determined by adding the number of adverse prognostic factors present at diagnosis. It was therefore possible to identify six

Table 4.11. Prognostic-factor models developed for Hodgkin's lymphoma.

Authors	Gobbi *et al.*	Proctor *et al.*	Straus *et al.*
Population analyzed			
	$n = 586$	$n = 93$	$n = 185$
	Stage I–IV	Stage I–IV	Stage II–IV
Prognostic factors used in the model			
Clinical	Age	Age	Age
	Sex	—	—
	Stage	Stage	—
	Histology	—	—
	B symptoms	—	—
	Bulky mediastinal	Bulky mediastinal	Bulky mediastinal
	—	—	Inguinal nodes
Biological	ESR	—	—
	Hemoglobin	Hemoglobin	—
	Albumin	—	—
	—	Lymphocyte count	—
	—	—	LDH
			Marrow involvement

Table 4.12. Prognostic factors for freedom from progression (FFP) in International Index patients.

Factors	Relative risk	*p*-value
Serum albumin < 40 g/L	1.49	<0.001
Hemoglobin < 105 g/L	1.35	0.006
Male sex	1.35	0.001
Stage IV	1.26	0.011
Age ≥ 45 yr	1.39	0.001
White cell count $\geq 15 \times 10^9$/L	1.41	0.001
Lymphocyte count $< 0.6 \times 10^9$/L or $< 8\%$ of white cell count	1.38	0.002

groups of patients (score 0, 1, 2, 3, 4, $\geq$5) who had FFP of disease at 5 years ranging from 84% (for score 0) to 42% (for score $\geq$5) (Fig. 4.11a, c). This International Prognosis Score (IPS) was also predictive for OS (Fig. 4.11b). However, only 13% of patients included in this analysis were at a limited stage and the IPS failed to identify the lower-risk groups reliably.

Furthermore, a score of 4 or more was still associated with a 47% FFP and 59% OS at 5 years, demonstrating the limits of the IPS in identifying very-high-risk patients.

Analysis of prognostic factors at diagnosis enables the assignment of patients to different therapeutic groups, and the definition of therapeutic strategies based upon individual risk. In Europe, the German Hodgkin Study Group (GHSG) stratifies patients according to stage and four prognostic factors (Table 4.13), defining three therapeutic groups (early, early unfavorable and advanced stages). The European Organisation for Research and Treatment of Cancer (EORTC) defines prognostic groups for localized sub-diaphragmatic stages with favorable (no adverse factor) or unfavorable (one or more adverse factors) outcome (Table 4.14), whereas the IPS is used to identify advanced HL with high risk of relapse. Most of these prognostic scores were established from patients treated before the last decade, and recent data have demonstrated that they lose predictive power with improved treatment, emphasizing the need for new prognostic factors.

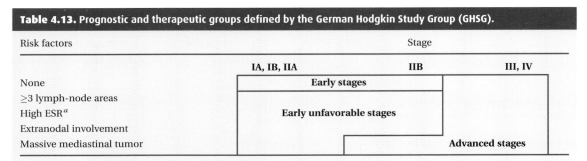

Table 4.13. Prognostic and therapeutic groups defined by the German Hodgkin Study Group (GHSG).

Risk factors	Stage		
	IA, IB, IIA	IIB	III, IV
None	Early stages		
≥3 lymph-node areas			
High ESR[a]	Early unfavorable stages		
Extranodal involvement			
Massive mediastinal tumor			Advanced stages

[a] Erythrocyte sedimentation rate (≥ 50 without or ≥ 30 with B symptoms)

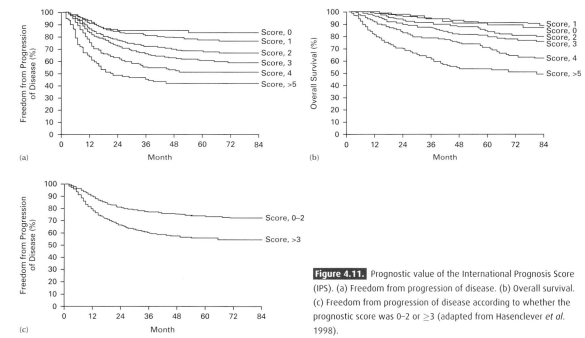

Figure 4.11. Prognostic value of the International Prognosis Score (IPS). (a) Freedom from progression of disease. (b) Overall survival. (c) Freedom from progression of disease according to whether the prognostic score was 0–2 or ≥3 (adapted from Hasenclever et al. 1998).

Histological factors

The prognostic value of the classification established in 1966 by Lukes and Butler has been analyzed in many studies. They demonstrated that the lymphocyte-depleted subtype of HL was associated with a worse outcome. The number of patients suffering from this subtype is very low, and histologic classification of HL has been reconsidered in the REAL classification, separating lymphocyte-predominant HL from classical HL. Up to 70% of the classical HL population suffer from nodular sclerosis, and can be separated into two subgroups. Nodular sclerosis subtype 2, with areas depleted of lymphocytes and a large

number of pleomorphic Hodgkin's and Reed–Sternberg (HRS) cells, has been found to be associated with a decreased survival independently of stage. Other groups did not confirm this prognostic value.

Some markers such as Ki67, p53, Rb, bcl-2 and LMP-1 expressed by HRS have been analyzed and correlated with outcome. Such studies have yielded conflicting results, they were retrospective and they included too few patients to support any definitive conclusion. Some groups have focused on non-malignant cells and have demonstrated a negative prognostic impact of CD8 granzyme B-positive T cells or eosinophilic infiltrates.

Table 4.14. Prognostic and therapeutic groups for sub-diaphragmatic stages I–II defined by the European Organisation for Research and Treatment of Cancer.

Risk factors	Stage	
	IA, IB	**IIA, IIB**
None	**Favorable stages**	
≥4 lymph-node areas		
High ESR[a]	**Unfavorable stages**	
Age ≥ 50 years		
Massive mediastinal tumor		

[a] Erythrocyte sedimentation rate (≥ 50 without or ≥ 30 with B symptoms)

Other biological factors

In the last decade, new biological parameters have been investigated as predictors of prognosis. CD30 is consistently expressed by HRS cells, and soluble CD30 was found to have independent prognostic significance in a number of studies. Soluble CD30 seemed to correlate with tumor burden and lymphocyte-depleted HL. VCAM-1 and ICAM-1 are adhesion molecules, and soluble forms could have prognostic significance. Several cytokines such as IL-2, IL-6, IL-7, IL-8, IL-10, IL-12, IL-13, TNF-α, secreted by both HRS cells and lymphoid cells surrounding HRS cells, have also been evaluated but their prognostic value needs to be specified.

Treatment-related prognostic factors

Dose intensity and time to complete response

Survival of patients with HL is closely related to reaching CR at the end of treatment, and stable and progressive disease (refractory disease) are associated with a poor survival. In a retrospective analysis, the dose delivered in the first three cycles of chemotherapy was the main factor predicting CR and outcome, demonstrating the importance of dose intensity in HL treatment. Moreover, early CR, usually assessed after 3–4 cycles, is also shown to be predictive of a better outcome.

Positron emission tomography using ¹⁸F-fluorodeoxyglucose (FDG-PET)

As with DLBCL, gallium-67 (^{67}Ga) scintigraphy has been replaced by FDG-PET in the assessment of response to chemotherapy. Most of the studies demonstrating the prognostic value of FDG-PET for post-treatment evaluation include both DLBCL and HL, and in this situation negative predictive value seemed to be higher in HL than in DLBCL. Early prognostic value of FDG-PET has also been demonstrated in early response assessment, where it correlated independently with PFS and OS, especially for advanced-stage patients. Prospective studies evaluating the impact of interim FDG-PET in patient management are now awaited. But because ASCT is not usually used in front-line therapy, the predictive value of FDG-PET before high-dose chemotherapy and ASCT in HL has not been systematically evaluated.

Prognostic factors at relapse

Many studies have analyzed prognostic factors of patients with refractory or relapsed HL. The length of remission after first-line chemotherapy has been shown to be an important prognostic factor. Using conventional salvage therapy, virtually no patient with primary progressive disease (10% of patients) survives after 8 years, contrasting with projected 20-year survivals of 11% and 22%, respectively, for patients relapsing within 12 months of CR (15% of patients) and more than 12 months after CR (15% of patients).

FURTHER READING

A predictive model for aggressive non-Hodgkin's lymphoma. The International Non-Hodgkin's Lymphoma Prognostic Factors Project. *N. Engl. J. Med.* **329** (1993), 987–994.

Dave, S. S., Wright, G., Tan, B. *et al.* Prediction of survival in follicular lymphoma based on molecular features of tumor-infiltrating immune cells. *N. Engl. J. Med.* **351** (2004), 2159–2169.

Ferreri, A. J., Blay, J. Y., Reni, M. *et al.* Prognostic scoring system for primary CNS lymphomas: the International Extranodal Lymphoma Study Group experience. *J. Clin. Oncol.* **21** (2003), 266–272.

Gascoyne, R. D., Aoun, P., Wu, D. *et al.* Prognostic significance of anaplastic lymphoma kinase (ALK) protein expression in adults with anaplastic large cell lymphoma. *Blood* **93** (1999), 3913–3921.

Hans, C. P., Weisenburger, D. D., Greiner, T. C. *et al.* Confirmation of the molecular classification of diffuse large B-cell lymphoma by immunohistochemistry using a tissue micro array. *Blood* **103** (2004), 275–282.

Hasenclever, D. and Diehl, V. A prognostic score for advanced Hodgkin's disease. International Prognostic Factors Project on Advanced Hodgkin's disease. *N. Engl. J. Med.* **339** (1998), 1506–1514.

Lossos, I. S., Czerwinski, D. K., Alizadeh, A. A. *et al.* Prediction of survival in diffuse large-B-cell lymphoma based on the expression of six genes. *N. Engl. J. Med.* **350** (2004), 1828–1837.

Patte, C., Auperin, A., Michon, J. *et al.* The Société Française d'Oncologie Pédiatrique LMB89 protocol: highly effective multiagent chemotherapy tailored to the tumor burden and initial response in 561 unselected children with B-cell lymphomas and L3 leukemia. *Blood* **97** (2001), 3370–3379.

Reiter, A., Schrappe, M., Tiemann, M. *et al.* Improved treatment results in childhood B-cell neoplasms with tailored intensification of therapy: a report of the Berlin–Frankfurt–Munster Group Trial NHL-BFM 90. *Blood* **94** (1999), 3294–3306.

Rosenwald, A., Wright, G., Chan, W. C. *et al.* The molecular use of profiling to predict survival after chemotherapy for diffuse large-B-cell lymphoma. *N. Engl. J. Med.* **346** (2002), 1937–1947.

Rosenwald, A., Wright, G., Wiestner, A. *et al.* The proliferation gene expression signature is a quantitative integrator of oncogenic events that predicts survival in mantle cell lymphoma. *Cancer Cell* **3** (2003), 185–197.

Solal-Céligny, P., Roy, P., Colombat, P. *et al.* Follicular lymphoma international prognostic index. *Blood* **104** (2004), 1258–1265.

Straus, D. J., Gaynor, J. J., Myers, J. *et al.* Prognostic factors among 185 adults with newly diagnosed advanced Hodgkin's disease treated with alternating potentially noncross-resistant chemotherapy and intermediate-dose radiation therapy. *J. Clin. Oncol.* **8** (1990), 1173–1186.

Thieblemont, C., Bastion, Y., Berger, F. *et al.* Mucosa-associated lymphoid tissue gastrointestinal and nongastrointestinal lymphoma behavior: analysis of 108 patients. *J. Clin. Oncol.* **15** (1997), 1624–1630.

Zucca, E., Conconi, A., Pedrinis, E. *et al.* Nongastric marginal zone B-cell lymphoma of mucosa-associated lymphoid tissue. *Blood* **101** (2003), 2489–2495.

5 CLINICAL TRIALS IN LYMPHOMA

Thomas M. Habermann and Susan M. Geyer

INTRODUCTION

Clinical trials are the backbone of the development and advancement of therapeutic interventions. The pace of development of new agents, the costs of data management, inclusion of quality-of-life assessments, symptom-control assessments and the evaluation of biologic correlates all present significant challenges for the future development of new therapeutic regimens. As these therapeutic regimens become increasingly targeted and our understanding of lymphoma deepens, the identification and assessment of relevant endpoints, be they clinical (e.g. physical examination, radiologic) or biologic (e.g. immunologic, genetic, metabolic etc.), also becomes increasingly complex. In turn, the more complex our endpoints and the more targeted our regimens, the more challenges are presented when designing and conducting clinical trials and analyzing and interpreting their results. While the field of clinical trial design is too broad and widely discussed to adequately give full discussion in this chapter, the reader is referred to more general references on this area. Given the complexity of issues when designing, monitoring, interpreting and analyzing data for a clinical trial, statistician input and collaboration is of paramount importance. This chapter focuses on the principles behind and details of clinical trials from the clinician perspective. As such, we discuss the fundamental considerations when designing trials as well as outline the types of trials typically conducted in clinical research.

BACKGROUND

The practice and science of clinical trials and research is in its relative infancy. Until 1750, the thinking was that of Galen, who attained an authority that remained unchallenged. Medicine had a long tradition of physicians as trusted advisors to patients, treatment choices were based not on investigation but rather on uncontrolled experimentation. One of the earliest and most commonly cited examples of clinical experiments to evaluate therapeutic interventions was the treatment of scurvy with oranges and lemons. The comparison of results from these clinical trials was primarily with those in the literature, with other historical controls, or with those of concurrent trials. The first strictly controlled clinical trial through random assignment of patients to treatment groups was not reported until 1931, in the examination of tuberculosis patients. A subsequent trial in tuberculosis patients was also the first to use random numbers to assign patients to experimental versus control groups, and it was demonstrated that streptomycin plus bed rest was superior to bed rest alone.

Since then, the practice and development of clinical trials has expanded greatly. In the United States, controlled clinical trials were first conducted by the National Cancer Institute (NCI) under Gordon Zubrod. Zubrod was one of the key individuals in the formation of the Eastern Solid Tumor Group (now the Eastern Cooperative Oncology Group, ECOG), which published the first randomized trial in solid malignancies in the USA, comparing nitrogen mustard and thiophosphamide.

In today's research environment, a primary focus in the development and conduct of clinical trials is the safety and protection of the patient involved in such research. This is of primary importance as we continue to refine and explore new methods for clinical trial design and analysis.

Lymphoma: Pathology, Diagnosis and Treatment, ed. Robert Marcus, John W. Sweetenham and Michael E. Williams. Published by Cambridge University Press. © Cambridge University Press 2007.

INFORMED CONSENT

The unprecedented growth in discovery has resulted in a dominant role for clinical research, and this in turn has emphasised the process of informed consent. The National Cancer Institute (NCI) and the Food and Drug Administration (FDA) in the USA, and the European Union Clinical Trials Directive legislation, have all structured and strengthened the elements of this process. Safeguards must be in place for patients who enter clinical trials. Informed consent is one of the key aspects.

The key elements of informed consent are outlined in Table 5.1. Additional points that need to be brought to the patient's attention include unforeseeable risks to the patient, embryo or fetus; circumstances in which the subject's participation may be terminated by the investigator without the patient's consent; the number of patients; additional costs which may result from study participation; consequences of withdrawal; and a statement that new findings may relate to the patient's willingness to continue study participation. The consent form must be signed and dated by the patient or patient's representative, and a copy must be given to the patient or the patient's representative.

The investigator must not unduly influence participation and/or continuation on a protocol, and should fully inform the subject or the subject's representative of all pertinent aspects of the trial. The language used in the oral explanation and in the written consent form should be non-technical, practical and understandable to the participant. If the patient or patient's representative is unable to read, an impartial witness should be present during the informed consent discussion and should sign and date the consent form along with the patient, if the patient is capable.

ENDPOINTS

To effectively develop, implement and analyze a clinical trial, it is critical to establish clearly the questions to be evaluated. A clear statement of the research question and the motivation for conducting the clinical trial leads to a clear definition of the endpoints to be evaluated in the trial. While intuitive, this is important in order to ensure that the endpoints actually address the goals of the trial. These goals and corresponding endpoints must also match the phase and type of trial.

Table 5.1. Informed consent.

Involves research
Purpose
Duration
Procedures (experimental or not)
Treatment(s)

Description of risks or discomfort
Must include all that are listed in the model
  consent form
Inconvenience

Description of benefits
Reasonable expected benefits
Benefits to society
Must include all that are listed in the model
  consent form

Description of the extent of confidentiality of records
If results are published, patient identity remains
  confidential
Individuals who have access to the medical records:
  monitors/auditors, IRB, regulatory authorities,
  sponsor(s), drug company/ies
Explanation regarding compensation and/or whether
  treatments are available if injury occurs

Voluntary participation
Refusal to participate involves no penalty
May discontinue at any time without loss of benefits
Alternative procedures or treatments

Contacts for
Research-related questions
Information regarding subject's rights
Research-related injury

Overall, the choice of the primary endpoint is critical to answering the primary research question, and typically drives the sample-size and power considerations. The ultimate goal in treating lymphoma patients is to extend their survival and improve their quality of life. Since overall survival is an endpoint that is not always easily evaluated in the constrained timeframe of a clinical trial with subsequent treatment options available, surrogate endpoints are often used to determine efficacy. Surrogate endpoints for clinical activity such as response and progression-free survival are the most typically used in evaluating efficacy of experimental regimens. Secondary endpoints to be evaluated are also defined a priori, but power considerations for these analyses do not usually impact on the determination of sample size. However, the sample size of the trial may be increased moderately to power specific secondary endpoint analyses of critical interest.

Defining the endpoints used to answer the research questions is best achieved when considering the treatment interventions to be evaluated, as well as the targeted patient population. For example, in the case of some of the novel therapeutic regimens being considered, the agents may have cytostatic rather than cytotoxic effects. In the past the focus has been on cytotoxic agents and high-dose therapies, but newer biologic agents have a range of targets including cell surface markers, modulators of signal transduction pathways, angiogenesis inhibitors, growth factor receptor inhibitors, potentiators of apoptosis and modulators of gene expression. They may include cellular therapy, gene therapy and vaccine therapy, and the application of clinical trials to these interventions presents new challenges and opportunities. With these cytostatic agents, the standard endpoint of clinical response may not be sufficient to determine efficacy. Instead, the proportion of patients who have not progressed or relapsed within a specified timeframe may be used, or other endpoints more appropriate to capture the effects of a cytostatic agent. In addition, evaluation of immunotherapeutic regimens may require similar alternative endpoints in order to evaluate efficacy.

OUTCOME DATA

After determining the primary and secondary endpoints of interest for the clinical trial, it is important to identify the variables and resulting outcome data necessary to assess the trial aims. Outcome measures will vary depending on the endpoints and the phase of the trial, and they may use qualitative (categorical), quantitative (measurement) or time-to-event data. An example of a qualitative measure is the classification of response, where changes in tumor measurements define complete response (CR), partial response (PR), stable disease (SD) and progressive disease (PD). For patients with more refractory and/or aggressive disease, the overall response rate may be of interest. For newly diagnosed and/or more indolent disease,

where the overall response (CR and PR) rates are typically high with standard treatment, and thus where a complete response is more interesting, the CR rate may instead be used as a primary measure of efficacy.

Quantitative endpoints focus on continuous measures of effect. Examples of this are outcomes such as changes or percentage changes in quality-of-life scores, immunologic parameters, or other biologic parameters that can measure clinical effect or adverse reactions. Time-to-event data can also be defined in many different ways, depending on the needs of the trial, and it is important to define what constitutes an event as well as the time from which this is measured (e.g. study entry, diagnosis). Time-to-event measures include event-free survival (i.e. time to an event defined as progression, relapse and/or death), overall survival (i.e. time to death from any cause) and even time to engraftment. Time-to-event measures must take account of the fact that not all patients will have had an event at the time of analysis, but having followed them for a certain time you know that they are event-free at least until that time. Statistical methods are used in the estimation and analysis of this type of data to account for some patients not obtaining endpoints.

Overall, outcome data can take many different forms to accommodate the endpoints and goals of the clinical trial. What is important is to adequately define these endpoints when designing the trial and carefully to consider how effectively these outcome data can be collected on all patients who will enroll onto the trial. This is a bigger logistical concern in the context of multi-institution clinical trials, where standards and instrumentation may differ.

EVALUATING TREATMENT EFFECT

In assessing and determining efficacy in clinical trials, the classification of the treatment effect on patients is critical not only for identifying the clinical response rate, but also in defining progression and thereby time to progression or progression-free or event-free survival. The definition of response is disease-dependent and differs in different diseases, such as leukemia versus lymphoma. These definitions also evolve over time as new technologies develop to evaluate the existence of and changes in the disease. The addition of computerized axial tomography (CT scan), for example, changed how lymphoma was assessed and measured, and now functional imaging – such as positron emission tomography (PET) scans – is replacing and/or complementing the CT scan in lymphoma.

In 1999, an International Working Group (IWG) developed recommendations for response assessment for non-Hodgkin's lymphoma (NHL) that were adopted internationally by study groups, industry, regulatory agencies and, subsequently, by clinical trial groups for Hodgkin's lymphoma. Despite the publication of standardized response criteria for NHL, an examination of current trial parameters from nine international lymphoma study groups – by the working group for quality management (WG-QM) of the Competence Network Malignant Lymphoma – found differences in how response was defined; in some cases the definition was missing. This finding led to an international project to harmonize trial parameters for malignant lymphoma. Revised response criteria for malignant lymphomas from the members of the International Harmonization Project (IHP) of the Competence Network Malignant Lymphoma were first reported at the American Society of Hematology in December 2005. These response criteria incorporate functional imaging via the PET scan.

PRECISION AND ERROR CONTROL

Two key aspects related to the precision of clinical trial design are interval estimates of the primary endpoint, referred to as confidence intervals (CI), and the similarity of the study sample to the population to which the results apply. A confidence interval is a point estimate ± a margin of error that depends on the degree of confidence one desires to place on the true value being within the interval. Typically, 95% confidence intervals are calculated, but other confidence levels are also useful. There is a trade-off between level of confidence and the width of the interval, where the wider the interval, the higher the confidence level that the true value is within that interval. Another determinant of confidence interval width (and thereby precision of the estimate) is sample size: the larger the sample, the greater the precision and thus the narrower the confidence interval. It is important to note that in the context of clinical trials, multi-stage designs can require different methods of calculating confidence intervals to avoid bias.

A broader aspect of precision is the degree to which the patients eligible for the study are similar to the target population of interest. The eligibility criteria determine the study population, which is typically a subset of the target population. A trade-off exists based on restrictive versus broad criteria. The advantages of restrictive eligibility criteria are that the patients are more homogeneous, smaller sample sizes may be required, and there is a reduced likelihood of confounding factors. Disadvantages are that the results may not be able to be generalized to the target population and fewer patients may be eligible, which may translate to a longer study duration or non-feasibility of the enrollment goal. In general, eligibility criteria should be loosened as the phase of the trial increases and trials become larger. Phase I trials are usually the most restrictive, because patients should not be enrolled in a dose-finding trial if there is an alternative treatment that is known to be effective. Such a trial may span multiple histologies if tolerability is the key determinant of dose level, but the criteria can be restrictive in terms of who would be eligible to receive this experimental regimen. Phase II trials are often conducted in the target population of interest, but are often more restricted to ensure a baseline level of health and some homogeneity, to better evaluate initial evidence of activity. This is an important reason why results from phase II trials should not be used to change clinical practice. Phase III studies are typically the most liberal in terms of eligibility criteria, as these are usually large trials that are intended to evaluate regimens against standard of care, and their results can affect clinical practice. Because of this, it is critical to design the eligibility criteria to ensure that patients entered into the clinical trial are similar to or representative of the target population, so that the results can be generalized to the patient population of interest.

In lymphoma, histology is the most important entry criterion. In 1982 the Non-Hodgkin's Lymphoma Pathologic Classification Project proposed a morphologic system that was representative of at least six previous classification systems. The Working Formulation had three major subdivisions: low grade, intermediate grade and high grade. A classification system that was based on immunohistochemistry, cytogenetics and molecular genetic characteristics was developed, the Revised European–American Lymphoma classification (REAL). The World Health Organization classification is now the accepted system internationally. This allows for cross-interpretation of study populations in different studies. However, two phase III trials in aggressive lymphoma demonstrated that phase II trials did not predict superiority of other agents over CHOP. At least one factor was the heterogeneity in the individual study populations. Shipp and colleagues developed the International Prognostic Index (IPI), encompassing diffuse large B-cell lymphoma, to address the issue of heterogeneity in patient study populations. This study defined the lymphoma populations of aggressive lymphomas. Subsequent studies have demonstrated the utility of the IPI in other lymphoma histologies, such as peripheral T-cell lymphoma. It has been demonstrated to have value in virtually all non-Hodgkin's lymphomas. Initially developed for the follicular lymphomas, an adaptation called the FLIPI has replaced the IPI and better differentiates groups of patients.

Closely related to the issue of precision is that of error rates and how to control these errors. In clinical trials there are two types of error for which we control: type I and type II. A type I error is defined as the probability of concluding that a treatment effect or difference exists when in truth it does not. The type II error is the probability of concluding that a treatment effect or difference does not exist when in truth it does. The level of acceptable error rates will depend on the phase of the trial. The closer the study is to results that will be generalized to the target population, the stricter the acceptable levels are for the rates of type I and type II errors. These predefined constraints on error rates affect the resulting sample size for the clinical trial, and by definition affect the power of the study. Power is defined as the probability of concluding that a treatment effect or difference exists when it truly does exist, which is 1 − type II error rate (e.g. type II error rate of 0.10 translates to 90% power). The constraint on the type I error rate also affects the decision rule to be used when determining if the results are significant. In lay terms, this translates to the strength of evidence we need to see to reject our assumption that the null hypothesis is true. The *p*-value is the probability of seeing an effect as large or larger by chance alone, given that the null hypothesis is true.

In addition to the need to constrain type I and type II error, it is also important to control potential inflation of the type I error through multiple interim analyses or "looks" at the primary endpoint. Each of these

considerations affects the study design and corresponding sample size required to evaluate the primary endpoint of interest. These complexities of clinical trial design, and the need to address various aspects of constraining these probabilities of making type I or II errors, further supports collaboration with statisticians in the development of clinical trials. Additional trial design issues are discussed in more detail below. Table 5.2 lists some of the key terms used.

PHASE I TRIALS

The primary aim of a phase I trial is to determine the dose to be recommended for evaluation in further study (Fig. 5.1). Historically, the assumption has been that "more is better" and thus the recommended dose level is defined by the maximum tolerated dose (MTD) of an agent. When tolerability is a determinant of the recommended dose level, the toxicities to be considered as excessive (dose-limiting toxicities, DLT) must also be defined. In the context of lymphoma trials, it is critical to take care in defining what constitutes a DLT. Leaving it open to any severe (grade 3 or greater) toxicity can mean that events such as grade 3 leukopenia may be counted as a DLT and thus affect the dose escalation decisions. It is prudent carefully to restrict what constitutes a DLT; often these are restricted to non-hematologic toxicities, but they can include time to engraftment (e.g. failure to engraft by the absolute neutrophil count [ANC] by 28 days could be considered a DLT). The timeframe for which observed toxicity will be considered in the dose escalation decisions should also be defined. When determining the study duration, it is important to consider not only how long it takes to accrue a cohort of patients, but also how long each cohort needs to be evaluated, as defined by the specified toxicity observation period. Even though a regimen may be given continuously until a patient progresses, or even when the regimen is given for 6 months, it is not uncommon for only the first one to two cycles to be considered when deciding whether or not DLT was observed, and thus whether or not the next cohort can be accrued to the next dose level.

The most commonly used phase I trial design is the standard cohort-of-three design. Patients are entered in a stepwise fashion in cohorts of three, with up to six patients per dose level, in order to determine the

Table 5.2. A glossary of terms.

Confidence interval	A range of values calculated from the sample observations that are believed with a particular probability to contain the true parameter value. These convey information that the p-values do not.
Cox regression model	The most widely used statistical model in clinical research. This is used when the analysis of a clinical trial is based on the time to an event. It models the hazard function on a set of explanatory variables rather than the mean.
Event-free survival	Time to event as determined by relapse, progression or death.
Hazard function	The probability that an individual experiences an event (death, impairment etc.) in a small time interval. It is a measure of how likely an individual is to experience an event, or a function of the age of an individual.
Intent-to-treat analysis	All patients entered in a clinical trial are analyzed together as representing that treatment, whether or not they completed or ever received the treatment. This prevents possible bias from many components.
Interim analysis	An analysis, preferably conducted by an independent data-monitoring committee, to assess whether the ongoing trial can realistically be expected to answer the primary question, taking into account the inclusion rate, adverse events, previous experience and the statistical significance as compared to the defined statistical guidelines in the trial.
Kaplan–Meier estimator	A procedure for estimating the survival function for a set of survival times, some of which may be censored observations. For example, the probability of a patient surviving 2 years after a treatment can be calculated as the probability of surviving 1 year given that the patient survived the first year.
Overall survival	Time to death from any cause.
Power	The probability of rejecting the null hypothesis when it is false.
P-value	An index measuring the strength of the evidence against the null hypothesis. It is not the probability that the specified hypothesis is true.
Primary endpoint	In lymphoma, the primary endpoints are overall survival and progression-free survival.
Randomization	The key features of randomization are that the treatment assignment is based on chance alone, the patient characteristics are balanced or equivalent, and the randomization process provides the foundation for the statistical tests that are used.
Sample size	The number of patients to be included in a study so that the study has a particular power to detect an effect.
Secondary endpoints	The secondary endpoints in lymphoma include event-free survival, time to progression etc.
Significance level	The level of probability at which it is agreed that the null hypothesis will be rejected. This is conveniently set at 0.05. P-values need to be much smaller than 0.05 before they can be considered to provide strong or conclusive evidence against the null hypothesis.
Significance test	A statistical procedure that results in a p-value relative to a hypothesis.

MTD. If no DLT is observed, then the next cohort of three patients is treated at the next dose level. If moderate toxicity (usually one patient with DLT) is observed, another cohort of three patients may be treated at that dose level, for a maximum of six patients. If significant toxicity is observed (usually defined as two or more patients with DLT), the MTD will have been exceeded. A subsequent cohort of three patients may be accrued to the previous dose level if six patients had not yet been treated, to ensure it is the MTD. Accrual must be stopped after each cohort of three patients is enrolled at a dose level in order to assess toxicity before proceeding to the next dose level. This type of trial design was utilized to study dose escalation of ProMACE–CytaBOM in DLBCL, resulting in a phase II study utilizing a 200% dose.

Preclinical Initial studies on in vitro samples and/or animal studies to obtain information on dosing and mechanisms of action.

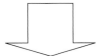

Phase I Trials to identify a recommended dose level to be evaluated in subsequent larger trials. This is often based on tolerability of the regimen, but can also be based on biologic markers.

Phase II Trials used to obtain initial evidence of efficacy, and typically incorporate a decision rule of what evidence is required to declare it promising vs. not. These are not definitive trials on efficacy of the regimen. Also used to obtain more information on toxicity profile of the regimen.

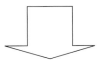

Phase III Trials that compare experimental regimen(s) to the standard of care; these trials are typically large, randomized trials whose outcomes can influence clinical practice.

Figure 5.1. Progression of clinical trial research

Alternatives to the standard cohort-of-three design for phase I trials include the continual reassessment method (CRM) and the accelerated titration method. In brief, the CRM approach utilizes the investigator's prior beliefs and the observed data to develop a model for determining the probability of unacceptable toxicity at a given dose level. This method uses data from each treated cohort to choose the dose for each successive cohort. Advantages of this method include that the MTD may be determined more quickly and accurately, but disadvantages are that it is more complicated and potentially difficult to implement. Also, the performance of this design depends on the accuracy of the model, and an incorrect model can cause problems, with too many patients treated at high dose levels or an inaccurate estimate of MTD.

In the accelerated titration method there are different schedules for accelerated dose escalation. In brief, one schedule evaluates one patient at a dose level until a certain (sub-DLT) level of toxicity is observed, after which it reverts to a standard cohort-of-three design. Another schedule allows for intrapatient dose escalation, using either a standard or a CRM escalation plan. Advantages of this approach are that it can require fewer patients, and specifically fewer patients at potentially sub-optimal levels, and that when dose escalation is done within patients no patient is under-treated. Disadvantages are that dose levels are potentially evaluated with very few patients, and for the intrapatient dose escalation there are ethical considerations concerning dosing patients until toxicity.

The designs that have been discussed focus on the determination of a recommended dose level based on MTD. In the current research environment, with more targeted therapies and/or immunotherapies, higher dose levels may not necessarily be associated with greater probability of response. The dose–response curve may not show a consistent increase, but rather may be parabolic or some other shape, with the curve reflecting decreasing efficacy at higher dose levels. In such a case, the phase I trial may be designed to determine both a recommended dose level based on tolerability (as assessed through determination of the MTD) and also some measure of efficacy or biologic response. Recent designs have been developed that use a CRM approach, where the possible outcomes are no efficacy and no toxicity, efficacy and no toxicity, or severe toxicity. These types of models are attractive in that they directly incorporate some measure of efficacy (usually as measured through some biologic parameter) in the dose escalation decisions. However, these designs also require that the biologic efficacy information be obtained relatively quickly in order to be used in the dose escalation decision-making process. In practice, many of these endpoints are batched and/or analyzed at the end of the study. An alternative is to conduct the study with dose escalation decisions determined by MTD rules, and utilize the biologic efficacy data at the end of the study to help determine the overall recommended dose level. This may require a specified number of patients at the MTD and sub-MTD dose levels to ensure sufficient samples for this type of evaluation by dose level.

Finally, there is the scenario where it is of interest to determine the recommended dose level only, based upon some biologic or immunologic outcomes. This is often the case in regimens where previous studies have determined the MTD to be higher than the dose levels of interest in the proposed dose-finding trial, and only changes in these correlative outcomes are of interest in determining the recommended dose level. This is the only situation in which multiple dose levels may be simultaneously evaluated, and where patients may be randomized to dose levels. In all other phase I scenarios, it is completely inappropriate to do so, and each dose level must be evaluated sequentially. However, there are other approaches that can be taken that reflect those of the tolerability-based phase I dose-finding trials but in which the trial takes into account a previously specified measure of biologic response.

Overall, there are many issues to consider when designing phase I clinical trials. Since these are dose-finding trials, often with no data yet on efficacy, there is no promise that these regimens will be effective. This affects the types of patients who are ethically eligible for these trials. Also, it is important to note that phase I trials are for determining recommended dose levels, not for concluding initial evidence of efficacy. While phase I trials can provide useful preliminary data on efficacy, there are still limited numbers of patients treated at a dose level. Finally, it is important to note that even though individual agents have been evaluated in the phase I setting, if their combination has not, and this is the regimen of interest, this too must be evaluated in the context of a phase I trial. At a minimum, this tolerability assessment can be combined with a phase II trial, where the phase II portion of the trial would be accrued at the determined MTD.

PHASE II TRIALS

The goals of a phase II trial are to assess therapeutic activity, to further characterize toxicity of the regimen, and to determine if the treatment warrants further investigation in a phase III trial. Phase II trials

are typically the first formal evaluation of efficacy of an experimental therapeutic regimen. With limited resources and the number of new agents available for evaluation in lymphoma, well-designed phase II trials are even more important. Therefore, sample sizes are constrained to reduce the number of patients who are exposed to a potentially ineffective or even toxic regimen, but a sufficient number of patients is required to effectively evaluate evidence of efficacy. Phase II trials are not definitive evaluations of efficacy, but rather identify those regimens worthy of further study in the phase III setting.

To evaluate efficacy in the phase II setting, decision rules are established for the level of evidence required to indicate that the regimen is promising. Typically, the outcome measures for documentation of efficacy are dichotomized as "successes" or "failures," where each is defined dependent on characteristics of the regimen and/or target patient population. In the context of lymphoma trials, this is most often the incidence of a clinical response (partial or complete) to treatment, although in some settings it may be more relevant to focus specifically on the incidence of complete responses or other definitions of "success." Accounting for constraints on type I and type II error rates and what true success rate one would expect if the regimen was not effective (p_0) versus what one would expect if it truly was effective (p_a), a required sample size and decision criteria are established.

Multiple possible methods for developing phase II trials exist. The focus in this review is on the broader issues to be considered when designing a phase II study. A primary consideration is whether or not to include one or more interim analyses, or "stages." A one-stage phase II trial accrues patients as rapidly as possible and then evaluates all endpoints at the end of the trial. The primary drawback to the one-stage design is that there is no formal opportunity for stopping the trial early. This can be more problematic if results on the first patients are available and investigators make early conclusions based on these observations without the benefit of a-priori criteria based on probabilistic rules. One-stage designs are best used when the sample sizes are moderately small and/or when the primary endpoint requires a relatively long follow-up to fully evaluate it (e.g. response rate by one year, if late responses are typical and should not be missed). However, this design is a concern when a large number of patients is required, where many patients may be treated with a regimen that does not have any evidence to date of potential therapeutic benefit.

Because of these considerations, a multi-stage trial is often the most appropriate method for evaluating efficacy of these experimental regimens. Most often, two-stage phase II designs are used, in which one interim analysis is conducted to permit early stopping for futility and/or toxicity. These designs require that accrual be temporarily suspended at each stage to fully evaluate those patients before proceeding to the next stage. This can cause concern regarding momentum of the trial and timeliness of the study duration, and modifications to these designs are sometimes used where the interim analyses are conducted but accrual is not halted (note that only the first n_1 patients required for the interim analyses are included to evaluate the corresponding decision criteria at that stage). If accrual is expected to be rapid, there is not much information on the toxicity profile for this regimen, and/or the primary endpoint can be evaluated in a relatively short timeframe, then it is recommended to temporarily halt accrual between stages to allow for the interim analyses. A general rule of thumb is to estimate how useful an interim analysis would be if accrual was not halted. If all patients required for the trial will be accrued by the time results from an interim analysis are available, then it is prudent to impose a halting of accrual between stages.

Designs such as the Simon optimal or Simon minmax are commonly used, and these provide a rule for stopping in the event of early evidence of lack of efficacy. The Fleming multi-stage design also provides decision criteria to stop accrual when sufficient evidence indicates lack of activity, but in addition provides an upper stopping limit, where accrual may be stopped for positive results. If there is sufficient early evidence that the regimen is effective, it is often not of interest to halt accrual, and accrual can be permitted to continue. This can allow a more complete evaluation of the toxicity profile in these patients, as well as more precision in estimating the primary endpoint. What this upper stopping limit can provide is a rule whereby it is possible to report out the early evidence of the positive results. Without such a rule, it is inappropriate to report out efficacy results before the study has completed accrual.

RANDOMIZED PHASE II TRIALS

When more than one experimental therapeutic regimen is to be evaluated, a randomized phase II study design provides a venue for simultaneously assessing the efficacy of these regimens in the same patient population. Since phase II trials are not comparative trials, the purpose of a randomized phase II trial is to simultaneously evaluate multiple experimental regimens independently. A study design and corresponding decision criteria are generated for each treatment arm, where multiple treatment arms can utilize the same study design and criteria as appropriate. The benefit of these trials is not only in evaluating multiple experimental treatments simultaneously but also in reducing potential patient selection biases.

Despite the fact that randomized phase II trials are underpowered for direct comparisons between arms, the success rates between arms can be informally evaluated together to identify the most promising regimen to be carried forward to the phase III setting. This screening design approach simultaneously screens two or more regimens to identify the most promising. However, this is not a definitive trial for establishing efficacy of one treatment over another, because of a lack of power to make this determination. Instead, this screening design approach can be used to identify the most promising regimen to take forward into the phase III setting.

It should be noted that for these phase II screening trials, the calculation of sample size has special considerations depending on the primary efficacy endpoints (e.g. response, survival). The biggest difference in calculating sample sizes for standard versus screening phase II trials is that in the screening trial setting, the type I error is typically not constrained. By definition, the type I error is the probability of concluding that one regimen is more promising than the other(s) when in truth they are equivalent. In the context of a screening trial this type of error is not seen as a problem, since it does not necessarily matter which one goes forward to the phase III setting if the regimens are truly equivalent.

PHASE III TRIALS

While efficacy may be formally evaluated in the context of phase II trials, these should not be considered definitive trials but simply preludes to the phase III trial. In the phase III setting a randomized controlled clinical trial can potentially affect clinical practice in the care of patients. The phase III setting is where the standard of care is evaluated, typically through the comparison of standard treatment to one or more experimental regimens of interest. If the standard of care for a target population is no treatment or a "wait and watch" approach, the control arm can be no treatment or a placebo control. The decision on whether or not to use a placebo and/or blinding of the assigned treatment depends on the potential for bias in the results. The patient and/or the treating physician may be blinded to the true treatment received, as necessary.

The design of the phase III trial will be determined first of all by the overall goal, whether the intention is to assess superiority, equivalence or non-inferiority. In the most common type of phase III clinical trial an experimental regimen is evaluated to determine if it is superior to another regimen, typically the standard of care or control arm. In this case, it is of interest to test the null hypothesis that the treatment arms are equivalent. However, there is increasing interest in evaluating the equivalence or non-inferiority of one regimen to another. This is often the case when an active standard of care exists, where the goal may be to ensure that an experimental regimen, which is possibly less toxic, easier to administer and/or more cost-effective, is at least as efficacious as the standard treatment. In equivalence trials, the trial tests the null hypothesis that there is a difference in the efficacy between treatment arms. For non-inferiority trials, it is of primary interest to ensure that the experimental regimen is not worse than the standard of care. The experimental regimen(s) may be superior, but this design focuses on evaluating only if it is at least as effective as the standard treatment.

Once the overall goals of the phase III trial have been defined (superiority versus equivalence or non-inferiority), then there are still many other factors to consider in the design of the trial. The most common is the single-factor trial, where we evaluate and compare the primary endpoint between two treatment arms. This is the most straightforward design, with patients randomized to one of two treatment groups, and the endpoints of interest compared at the end of the trial. There are other special designs that can be used in the phase III setting, including multi-factor (or multiple treatment arm), crossover and factorial

designs. The advantage of a multi-factor design is that it addresses multiple treatment questions in the context of one clinical trial. An example of this type of trial is one in which patients are randomized to an initial treatment. A specific example is the SWOG 8516 study, in which CHOP was compared with three other regimens that had sufficient evidence of promising efficacy in the phase II setting: MACOP-B, m-BACOD and ProMACE–CytaBOM. The trial demonstrated that all arms were equivalent, and therefore CHOP remained the standard of care.

In the crossover design, every patient gets each intervention but they are randomized in terms of the order in which they receive the interventions. These types of designs are best used when there is a short duration of effect of the treatments (to avoid carry-over effects and bias), and the patients are in a relatively stable condition where they can complete both treatments. A classic example of such a trial in a B-cell malignancy was the interferon versus pentostatin trial in hairy cell leukemia. Pentostatin had demonstrated a higher CR rate in previously performed phase II studies, but in the subsequent phase III trial, when 159 patients were randomized to interferon and 87 crossed over to pentostatin, the latter patients had a similar survival curve to that observed in patients initially treated with interferon and then crossed over to pentostatin. An advantage of this type of design is that each patient essentially serves as their own control, and can potentially reduce the required sample size. This design is most suited to chronic conditions, but for lymphoma patients the response may depend on the order in which the different therapies are given. It is possible to use crossover studies to evaluate interventions to ameliorate side effects or conditions that affect lymphoma patients, but generally not in attempting to improve overall survival or other measures of disease control.

The factorial design can also be used when there are two or more different comparisons to be made and the treatments can be combined. For example, one may wish to determine if the addition of an agent makes therapy more effective, and also to assess whether a shorter duration of therapy is as effective as the standard duration (e.g. 4 versus 6 months). For this hypothetical example, there are two treatment questions of interest, and they can be combined as in a two-by-two table, with patients randomized to receive one of the four combined treatment possibilities. This is the only clinical trial that is designed to formally evaluate interactions between two treatment interventions. In this setting, an interaction means that the effect of one intervention depends on the level of another intervention. While the ability to assess the existence of a treatment interaction can be of interest, this type of trial design also introduces a level of complexity that can make implementation and conduct logistically difficult. In addition, the existence of a treatment interaction can require a much larger sample size to fully evaluate treatment effects.

Another major consideration in the design of phase III clinical trials is the need for interim analyses of the data. Formal interim analyses of the primary endpoint need to be defined a priori when designing the trial. Beyond the decision on the number of interim analyses and the timing of these analyses, it is important to determine in the design how to control for the potential inflation of the type I error rate arising from these interim looks at the data (i.e. the increased possibility of rejecting the null hypothesis when it is in fact true, due to the additional analyses of the hypotheses). To account for this in the development of the trial design, we choose what is called an α (or type I error) spending function; this essentially takes into account the multiple tests of the primary endpoint. These spending functions range from simple to complex. One of the more straightforward is that proposed by Pocock, which essentially divides the targeted type I error rate, α, by the number of looks, k. This approach uses the same p-value cutoff for all analyses: if the p-value is less than α/k then it is statistically significant. This approach is easy to use and understand, but the cutoff at the final analysis can be quite small. Other more complex approaches are more commonly used, the most common being the O'Brien–Fleming method. This approach uses a more complicated statistical algorithm to determine the p-value cutoffs to be used for each analysis, where the cutoffs to determine statistical significance increase as more patients are accrued and one gets closer to the final analysis. This approach, although more complicated in its calculations, is the more intuitive. Recall that the p-value from the test statistic of interest is the probability of seeing as extreme a result if the null hypothesis was indeed true. The earlier the interim analysis, the smaller the p-value cutoffs; i.e. the fewer the patients accrued and data

analyzed, the stronger the evidence has to be to reject the null hypothesis.

As discussed above, the purpose of the phase III trial is a comparative randomized controlled trial to evaluate two or more treatment interventions. The choice of primary endpoint to formally compare between treatment groups will depend on the overall goals of the study. These primary endpoints may be focused on efficacy, such as progression-free survival, overall survival or even response rates. However, it is also possible to focus on tolerability-based endpoints, such as the incidence of a specific severe toxicity, if that is what is truly needed to differentiate and determine the best treatment intervention. Although the choice of primary endpoint is flexible, the most commonly used endpoint in the phase III setting for lymphoma studies is progression-free or overall survival. Given that phase III trials are used to help define clinical practice for these patients, it is thus important to focus on the endpoints of ultimate interest when caring for these patients. One can argue that overall survival as well as quality of life is the ultimate goal when treating patients, but endpoints such as progression-free survival are useful surrogates. The choice of endpoint will depend on the target patient population and the ability to conduct and analyze the trial in a reasonable timeframe. For example, overall survival may best be used when evaluating treatment options for aggressive lymphoma histologies, but for indolent histologies this endpoint may take too long to adequately evaluate with sufficient power. In that setting, it is probably better to focus instead on progression-free survival.

The important part of this process is ultimately to fully define the primary endpoint to be used in comparing the effect of the treatment groups. For example, overall survival is typically defined as the time from study entry to death due to any cause. If it is of interest to evaluate survival from time of diagnosis, this is valid for studies focused on newly diagnosed patients, where lead-time biases and the potential impact of any prior therapies are unlikely to present a problem. In defining progression-free survival, the event of interest is often inclusive of both disease progression and true relapse (disease recurrence after a complete response). Again, the key to time-to-event analyses is to effectively and consistently define what constitutes an event, as well as the date from which the time will be calculated (e.g. study entry or diagnosis). In the analysis of these time-to-event endpoints between treatment arms, the differences are typically expressed in terms of a hazard ratio (HR), which is the ratio of the event rates on each arm. Many considerations are required when determining sample size based on a time-to-event endpoint, such as the anticipated accrual period, minimum length of follow-up on all patients, expected loss to follow-up, and of course the number of events expected or median time to the event of interest. Kaplan–Meier methods and/or Cox regression models and corresponding logrank or Wald statistics are most often used to evaluate and compare time-to-event endpoints between treatment arms. These methods formally account for the possibility that not all patients will have had the event of interest at the time of the analysis, but we may want to incorporate the important information that they have been event-free up until their last evaluation.

Randomization is the key component of the phase III trial. There are different methods of randomization, and other relevant issues include stratification and the different time points at which patients are randomized to various treatments. Randomization is a controlled assignment of patients to treatment arms, used to produce comparable groups, and it removes the potential for bias in treatment allocation, thus supporting the validity of statistical tests of significance. Patients are randomized at a time as close as possible to the initiation of treatment, in order to avoid death, clinical deterioration, complications, ineligibility or a change of mind regarding participation in a clinical trial. Since clinical trials are based upon an intent-to-treat analysis, this limits further variability.

The randomization method used will also depend on whether or not it is necessary to stratify. Stratification is a process used to insure treatment arms are well balanced with respect to important baseline prognostic factors, and it helps reduce the potential for confounding variables when analyzing the data. Stratification prevents chance imbalances on important factors that can affect the interpretation of the primary endpoint between treatment arms. *Post hoc* methods to adjust for these imbalances are less credible. Examples of stratification factors in lymphoma clinical trials are IPI and histology (if conducted across multiple histologies). In multicenter studies, it is also useful to stratify

on center to account for inherent differences between treating sites.

In a phase III setting, rather than randomizing patients to different initial treatments, all patients may be given the same initial regimen and are only randomized to different additional therapies at the maintenance stage. This second randomization asks a different question. Patients who are eligible to be randomized to maintenance therapy are separated in time and by response, usually a CR or PR; therefore, not all of the patients who entered the study initially will undergo the second randomization, as they may need to be responding to be eligible. With the time separation, long-term questions about the first randomization may be difficult to answer. Patient selection biases are introduced because patients in the second randomization can be different. Interactions of the different treatments make the interpretations complex. If patients are randomized up-front, then patients dropping out can present major issues since patients are analyzed according to the initial randomization on an intent-to-treat basis. Comparing only those patients who received the assigned treatment is not valid since baseline characteristics are balanced only at the time of the randomization and the benefits of randomization are lost. To compare induction treatments without the confounding effect of maintenance, analyses cannot simply exclude all patients randomized to a maintenance treatment, because the proportion of non-responding patients relative to the whole population could be higher and underestimate the event-free and overall survival. Statistical modeling approaches exist to address these issues and achieve unbiased estimates, as was recently applied to the ECOG E4494 trial. This DLBCL trial initially randomized patients to R-CHOP (rituximab CHOP) versus CHOP, followed by a second randomization to rituximab versus observation.

CONCLUSION

The goal of clinical trials is to determine which regimens work, which regimens do not work, and how to lead to new innovations and approaches. Lymphoma is a heterogeneous disease. A significant number of new agents are being developed with different mechanisms of action, molecular targets and responses. International standardization of definitions of disease, response assessment and statistical interpretation are essential in the international world that we live in. Clinical trials are only one application that will lead to our understanding of therapeutic efficacy in lymphoma, but clinical trials determine the standard of care and future therapeutic directions.

FURTHER READING

General reviews

Everitt, B. S. *Medical Statistics from A to Z: a Guide for Clinicians and Medical Students* (Cambridge: Cambridge University Press, 2003).

Friedman, L. M., Furberg, C. D. and DeMets, D. L. *Fundamentals of Clinical Trials* (New York, NY: Springer-Verlag, 1998).

Green, S., Benedetti, J. and Crowley, J. *Clinical Trials in Oncology* (Boca Raton, FL: Chapman & Hall/CRC, 2003).

Hill, A. B. Memories of the British streptomycin trial in tuberculosis. *Control. Clin. Trials* **11** (1990), 77–79.

Piantadosi, S. *Clinical Trials: a Methodologic Perspective* (New York, NY: Wiley, 1997).

Pocock, S. J. *Clinical Trials: a Practical Approach* (Chichester: Wiley, 1983).

Spilker, B. *Guide to Clinical Trials* (New York, NY: Raven Press, 1991).

Lymphoma-specific

Cheson, B. D., Pfistner, B., Juwied, M. E. *et al.* Revised response criteria for malignant lymphomas. From the members of the International Harmonization Project (IHP) of the Competence Network Malignant Lymphoma. *Blood* **106**(S) (2005), 10a.

Fisher, R. I., Gaynor, E. R., Dahlberg, S. *et al.* Comparison of a standard regimen (CHOP) with three intensive chemotherapy regimens for advanced non-Hodgkin's lymphoma. *N. Engl. J. Med.* **328** (1993), 1002–1006.

Flinn, I. W., Kopecky, K. J., Foucar, K. *et al.* Long-term follow-up of remission duration, mortality, and second malignancies in hairy cell leukemia patients treated with pentostatin. *Blood* **96** (2000), 2981–2986.

Gordon, L. I., Andersen, J., Habermann, T. M. *et al.* Phase I trial of dose escalation with growth factor support in patients with previously untreated diffuse aggressive lymphomas: determination of the maximum tolerated dose of ProMACE–CytaBOM. *J. Clin. Oncol.* **14** (1996), 1275–1281.

Habermann, T. M., Weller, E., Morrison, V. A. *et al.* Rituximab-CHOP versus CHOP alone or with maintenance rituximab in older patients with diffuse large B-cell lymphoma. *J. Chin. Oncol.* **24** (2006), 3121–3127.

A predictive model for aggressive non-Hodgkin's lymphoma. The International Non-Hodgkin's Lymphoma Prognostic Factors Project. *N. Engl. J. Med.* **329** (1993), 987–994.

Solal-Céligny, P., Roy, P., Colombat, P. *et al.* Follicular lymphoma international index. *Blood* **104** (2004), 1258–1265.

Phase I, II and III trials

Bryant, J. and Day, R. Incorporating toxicity considerations into the design of two-stage phase II clinical trials. *Biometrics* **51** (1995), 1372–1383.

Conaway, M. R. and Petroni, G. R. Bivariate sequential designs for phase II trials. *Biometrics* **51** (1995), 656–664.

Green, S. and Dahlberg, S. Planned versus attained design in phase II clinical trials. *Stat. Med.* **11** (1992), 853–862.

Hunsberger, S., Rubinstein, L. V., Dancey, J. and Korn, E. L. Dose escalation trial designs based on a molecularly targeted endpoint. *Stat. Med.* **24** (2005), 2171–2181.

Liu, P.-Y., Dahlberg, S. and Crowley, J. Selection designs for pilot studies based on survival. *Biometrics* **49** (1993), 391–398.

Sargent, D. J. and Goldberg, R. M. A flexible design for multiple armed screening trials. *Stat. Med.* **20** (2001), 1051–1060.

Simon, R., Wittes, R. E. and Ellengerg, S. S. Randomized phase II clinical trials. *Cancer Treat. Rep.* **69** (1985), 1375–1381.

Thall, P. F. and Russel, K. E. A strategy for dose-finding and safety monitoring based on efficacy and adverse outcomes in phase I/II clinical trials. *Biometrics* **54** (1998), 251–264.

Zhang, W., Sargent, D. J. and Mandrekar, S. An adaptive dose-finding design incorporating both toxicity and efficacy. *Stat. Med.* **25** (2006), 2365–2383.

Intrepretation

Cox, D. R. Regression models and life-tables. *J. Roy. Stat. Soc. Ser. B* **34** (1972), 187–200.

Kaplan, E. and Meier, P. Nonparametric estimation from incomplete observations. *J. Am. Stat. Assoc.* **53** (1958), 457–481.

Lunceford, J. K., Davidian, M., Tsiatis, A. A. *et al.* Estimation of survival distributions of treatment policies in two-stage randomization designs in clinical trials. *Biometrics* **58** (2002), 48–57.

O'Brien, P. C. and Fleming, T. R. A multiple testing procedure for clinical trials. *Biometrics* **35** (1979), 549–556.

Therneau, T. M. and Grambsch, P. M. *Modeling Survival Data: Extending the Cox Model* (New York, NY: Springer-Verlag, 2000).

Neil L. Berinstein

INTRODUCTION

There has been significant progress in developing immunotherapeutics for non-Hodgkin's lymphoma (NHL). The first monoclonal antibodies for treatment of cancer were approved for the non-Hodgkin's lymphoma indication in 1997. This has led to a burst of development and expansion of various forms of passive immunotherapy, targeted therapy and active immunization. In fact a whole new paradigm of cancer management is evolving based upon these seminal observations and advances. This chapter will review important principles of both active and passive immunotherapy, focusing mainly on non-Hodgkin's lymphoma.

TUMOR ANTIGENS

Tumor antigens are of fundamental importance to both passive and active immunotherapy strategies. The existence of tumor antigens enables immunotherapeutic approaches to be specific to the tumor and ideally not directed to normal cells. The favorable toxicity profile that results is one of the major attractions of immunotherapeutic approaches. Thus the tumor antigen will be an important factor in determining the specificity and the toxicity profile of the approach. The success of the immunotherapeutic strategy will depend to a large extent on the features of the tumor antigen target.

Features and types of tumor antigens

Whereas the innate immune system is not for the most part antigen-specific, the adaptive immune response mediated by B and T lymphocytes has a level of specificity built in and is directed towards antigenic targets. In the case of tumor immunology,

these antigenic targets are termed "tumor antigens" (Table 6.1). The tumor antigens arise as part of the oncogenesis process and may distinguish tumor cells from normal cells to varying degrees. At one extreme the tumor antigen may be unique to the particular tumor that it arose in and be highly tumor-specific. Examples of such tumor antigens could be mutations arising in specific proto-oncogenes (e.g. *RAS*) that are important in driving the tumor. These mutations may be different from tumor to tumor yet will be propagated in all of the cells of a particular tumor. These types of tumor antigen are called "tumor-specific" antigens. The immunoglobulin idiotype protein is an example of a tumor-specific antigen found in hematologic malignancies such as B-cell lymphoma. On the other hand, aberrant protein expression within a cell may arise as a result of the oncogenesis process and result in expression of protein targets that are more universally expressed from tumor to tumor. Proteins that are physiologically transiently expressed or that are shut off in mature adult tissues may be dis-regulated. Such proteins may be important in the differentiation of the tissue, either embryonically or in earlier stages of differentiation. These types of tumor antigen are termed "tumor-associated antigens," and include differentiation antigens or oncofetal antigens. Lymphoid differentiation antigens, expressed physiologically in mature lymphoid cells, can be considered tumor-associated antigens because of the high level of lineage restriction of these lymphoid differentiation antigens to the lymphoid system. Another class of tumor-associated antigen includes proteins from viruses that may contribute to the pathogenesis of certain malignancies (e.g. EBV, HPV and hepatitis C). The EBV (Epstein–Barr virus) is of special interest for hematologic malignancies because it is found in many B-cell malignancies as well as Hodgkin's lymphoma.

Lymphoma: Pathology, Diagnosis and Treatment, ed. Robert Marcus, John W. Sweetenham and Michael E. Williams. Published by Cambridge University Press. © Cambridge University Press 2007.

Table 6.1. Common lymphoid tumor antigens.

Tumor-specific antigens	Malignancy
Immunoglobulin idiotype	B-cell lymphoma
T-cell receptor idiotype	T-cell lymphoma

Tumor-associated antigens	Malignancy
Differentiation antigens	
CD19	B-cell lymphoma
CD20	B-cell lymphoma, lymphocyte-predominant Hodgkin's lymphoma
CD22	B-cell lymphoma
CD10	B-cell lymphoma
CD5	Chronic lymphocytic leukemia, small lymphocytic lymphoma
CD52	B-cell lymphoma, T-cell lymphoma
CD25	T-cell lymphoma, Hodgkin's lymphoma
CD15	Hodgkin's lymphoma
CD30	Hodgkin's lymphoma, anaplastic T-cell lymphoma
Functional antigens	
CD40	
CD80	
Transforming antigens	
Cyclin D1	Mantle cell lymphoma
c-myc	Burkitt's lymphoma, other B-cell lymphoma
bcl-2	B-cell lymphoma
bcl-6	B-cell lymphoma
p53	B-cell lymphoma
Other	
Telomerase	B-cell lymphoma
Viral: EBV	Burkitt's and other B-cell lymphoma, Hodgkin's lymphoma

In lymphoid malignancies there are several differentiation antigens that can be used for immunotherapy purposes, including CD19, CD22 and CD20. In Hodgkin's lymphoma the CD15, CD30 and CD25 differentiation antigens similarly are overexpressed in the malignant Reed–Sternberg cells. All of these differentiation antigens may be particularly useful targets for immunotherapy because they are highly restricted to the lymphoid lineage, although there is expression in normal lymphoid as well as malignant cells.

Tumor antigens can be expressed in any cellular compartment, but expression on the cell surface is a prerequisite for targets for passive immunotherapy with monoclonal antibodies. In addition, there are a number of other features of the protein that may determine its degree of suitability as a monoclonal antibody target or the type of monoclonal antibody approach that might be optimal. For example, antigens that internalize when bound by a monoclonal antibody will be more suitable targets for passive immunotherapy approaches that deliver a cytotoxic drug or toxin to the cell for inducing cell death. Antigens that are stably expressed on the cell surface may be best suited for immunotherapy approaches that rely on the immune system (antibody-dependent cellular cytotoxicity and complement-mediated lysis) to induce cell death, or for approaches delivering radiation. Antigenic targets that are attached to intercellular signaling pathways that mediate cell proliferation or sensitivity to apoptosis may be best suited for immunotherapy approaches that are directed at interfering with autocrine growth factor/growth factor receptor interactions. The level of shedding of the tumor antigen into the circulation may be an important factor: it may interfere with the ability of a monoclonal antibody to reach its target, and in the case of antibodies that deliver targeted radiation it may predispose to unwanted toxicities.

Intracellular tumor antigens, as well as cell-surface tumor antigens, may be targets in active immunization. Because 80–90% of a cell's protein expression is limited to various intracellular compartments, a much larger selection of tumor antigens may be considered for active vaccination approaches. Targets for active vaccination approaches must be processed and presented on major histocompatibility complex (MHC) proteins. This processing and presentation must occur both on the tumor cells and also on normal antigen-presenting cells (APC). The processing of intracellular proteins is mediated by the proteosomes, and there may be different patterns of proteosome expression in tumor cells and antigen-presenting cells. Thus it is important to demonstrate that similar epitopes can be processed and presented similarly in both cell types. In order for the intracellular tumor antigen to be recognized by T cells, the tumor cells must express MHC complexes. Whereas most intracellular proteins are processed and presented through a class-I-mediated pathway involving the endoplasmic reticulum and the proteosome, tumor antigens that are secreted may be taken up by the exogenous pathway and processed by the endosome into MHC class II molecules. These different processing features of the tumor antigen may influence the quality of the immune response that is generated in an active vaccination approach. In the former example the immune response may consist predominantly of CD8 T cells, whereas in the latter it may be primarily CD4, or a more balanced immune response to that tumor antigen, involving both CD4 and CD8 T cells. Finally, another consideration for selecting intracellular antigens for active vaccination approaches is based on the level of tolerance to that particular tumor antigen. There may be high levels of central tolerance to tumor antigens that have been expressed in embryonic or adult thymic tissues, and specifically thymic endothelial cells. Thus it is important to demonstrate that T cells can be detected in the periphery that have the right T-cell receptor to

Table 6.2. Preferred characteristics of tumor-associated antigens.

Overexpression in tumor cell
Absent expression in critical organs
Expression in >30% of a particular tumor type
Expression in multiple different types of tumors
Expression in early and late stages of cancer
  – expression in pre-malignant tumour
  – expression in tumor stem cells
Contributes to pathogenesis of tumor
Minimal splice variants or homologous gene family
  members
Cell-surface expression for monoclonal antibody targets
Immunogenic for vaccine targets

Table 6.3. Current bioinformatic tools to identify tumor antigens.

Lymphoma Leukemia Molecular Profiling project	llmpp.nih.gov/ lymphoma
SEREX	www2.licr.org/ CancerImmunomeDB
SAGE	www.ncbi.nlm.nih.gov/ projects/SAGE

recognize and that become activated by processed and presented epitopes from the tumor antigen.

Criteria that should be considered when selecting antigenic targets for either passive or active immunotherapy are listed in Table 6.2. Approaches to identify useful antigenic targets for cancer immunotherapy are complex and involve screening and validation steps (Fig. 6.1). The list of tumor antigens that can be used for cancer immunotherapy is expanding, and some more highly restricted and suitable targets are becoming available. Various electronic databases highlighting antigens identified by SEREX or protein or RNA expression approaches, including databases specifically focusing on hematologically restricted antigens, are now available to the public (Table 6.3).

MONOCLONAL ANTIBODIES

Types of monoclonal antibodies

The first monoclonal antibodies studied in the clinic were murine. These included murine antibodies to

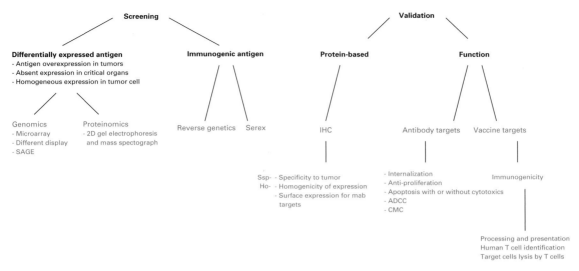

Figure 6.1. Steps for identification of new tumor antigens. Identification of new tumor antigens involves both a screening and a validation step. The initial screening can be performed either by looking for antigenic targets that are differentially expressed in the tumor cell or, in the case of cancer vaccines, looking for immunogenic antigens. Either genomics or proteinomics approaches can be used to identify differentially expressed antigens. For vaccine targets, immunogenic antigens can be identified by reverse genetics or SEREX approaches. To confirm that useful antigenic targets have been identified, several validation steps must be performed. Protein validation involves demonstrating that the antigenic target is indeed expressed specifically in primary tumor samples and not in normal cells by using immunohistochemical analyses. Several different assays can be employed for functional validation and the choice of assays depends upon whether one is trying to identify antibody targets or vaccine targets.

the idiotype (anti-idiotype antibodies), anti-CD19, anti-CD22 and anti-CD10 monoclonal antibodies. Even the initial versions of the anti-CD20 antibodies were murine (anti-B1, 1F5). Because these monoclonal antibodies were entirely a foreign murine protein, they elicited human anti-murine antibody responses (HAMA) in many patients. These immune responses had the effect of neutralizing the therapeutic activity of the antibody therapy. In addition, the murine protein had a relatively short half-life (24–48 hours) in humans. Because of this it was difficult to build significant levels of antibody in the serum of treated patients. Finally, because these antibodies contained murine constant regions, interactions with human complement and human Fc receptor regions on Fc receptor bearing cells were less than optimum and limited the full potential of the immunologic anti-tumor response.

To enhance the properties of therapeutic monoclonal antibodies, more fully human monoclonal antibodies were developed. The first generation of these antibodies consisted of chimeric antibodies, in which the murine constant region was exchanged for a human constant region. With these monoclonals, human anti-murine antibody responses were decreased or eliminated and the serum half-life increased from approximately 3 to 7 days. Experimental data demonstrated improved antibody-dependent cellular cytotoxicity (ADCC) and complement-mediated cytotoxicity (CMC). Rituximab is an example of a chimeric monoclonal antibody.

Further improvements in the experimental methodologies yielded more fully humanized monoclonal antibodies, either through the process of CDR engraftment or by generation of hybridomas from human Ig transgenic mice. These monoclonal antibodies have been found to have characteristics very similar to chimeric monoclonal antibodies, with similar half-lives and effector function. From a theoretical standpoint these have less risk of HAMA responses. Campath-1H is an example of a humanized monoclonal antibody made by CDR engraftment.

Phage display technology is another approach to generating monoclonal antibodies. In this approach, univalent heavy chain and light chain or single chain Fv phages are screened for reactivity to antigens of interest. Higher-affinity phage-derived monoclonal antibodies can be obtained by generating phage libraries after immunization. This technology produces a large number of phage-derived clones to be screened. Single chain Fvs can be generated, and these may have special application in therapeutics, where their small size enhances penetration into tumor masses to deliver toxins, cytotoxics or biologically active molecules.

Mechanisms of anti-tumor activity by monoclonal antibodies

There may be several different mechanisms through which monoclonal antibodies can mediate therapeutic anti-tumor activity. In the mechanism of antibody-dependent cellular cytotoxicity (ADCC), the F(ab) part of the antibody binds to the antigenic target on the tumor cell and the Fc region of the antibody binds to Fc receptors expressed on host effector cells. These effector cells can be polymorphonuclear cells, NK cells or cells of the macrophage/monocyte lineage. Factors that determine the level of ADCC include the intrinsic susceptibility of the target cell to lysis, the level of antigenic expression on the cell surface, the isotype of the monoclonal antibody (IgG1 > IgG2a > IgG2b) and the state of activation of the effector cells. ADCC may be a dominant mechanism, which would explain why rituximab and other anti-CD20 monoclonal antibodies were ineffective in mice with knock-outs of FcR. Several monoclonal antibodies directed at antigens expressed on Hodgkin/Reed–Sternberg cells (anti-CD15, anti-CD30 and anti-CD25) were evaluated and found to be ineffective at mediating anti-tumor cytotoxicity on their own through immunologic mechanisms. The state of activation of the effector cells participating in immune cytotoxicity through ADCC mechanisms can be increased by various cytokines including interferon alpha, IL-2 and GM-CSF.

The importance of antibody-dependent cellular cytotoxicity has also been demonstrated by analysis of spontaneously occurring polymorphisms of the FcγIIIA receptor (FcγR) in patients with lymphoma. Two polymorphisms have been described which result in either a phenylalanine or a valine at amino acid position 158. The FcγRIIIA-158V has a higher affinity

for human IgG than the FcγRIIIA-158F. Two groups have shown that patients with the FcγRIIIA-158F had higher response rates to monotherapy with rituximab than patients with the phenylalanine polymorphism or heterozygotes. FcγRIIIA polymorphisms are not independent prognostic factors for the outcome of patients with indolent or aggressive lymphoma not treated with monoclonal antibody therapy. These data suggest that ADCC may be an important mechanism of anti-tumor activity for patients receiving rituximab.

Another mechanism of tumor cytotoxicity involves complement-mediated lysis (CMC). The classical pathway of complement can be activated by antibodies. The isotype of the monoclonal antibody is related to the level of CMC. There is in-vitro evidence to support this, and preclinical in-vivo experiments have shown that the protective affects of rituximab are diminished in mice deficient in C1Q. Three complement regulatory proteins have been described, including CD46, CD55 and CD59. These may inhibit the complement cascade at different steps of its activation. There is preclinical evidence to suggest that the sensitivity of follicular lymphoma cells to CMC may be related to the level of expression of complex regulatory proteins. In addition, sensitivity to CMC can be enhanced by neutralizing antibodies to CD55 and CD59. However, from a clinical perspective there are no clear data showing that the expression of complement regulatory proteins on tumor cells influences the clinical responses to antibodies such as rituximab.

Monoclonal antibodies may also work through a mechanism of intracellular signaling. This effect may be very much associated with the specific target antigen. In some situations the intracellular signaling may affect the sensitivity of the lymphoma cells to apoptosis. This mechanism may help explain the added activity of combinations of monoclonal antibodies and certain cytotoxic drugs, seen both in vitro and in clinical practice. The GELA group has demonstrated an approximately 15% survival improvement for elderly patients with first-line aggressive lymphoma who were treated with CHOP and rituximab compared to CHOP alone in a randomized phase III trial. Marcus and colleagues have demonstrated almost a doubling of the time to progression in patients with indolent lymphoma treated with the combination of CVP and rituximab in a randomized trial. Several other chemotherapy combinations have been significantly enhanced by the addition of rituximab in randomized trials, again suggesting that rituximab may predispose lymphoma cells to the cytotoxic effects of the chemotherapy combination.

Genetically enhanced monoclonal antibodies

Monoclonal antibodies can be genetically enhanced using a variety of strategies. Chimeric and humanized versions of monoclonal antibodies may have a number of advantages over their murine counterparts. More specifically, by making a monoclonal antibody more human, the serum half-life will be increased. This will result in greater accumulation of the monoclonal antibody in the serum and facilitate penetration into tumor sites. In addition, the immunogenicity of the monoclonal antibody will be reduced and human antibody responses to the mouse components of the antibody can be almost eliminated. Another major advantage of chimeric or humanized monoclonal antibodies is the potential enhancement of effector function. By using human constant regions, binding to human Fcγ receptors on certain cell types and C1Q will be increased. This will result in enhanced ADCC or CMC respectively.

Several genetically engineered anti-CD20 monoclonal antibodies are now being evaluated and compared to the chimeric anti-CD20 antibody rituximab. PRO70769 is a completely humanized IgG1 anti-CD20 monoclonal that has been shown to effectively deplete B-cell subsets in the blood and in lymphoid tissues. It is now being tested in a clinical trial in patients with rheumatoid arthritis, where it is expected to have advantages over rituximab with respect to immunogenicity after repeated injections in patients with autoimmune disorders.

IMMU-106 is another fully humanized anti-CD20 monoclonal antibody. This monoclonal has a human IgG1κ constant region and uses the same non-CDR variable regions as the humanized anti-CD22 monoclonal antibody epratuzumab. It has been shown to have the same antigen-binding specificity avidities and dissociation constant as rituximab, and it induces similar levels of apoptosis, ADCC and CMC. It was also effective in treating SCID mice containing B-cell lymphoma xenografts. It is expected that IMMU-106 should be comparable to rituximab but, being fully humanized, it may have pharmacokinetic

advantages. Clinical evaluation will need to establish whether there are any significant clinical benefits of this monoclonal antibody.

Three different human hybridomas were generated by immunizing humanized mice with CD20 transfected cells. All three bound strongly to CD20-positive cells, and all induced antibody-dependent cellular cytotoxicity. Two monoclonal antibodies, however, were more active in complement-mediated cytotoxicity and were able to lyse a range of rituximab-resistant targets including CLL targets. These two hybridomas had markedly slower off-rates to the CD20 antigen. One of these monoclonal antibodies, named HUMAX-CD20, is now undergoing phase I clinical evaluations. Preliminary results in abstract form have shown that this monoclonal antibody was effectively able to deplete circulating B cells in 40 patients with follicular lymphoma treated with four weekly infusions of varying dosage. The median half-life of the antibody after the fourth infusion was 342 hours, which is greater than the half-life of rituximab. Objective responses were seen in 12 of the 24 patients, and four complete responses and one unconfirmed complete response were documented. No dose-limiting toxicity was obtained. Further trials will be necessary to determine whether this antibody has clinical advantages over rituximab.

A fully humanized monoclonal antibody directed at CD30 is being evaluated in patients with Hodgkin's lymphoma. This antibody has been well tolerated at doses up to 15 mg/kg and some objective responses have been documented. It is too early to know whether this monoclonal will eventually be useful in Hodgkin's lymphoma, either to reduce the low but significant relapse rate or to allow the use of reduced doses of cytotoxics in front-line therapy and reduce long-term toxicity.

There are also a number of other strategies that can be used to further enhance the activity of these humanized monoclonal antibodies (Fig. 6.2). The regions in the human constant regions that are responsible for binding of the monoclonal antibody to C1Q and Fcγ-receptor-bearing cells, specifically FcγR1, FcγR2 and FcγR3, as well as FcRn, have been defined. Manipulation of C1Q binding could result in enhanced binding to complement and enhance complement-mediated cytotoxicity. Modification of binding to the different FcγRs could theoretically enhance phagocytosis or antibody-dependent cellular

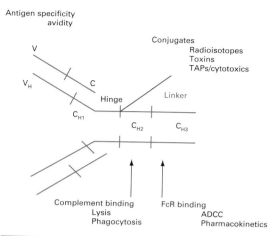

Figure 6.2. Modification of monoclonal antibodies. Monoclonal antibodies can be modified to enhance their anti-tumor activity in several different positions. The variable region of the light chain or heavy chain can be modified to enhance the binding to the antigen. Either the CH2 or CH3 regions of the heavy chain constant region can be modified to enhance complement binding or binding to Fc receptors. Monoclonal antibodies can be conjugated to radioisotopes, toxins or tumor-active prodrugs/cytotoxics.

cytotoxicity, and modification of the FcRn could result in significant alterations in the antibody half-life. It is also possible to manipulate the affinity of the binding of the monoclonal antibody to its antigenic target by manipulating amino acids in the CDR regions. It is expected that monoclonal antibodies with these modifications will soon start to be evaluated.

Antibody conjugates

Radiolabeled monoclonal antibodies

Monoclonal antibodies can be used to target cytotoxic substances to tumor cells bearing the antigen of interest. These cytotoxic substances can include radio-isotopes, toxins or tumor-active prodrugs (TAPs). In the area of non-Hodgkin's lymphoma several radio-labeled monoclonal antibodies have been evaluated and already two have been approved by the FDA for specific treatment indications for patients with non-Hodgkin's lymphoma.

The rapid progress of radioimmune conjugates in the field of non-Hodgkin's lymphoma has been facilitated by two major factors. Firstly, non-Hodgkin's lymphomas are characterized by a tumor-associated antigen target that has attractive features for radioimmuno-therapy. The CD20 antigen is highly specific for B cells and various B-cell lymphomas. It is a cell-surface trans-membrane protein that is homogeneously expressed on lymphoma cells and appears to be retained during tumor progression. It may play a role in calcium meta-bolism. It is not expressed on hematopoetic stem cells. In addition, CD20 does not shed into the circulation and does not internalize significantly, both particularly important features for targeting radiation.

The second important factor is that non-Hodgkin's lymphomas are for the most part radiosensitive. External beam radiation therapy is a major component of treatment of early stages of most non-Hodgkin's lymphomas, and local involved-field radiation therapy can reliably induce tumor regressions. The effective-ness of radiation therapy is limited by toxicities to normal tissues and by the inability to apply external beam radiation therapy as a systemic therapy.

There is even some evidence that non-Hodgkin's lymphomas may be even more sensitive to low-dose radiotherapy (LDR). The radiation from radioimmune therapy is approximately 2.5 orders of magnitude lower in intensity than external beam radiation ther-apy. In addition, it is continuous and decreases with time. The enhanced therapeutic effect of continuous low-dose radiation may be related to the ability of normal cells to repair sublethal DNA damage during cell-cycle arrest at the G2/M phase of the cell cycle. Lymphoma cells are less efficient at doing this because of deficient DNA repair mechanisms. Trials of low-dose external beam radiation therapy have demonstrated the effectiveness of LDR in patients with indolent lymphoma.

There are also some important considerations rele-vant to the choice of monoclonal antibody that will be used to target the radioimmunoisotope. Whereas for immunotherapy with naked monoclonal antibodies, humanized monoclonal antibodies provide benefits over their murine counterparts with respect to prolong-ing the serum half-life of the antibody, reduction of immunogenicity to the foreign protein and enhanced effector functions, some of these advantages are less important – and perhaps even undesirable – for radio-immunotherapy. In fact, for radioimmunotherapy a shorter serum half-life may provide less non-specific uptake and toxicity from the radioimmunoconjugate and is therefore desired. Murine monoclonal anti-bodies are thus preferred, to provide a relatively short serum half-life. The reduced effector function mediated by the antibody protein itself is probably

Table 6.4. Features of common radioisotopes used for radioimmunotherapy.

	^{90}Y	^{131}I
Half-life (days)	2.7	8
Mean B energy (keV)	939	192
Mean range in tissue (mm)	2.76	0.40
Non-tumor uptake	bone	thyroid

not significant for radioimmunoconjugates because the cytotoxicity is provided by the radioisotope. However, the potential increased immunogenicity of a murine antibody protein is a concern that can limit the effectiveness of this therapy, and in fact human anti-mouse reactions have been seen in patients undergoing treatment, particularly in early-stage disease settings.

Two different radionucleotides have been used in radioimmunotherapy for non-Hodgkin's lymphoma, in the form of ^{90}Y-ibritumomab tiuxetan (Zevalin) and ^{131}I-tositumomab (Bexxar). The different emission profiles of these two radioimmunotherapies are shown in Table 6.4. In general, ^{90}Y has a higher average energy and a longer mean path length in tissue. Its half-life is also shorter.

The administration of either Bexxar or Zevalin requires the initial blocking of antigenic targets within the circulation by a pre-infusion with an unlabeled anti-CD20 monoclonal antibody. In the case of Zevalin the chimeric monoclonal antibody rituximab is used for this purpose, and with Bexxar the same unlabeled murine anti-CD20 antibody is used. The unlabeled anti-CD20 monoclonal antibodies will bind both to circulating B lymphocytes and to Fc receptors throughout the reticuloendothelial system. Thus, either through depletion of B cells or through partial blocking of antigenic sites on these cells, the biodistribution of the subsequently administered radiolabeled monoclonal antibody is improved. This enhances the tumor-specific/non-specific cytotoxicity ratio. For the administration of Bexxar a dosimetric study is performed initially to calculate patient-specific therapeutic doses. The objective is to deliver a whole-body dose of 75 cGy in patients with platelets $> 150 \times 10^9$/L. In initial trials with Zevalin, initial tracer imaging/dosimetry doses were also administered.

The principal toxicities associated with radioimmunotherapy are hematologic, and they occur approximately 4–8 weeks after treatment. These are related to the effects of radiation on the bone marrow. In the pivotal trial with Bexxar, 18% of patients had grade IV neutropenia and 22% had grade IV thrombocytopenia. The incidence of grade IV neutropenia with Zevalin is approximately 10% and grade IV thrombocytopenia is approximately 3%. These toxicities are reversible, and the incidence of febrile neutropenia is relatively low. In addition, there is very little need for hematopoietic growth factor support or transfusions. Hypothyroidism has also been documented with Bexxar treatment in approximately 10% of subjects. The frequency of HAMA responses is higher with Bexxar and occurs more frequently when it is used earlier in the disease course. The incidence of myeloplastic syndrome and secondary leukemia does not appear to be greater than that expected as a background rate for the heavily pre-treated population.

Although Bexxar and Zevalin have now been approved by regulatory authorities for treatment of relapsed or refractory B-cell lymphoma, ongoing long-term toxicity data continue to be collected.

Radiolabeled monoclonals are also being developed for Hodgkin's lymphoma, where it was hypothesized that the "cross-fire effect" mediated by radiolabeled monoclonals would be useful to eliminate the low-frequency dispersed Reed–Sternberg cells. Initial approaches used either ^{131}I- or ^{90}Y-labeled anti-sera to ferritin. The limiting factors were the marked myelotoxicity and particularly thrombocytopenia. An ^{131}I-labeled anti-CD30 monoclonal is now being evaluated.

Conjugates of monoclonal antibodies with anti-tumor prodrugs and toxins

Another potential strategy to enhance the anti-tumor activity of monoclonal antibodies is to link these monoclonals to cytotoxic agents. The cytotoxic agent can be a tumor-active prodrug or a toxin. This approach differs from targeted radioimmunotherapy in that there is no bystander effect. In other words, only cells that bind the conjugate will be killed. With these TAP or toxin conjugates the strategy is to link the cytotoxic agent in a stable fashion to the monoclonal such that toxicity is limited to the cells that the monoclonal binds to. As long as the toxin or TAP does not become unbound, loose in the circulation, non-specific cytotoxicity is minimized. For this approach to be successful the antigen that is being targeted must have several features. As well as being highly specific for the tumor cell, the target must internalize or modulate when the monoclonal antibody binds to it. This feature of the target antigen would be considered to be undesirable in the case of naked monoclonal antibody therapy.

The features of the monoclonal antibody used in the conjugate are also important. Unlike targeted radioimmunotherapy, where a short half-life of the conjugate is desirable because of the potential non-specific toxicity, more important considerations for monoclonal antibody–toxin/TAP conjugates are the size of the conjugate and its immunogenicity.

Monoclonal antibodies have molecular weights of 150 kilodaltons, and this relatively large size may limit the ability of a monoclonal antibody conjugate to penetrate thoroughly into tumors. Truncated monoclonal antibodies may reduce this limitation and have better tumor penetration. Conversely, however, the smaller molecules may be cleared more rapidly by the kidneys.

Because the tumor-active prodrug or toxin itself may be recognized by the immune system as being a foreign protein, these conjugates may be relatively immunogenic. In fact, in earlier trials using murine monoclonal antibodies, HAMA responses were a major factor that limited efficacy. For this reason, in order to minimize the immunogenicity of the conjugate, it is more desirable to use humanized or CDR-engrafted antibodies for the targeting component.

Because the monoclonal antibody–TAP/toxin conjugate is designed to be highly specific, the cytotoxic agent that is used in the conjugate can be very potent. In fact, it may be possible to utilize cytotoxic agents that could not be considered for systemic therapy, because the toxicity of the cytotoxic will be limited (at least in theory) to cells that bind the conjugate. Several such highly potent TAPs have already been used in various immunoconjugates, including calicheamicin, maytansine derivatives and new-generation taxoids. Protein toxins such as diphtheria toxin, *Pseudomonas* exotoxin and ricin are also highly toxic and potentially attractive agents for these immunoconjugates.

The third important consideration for these monoclonal antibody–TAP/toxin conjugates is the linker strategy. Ideally the linker must be completely stable in the circulation but be efficiently cleaved once inside the cancer cell. There are three classes of

linkers that have been used in immunoconjugates to date: hydrazone linkers, peptide linkers and disulfide linkers. The choice of linker may depend upon the type of cancer being targeted and the cytotoxic agent being utilized.

Hydrazone linkers are stable except in acidic conditions. Inside the cell the hydrazone linker will therefore be cleaved in the low pH environment of the lysozome. This linker technology has been used in the Mylotarg immunoconjugate, which targets CD33 on myeloid blast cells and has been approved for use in the treatment of acute myeloblastic leukemia.

Peptide linkers are also designed for high levels of stability in the serum and can also be cleaved in lysozomes. There is some evidence that these linkers may be more stable than hydrazone linkers.

The third type of linker consists of disulfide moieties. These are cleaved through disulfide exchange with intracellular thiol groups in tumor cells. Concentrations of glutathione are much higher in tumor cells than in normal cells. In preclinical models disulfide linkers have proven to be superior in efficacy to several other linkers. An example of a monoclonal TAP with disulfide linkers which has been tested in the clinic is HuC242-DM1.

A monoclonal antibody–TAP conjugate named CMC-544 has been generated to CD22. It uses a humanized version of G5/44, the murine monoclonal antibody that recognizes CD22 and is internalized into B cells, conjugated using an acid-label linker to calicheamicin. The CMC-544 conjugate has been shown to be cytotoxic for BCL xenografts and more potent than its murine homologue or a homologue that used an acid-stable linker. This antibody conjugate has been selected for evaluation in a phase I clinical trial.

Monoclonal toxin conjugates and radiolabeled monoclonals are being evaluated in Hodgkin's lymphoma, where initial experimental data have suggested that there may be a benefit in adding additional effector mechanisms to enhance the therapeutic potential of monoclonal antibodies. Unfortunately the initial toxicities in several phase I trials evaluating anti-CD25 ricin conjugates and a saporin anti-CD30 conjugate have been prohibitive, with vascular leak syndrome, hepatic toxicities and induction of neutralizing human anti-toxin antibody responses.

The current generation of immunoconjugates has tremendous potential. Issues related to non-specific

Table 6.5. Cancer vaccine platforms.

Platform	Type of immune response
Autologous	
Autologous tumor cell	Th1 CD8
Dendritic cell	Th1 CD8
Heat shock protein	Th1 CD8
Idiotype protein	Th2
Generic	
Allogeneic tumor cell	Th1 CD8
Genetically modified tumor cell	Th1 CD8
Peptide	CD4 or CD8
Protein	Th2
DNA	Th1 CD8
Viral	Th1 CD8

include allogeneic tumor cell lines or vaccines containing commonly expressed tumor-associated antigens.

The platform used to present the antigen to the immune system may influence the character of the immune response. The platforms which present antigens to the class I processing pathway (discussed below) will promote Th1 and cytotoxic T-lymphocyte CD8 immune responses. Nonamer class I MHC-binding peptides are the best example of a platform that focuses the CD8 T-cell arm. On the other hand, protein or carbohydrate platforms will present antigens to the class II processing pathway and produce responses biased towards Th2. Some platforms, such as certain viral platforms and potentially dendritic cell platforms, will result in antigen presentation to both class I and class II pathways and generate broad CD4 and CD8 immune responses (Table 6.5).

Immunologic adjuvants
Adjuvants may enhance activation and maturation of antigen-presenting cells, and can also stimulate the chemotaxis of APCs or T cells, increase the proliferation of APCs and induce more rapid maturation of APCs. Adjuvants may be biologically based and act through specifically defined receptors on APCs, or they may be non-biologically based. Examples of non-biologically based adjuvants include alum, BCG and Friend's adjuvants. More specific biologic adjuvants include molecules that will bind to receptors on APCs

such as GM-CSF or toll-like receptors. In addition, activation of APCs through the CD40 pathway may also be an important strategy to provide the "second signal" required by APCs to become optimally activated. Agonist antibodies to CD40 or CD40 ligand reagents have both been shown to be effective in providing this second activating signal. Adjuvants may also play an important role in influencing the character of the immune activation. The optimal cancer vaccine adjuvant(s) have not yet been defined.

Immune modulators
There are several different strategies that can be used to enhance the magnitude and quality of the immune response generated by a cancer vaccine, and immunomodulators can act at several different points (Fig. 6.4). They can augment (1) the activation of antigen-presenting cells (in which case they are termed adjuvants: see above), (2) the activation of T cells or (3) the reduction of the T regulatory response. It is generally necessary to combine immunomodulation(s) with the vaccine platform to generate the optimal immune response that is sufficient to induce clinically relevant anti-tumor activity.

T-cell activation can also be augmented through several different strategies. Foremost amongst these is the use of co-stimulatory molecules, and it has been demonstrated that introduction of the B7.1 co-stimulatory molecule into tumor cells or APCs can enhance T-cell activation. T cells can be further activated by introducing a triad of co-stimulatory molecules (TRICOM) into the vaccine platform. These have been shown to further augment the frequency and avidity of tumor-specific T cells beyond that induced by vaccines incorporating B7.1 alone. Other co-stimulatory molecules, particularly of the TNF family (4-1BB ligand), can also augment T-cell activation.

T cells can be further enhanced with various cytokines. Cytokines such as IL-2 may increase the proliferation of T cells. More recent cytokines such as IL-18 may increase T-cell activation and proliferation without inducing activation-induced cell death. Interferon α is also an important cytokine that may have multiple effects on the immune system, including generation of increased numbers of memory T cells. IL-12 is a potent stimulator of Interferon γ and will enhance the activation of Th1, CD4 cells and CD8 T-cell responses. Approaches to eliminate

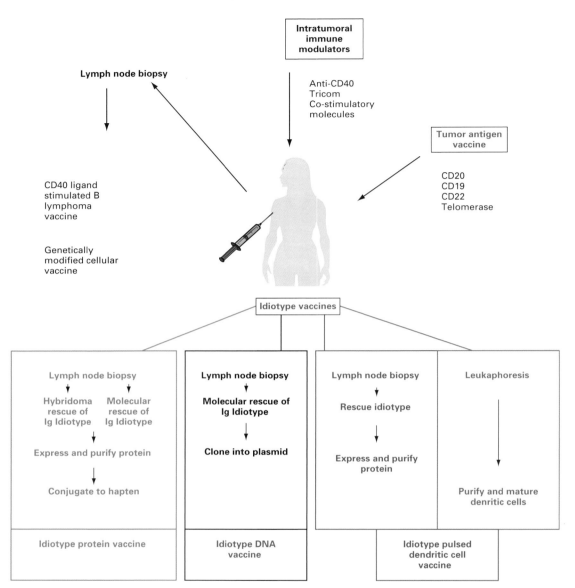

Figure 6.5. Types of lymphoma vaccines. The immunoglobulin idiotype tumor-specific antigen has been most extensively studied as a vaccine target for B-cell lymphomas. Idiotype vaccines can be produced using several different technologies. For all of these approaches a lymph node biopsy must be obtained to isolate the patient's B-lymphoma cells. Idiotype protein can be rescued either through hybridoma technology or by using molecular techniques from this lymph node. After rescue, the idiotype can be expressed as purified protein or a cDNA and cloned into a plasmid DNA vector. For optimal immunogenicity, the idiotype protein is conjugated to an immunogenic hapten such as KLH. The purified protein can also be used to pulse patient-derived dendritic cells that have been matured ex vivo. These pulsed dendritic cells can also be used as a patient-specific vaccine. Other techniques include obtaining patient biopsy material to develop an immunogenic cellular vaccine by activating the lymphoma cells with CD40 ligand or introducing immunogenic molecules such as cytokines or co-stimulatory molecules. Lymphoma tumor antigens (differentiation antigens) can be presented to the immune system in various platforms as generic vaccine approaches that do not require patient-derived material. Molecules that can activate lymphoma cells can also be introduced into malignant lymph nodes in vivo to enhance the immunogenicity of the lymphoma.

immunosuppressant cytokines may also further augment the level of T-cell activation. For example, antibodies to IL-10 or TGFβ have been shown in preclinical models to enhance T-cell activation.

T-cell activation can also be augmented by eliminating the inhibitory responses mediated through the CTLA4 receptor on T cells. Antibodies to CTLA4 enable the B7 co-stimulatory molecules to stimulate T cells selectively through CD28, resulting in T cells that can overcome tolerance. This has been shown in both preclinical tumor models and in initial early-phase clinical trials.

Another important approach to the optimal activation of tumor-specific T cells is to eliminate or reduce the regulatory T-cell inhibition of these cells. Although reagents that can selectively deplete T regulatory cells (and not effector T cells) have not yet been developed, positive results in preclinical models and some initial clinical trials have been achieved with approaches that are not entirely specific for T regulatory cell depletion. These include the use of the IL-2–diphtheria toxin conjugate (Ontak) that kills cells expressing the IL-2 receptor.

ACTIVE VACCINATION APPROACHES AGAINST NON-HODGKIN'S LYMPHOMA

Idiotype vaccines

The idiotype of surface immunoglobulin is an almost ideal antigenic target for immunotherapeutic approaches. It is highly lymphoma-specific and is a customized marker of each patient's lymphoma clone. Idiotype determinants are not shared between lymphomas (although some level of cross-reactivity has been documented) and the lymphoma's unique idiotype is not expressed on the patient's normal B cells. Thus specific immune responses directed at the idiotype would be expected to be highly lymphoma-specific and not to produce toxicities due to cross-reactivity. The only limitation is the need to identify and synthesize the idiotype vaccine for each individual lymphoma (Fig. 6.5).

Preclinical models

Active immunotherapy with idiotype vaccines has been evaluated in several different preclinical models. In these models the idiotype protein from syngeneic murine B-cell lymphoma was expressed through hybridoma technology and purified idiotype protein was then conjugated to an immunogenic carrier (KLH) and used as a vaccine by injection with incomplete Friend's adjuvant. Vaccinated mice were then challenged with the syngeneic tumor expressing the idiotype protein, and tumor formation and survival were monitored. Significant improvements in both tumor development and survival were seen after vaccination with the tumor-specific idiotype but not with idiotype protein from an unrelated B-cell lymphoma. This protection was associated with increases of humoral responses to the idiotype protein used in the vaccination. In addition, studies have shown that depletion of LY3/4 cells resulted in minor reductions in survival but depletion of LY2 T-helper cells significantly impaired survival of the vaccinated mice. These experiments provided the rationale for subsequent clinical evaluation of idiotype vaccination approaches.

Further variations of the idiotype vaccination approach have been studied. A GM-CSF-Id fusion protein was shown to be more immunogenic than the Id protein alone in preclinical murine models. Similar results were seen with two Id-chemokine (MCP-3 or IP-10) fusion proteins. Plasmid DNA immunogens linking the Id to GM-CSF or MCP-3 have also proven to be more immunogenic than the control DNA Id vaccine. Finally, in a preclinical murine model, a DNA vaccine linking the tumor-specific idiotype region to a foreign (human) constant region was more immunogenic and effective than the same vaccine containing a murine constant region. The importance of including a xenogeneic constant region in the vaccine was also demonstrated using an adenovirus-based idiotype vaccine.

Early-phase clinical trials with idiotype vaccines

Idiotype vaccination approaches have been evaluated in patients with recurrent indolent lymphoma in phase I/II clinical trials. The idiotype protein was rescued from a patient's autologous tumor by fusion of the patient's tumor cells with heterohybridomas. The secreted idiotype protein was purified and, after demonstration that the protein was identical to the patient's own tumor idiotype, the protein was conjugated to KLH and formulated for use as a vaccine.

Hsu reported on a study of 41 patients with recurrent indolent lymphoma who were vaccinated with their own idiotype proteins. The toxicity of this vaccination was mild, and only grade I or grade II constitutional symptoms including fatigue, myalgia, flu-like symptoms, fever and headaches, as well as local injection-site reactions, were documented. ELISA assays were used to document the patient's specific immune response to the idiotype protein or to KLH. All patients vaccinated had evidence of either a cellular or a humoral response to the KLH protein used as an immunogenic carrier. Approximately half of the patients had either a cellular or a humoral response to their own idiotype protein. Patients who had minimal disease at the time of vaccination were more likely to develop an immune response (15 of 21 patients) and patients with significant evidence of lymphoma at the time of vaccination were less likely (5 of 20 patients). Objective tumor regressions were seen in 2 out of 5 patients who had tumor present and who were found to have an immune response after idiotype vaccination. Of the 15 patients without evidence of tumor at the time of vaccination who had evidence of immune response, 13 remained free of tumor progression for variable lengths of time post-vaccination. There was a clear statistically significant association between the probability of survival and development of an immune response in these 41 patients. Encouraging results were also described in a phase II trial of 35 patients with indolent lymphoma treated with idiotype vaccination and GM-CSF adjuvant after entering a complete remission after ProMACE chemotherapy. Twenty of the initial 35 patients actually received the vaccine. Of these 20 patients, 11 had detectable PCR evidence of lymphoma in their peripheral blood after the chemotherapy and 8 of these patients became PCR-negative in the peripheral blood after vaccination. Nineteen of the 20 patients had evidence of the CD8 or CD4 T-cell response to their vaccine.

The Levy group reported on their experience of vaccinating a total of 136 patients with idiotype proteins, using a number of different formulations which included either a chemical adjuvant (Syntax adjuvant formulation), a cytokine adjuvant (GM-CSF) or autologous dendritic cells. Of 136 patients, 67% had evidence of either a humoral or a cellular immune response (or both) to the vaccine. Improvement of progression-free survival was associated with achieving a humoral anti-idiotype immune response to autologous idiotype. The most important predictors of outcome in this relatively large group of patients were a combination of humoral immune response and favorable $Fc\gamma R$ phenotype. These results are consistent with the importance of humoral immune response in mediating the anti-tumor activity of idiotype vaccines, as suggested by the initial preclinical trials.

Limitations to idiotype vaccine approaches

The preclinical and clinical trials are encouraging in that they suggest that vaccination with idiotype proteins can be immunogenic and can induce either humoral or cellular immune responses that are specific for the idiotype protein. In addition, there is some suggestion that clinical outcome may be related to the induction of a specific anti-idiotype immune response.

However, there are also some limitations from this initial data. Firstly, the overall approach is a highly customized autologous approach requiring manufacturing of an idiotype protein from patient-derived material. This is logistically difficult and may have commercialization limitations. In addition, although immune responses are generated in many patients, they are not generated in at least a third of patients. In addition, both cellular and humoral responses are generated in only a small subset of patients. The magnitude of the immune response can also be further optimized. Although there is a suggestion of some anti-tumor clinical activity, these initial results are difficult to interpret, as another interpretation of the clinical data is that patients in whom an immune response is generated are more likely to live longer because of their better performance status. Finally, the manufacturing approach used in the initial trials was very labor-intensive and time-consuming. A considerable amount of cell culture is necessary to generate and select hybridomas that secrete patient-specific idiotype protein.

Non-hybridoma idiotype vaccine approaches

There are several strategies that can be used to enhance the manufacturing of idiotype vaccines. Most of these involve molecular approaches. Polymerase chain reaction amplification (PCR) can be used to specifically amplify the idiotype region from patient-derived material. These amplified products can then be engineered into various expression cassettes and use to produce large amounts of specific protein, or they could be used as DNA expression vectors, as the vaccine itself. In fact, vaccination of patients with idiotype proteins generalized by molecular technology has been pursued, and an initial clinical trial with molecularly derived idiotype protein in patients with recurrent indolent lymphoma in combination with GM-CSF has demonstrated humoral and cellular response rates comparable to those seen using idiotype protein derived from hybridoma technology. In addition, the toxicity profile was similar and the success rate in producing the idiotype protein with these techniques was greater than 90%. The time to produce vaccine was considerably shorter than the time needed to produce vaccines through hybridoma technology. Given these data showing comparable immunogenicity and an approved manufacturing process, two phase III trials to evaluate idiotype vaccination using molecular production processes are under way. These trials will address whether time to progression can be increased in patients treated with vaccine after either standard first-line chemotherapy with cyclophosphamide, vincristine and prednisone or after rituximab monotherapy.

A strategy to overcome the complexities of manufacturing involves using a plasmid DNA vaccine containing the patient-specific idiotype. In this approach the patient-specific heavy chain and light chain variable regions are cloned into an expression vector containing murine heavy and light chain constant regions. It is expected that this may enhance the immunogenicity of the vaccine, since this has been shown in a mouse model by the inclusion of human constant regions with murine variable regions. In an early phase I study patients were vaccinated subcutaneously or with a combination of intramuscular and intradermal injections, using a bioinjector. Another research group has evaluated bioinjector vaccination with GM-CSF. Most patients in all groups showed humoral or T-cell responses to the foreign constant regions but not to the autologous idiotype regions. Although the manufacturing of the vaccine with this approach seems simpler, the results from this small non-randomized trial suggest that the idiotype-specific immune response may not be as good as that seen with protein-based vaccination.

One other approach designed to further enhance the immunogenicity of idiotype vaccine strategies involves pulsing autologous dendritic cells with idiotype protein. In preclinical models, dendritic-cell-based vaccines were immunogenic and effective in inducing protective T-cell anti-tumor responses. Two clinical trials using this approach have been completed in patients with recurrent indolent lymphoma. Patients were treated with a combination of dendritic cells pulsed with idiotype protein conjugated to KLH. Of ten patients with measurable disease, eight developed T-cell responses and four of these had objective clinical responses. In another trial, 25 patients with indolent lymphoma were treated with idiotype vaccines after initial chemotherapy. Immune responses occurred in 65% of these patients and 4 of 18 patients with measurable disease had objective responses. These results are encouraging from an immunogenic and clinical perspective but the applicability of this approach may be limited by the requirements both to produce autologous idiotype protein and to purify and mature autologous dendritic cells for each patient.

Cell-based lymphoma vaccines

Another vaccination approach that has been studied in murine lymphoma models involves using the lymphoma cell itself as an immunogen (Fig. 6.5). An advantage of this approach is that the patient-specific idiotype does not need to be rescued from the tumor. In addition, the potential problem of tumor escape from therapy by evolution of idiotype-negative variants is not a limiting factor. In order to make the lymphoma cells more immunogenic various molecules such as cytokines (IL-2, IL-12 or GM-CSF) or co-stimulatory molecules (such as B7.1, 4-1BB ligand) have been introduced into the lymphoma cells using various gene transfer techniques. There have not yet been any reports of clinical trials with these approaches.

Other vaccination approaches

Other approaches to generate anti-lymphoma immune responses have been considered (Fig. 6.5). A generic approach that would not involve the need to obtain patient-specific biopsy material would be to use lymphoma tumor-specific antigens (see Table 6.1) as an immunogen. These could be presented to the immune system in a variety of platforms including protein, peptide, dendritic cell or viral vaccine approaches. It is also possible to directly introduce immunogenic molecules such as cytokines, co-stimulatory molecules or CD40 ligand into lymphomatous lymph nodes. With this approach multiple different tumor-associated and specific antigens expressed by the lymphoma cell itself would be potential targets for the immune system. A limitation of this approach would be the need to overcome the strong immunoregulatory and suppressive factors present within the local tumor environment.

FUTURE PROSPECTS FOR IMMUNO-THERAPEUTIC APPROACHES DIRECTED AT HEMATOLOGIC MALIGNANCIES

There has already been significant progress in the development and integration of new forms of immunotherapy into the management of various lymphoid malignancies. Monoclonal antibodies such as rituximab and radiolabeled versions of anti-CD20 monoclonals are playing important roles in extending the well-being and in some cases survival of many patients with lymphoid malignancies. Many new monoclonal antibodies, including improved anti-CD20 monoclonals, antibodies recognizing tumor antigens distinct from CD20, genetically modified antibodies with improved pharmacokinetic or effector features, monoclonals conjugated to cytotoxic compounds for highly specific targeted delivery and radiolabeled monoclonals for non-Hodgkin's and Hodgkin's lymphomas are in the development stages. In addition, a whole new therapeutic modality – therapeutic cancer vaccines – holds the promise of harnessing memory immune responses that may eliminate minimal residual disease and prolong or prevent disease recurrences with negligible toxicity to the patient. Although it has taken more than two decades of research in this area before the first fruits were delivered, the future looks bright, with a rich crop of rationally based, highly specific and relatively non-toxic immune therapies that will further enhance the management of various lymphoid malignancies, both by improving outcome and by reducing treatment-related toxicities.

FURTHER READING

Borchmann, P., Schell, R. and Engert, A. Immunotherapy of Hodgkin's lymphoma. *Eur. J. Haematol. Suppl.* **75** (2005), 159–165.

DiJoseph, J. F., Popplewell, A., Tickle, S. *et al.* Antibody-targeted chemotherapy of B-cell lymphoma using calicheamicin conjugated to murine or humanized antibody against CD22. *Cancer Immunol. Immunother.* **54** (2005), 11–24.

Hernandez, M. C. and Knox, S. J. Radiobiology of radioimmunotherapy: targeting CD20 B-cell antigen in non-Hodgkin's lymphoma. *Int. J. Radiat. Oncol. Biol. Phys.* **59** (2004), 1274–1287.

Jaracz, S., Chen, J., Kuznetsova, L. V. and Ojima, I. Recent advances in tumor-targeting anticancer drug conjugates. *Bioorg. Med. Chem.* **13** (2005), 5043–5054.

McLaughlin, P., Grillo-Lopez, A. J., Link, B. K. *et al.* Rituximab chimeric anti-CD20 monoclonal antibody therapy for relapsed indolent lymphoma: half of patients respond to a four-dose treatment program. *J. Clin. Oncol.* **16** (1998), 2825–2833.

Morrison, S., Johnson, M. J., Herzenberg, L. A. and Oi, V. T. Chimeric human antibody molecules: mouse antigen-binding domains with human constant region domains. *Proc. Natl. Acad. Sci. USA* **81** (1984), 6851–6855.

Radvanyi, L. Discovery and immunologic validation of new antigens for therapeutic cancer vaccines. *Int. Arch. Allergy Immunol.* **133** (2004), 179–197.

Reff, M. E., Carner, K., Chambers, K. S. *et al.* Depletion of B cells in vivo by a chimeric mouse human monoclonal antibody to CD20. *Blood* **83** (1994), 435–445.

Teeling, J. L., French, R. R., Cragg, M. S. *et al.* Characterization of new human CD20 monoclonal antibodies with potent cytolytic activity against non-Hodgkin lymphomas. *Blood* **104** (2004), 1793–1800.

Timmerman, J., Czerwinski, D. K., Davis, T. A. *et al.* Idiotypic-pulsed dendritic cell vaccination for B-cell lymphoma: clinical and immune responses in 35 patients. *Blood* **99** (2002), 1517–1526.

Timmerman, J. M., Singh, G., Hermanson, G. *et al.* Immunogenicity of a plasmid DNA vaccine encoding chimeric idiotype in patients with B-cell lymphoma. *Cancer Res.* **62** (2002), 5845–5852.

Weng, W. K., Czerwinski, D., Timmerman, J., Hsu, F. J. and Levy, R. Clinical outcome of lymphoma patients after idiotype vaccination is correlated with humoral immune response and immunoglobulin G Fc receptor genotype. *J. Clin. Oncol.* **22** (2004), 4717–4724.

Ziller, F., Macor, P., Bulla, R., Sblattero, D., Marzari, R. and Tedesco, F. Controlling complement resistance in cancer by using human monoclonal antibodies that neutralize complement-regulatory proteins CD55 and CD59. *Eur. J. Immunol.* **35** (2005), 2175–2183.

Part II

LYMPHOMA SUBTYPES

Stephanie Sasse and Andreas Engert

Pathology: Andrew Wotherspoon
Molecular cytogenetics: Andreas Rosenwald and German Ott

INTRODUCTION

Hodgkin's lymphoma (HL) is a malignant lymphoma. The classical variant (cHL) is characterized by the presence of mononucleated Hodgkin and multinucleated Reed–Sternberg (HRS) cells, while lymphocytic and histiocytic (L&H) cells ("popcorn cells") are pathognomonic for nodular lymphocyte-predominant HL (NLPHL). After the first description of patients suffering from enlarged lymph nodes and spleen by Thomas Hodgkin in 1832, it took more than 150 years finally to prove the malignant character of these pathognomonic cells and to show their origin from a germinal-center B cell in the majority of cases. Many questions concerning the pathogenesis of Hodgkin's lymphoma are still unanswered; an important step in the pathogenesis of classical HL seems to be the constitutive activation of the NF-κB pathway.

The prognosis of patients with HL depends on the stage of disease and clinical risk factors. The development of stage- and risk-adapted treatment regimens based on modern polychemotherapy and radiotherapy has improved the outcome dramatically over the past few decades. Current strategies aim at reducing therapy-associated complications while maintaining high cure rates.

EPIDEMIOLOGY

HL has an annual incidence of 2–3 per 100 000 in Europe and the USA, and accounts for approximately one-sixth of all lymphoma. Slightly more men than women are affected. In industrialized countries the onset of disease shows a bimodal distribution, with a first peak in the third decade and a second, much smaller, peak after the age of 60.

CLINICAL PRESENTATION

Indolent swellings localized to the cervical or supraclavicular region are the first symptoms of disease in 60–70% of patients. Axillary lymph nodes are observed in about 30%. Almost two-thirds of patients with newly diagnosed classical HL have radiographic evidence of intrathoracic involvement. Bone marrow involvement occurs in fewer than 10% of newly diagnosed patients. Details of organ involvement at diagnosis are given in Table 7.1.

About 40% of patients, especially those with initial abdominal involvement or advanced-stage disease, demonstrate B symptoms. Other symptoms comprise pain at the site of nodal involvement shortly after drinking alcohol, pruritus or fatigue.

In contrast to cHL, NLPHL normally begins as a localized, slowly growing and rather benign entity with participation of only one peripheral nodal region.

DIAGNOSIS

In our view an excision biopsy of a suspicious lymph node is indispensable for the diagnosis of Hodgkin's lymphoma.

PATHOLOGY

Nodular lymphocyte-predominant Hodgkin's lymphoma (NLPHL)

The lymph node shows a lymphoid proliferation with a nodular growth pattern. In most cases this is prominent, but in some cases the nodularity may be difficult to discern. A proportion of cases will have areas of preserved normal nodal architecture with

Table 7.1. Anatomic sites of disease involved in untreated patients with Hodgkin's lymphoma.

Anatomic site	Involvement
Waldeyer's ring	1–2%
Cervical nodes	60–70%
Axillary nodes	30–35%
Mediastinum	50–60%
Hilar nodes	15–35%
Para-aortic nodes	30–40%
Iliac nodes	15–20%
Mesenteric nodes	1–4%
Inguinal nodes	8–15%
Spleen	30–35%
Liver	2–6%
Bone marrow	1–4%
Total extranodal	10–15%

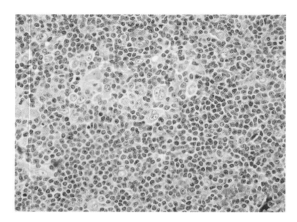

Figure 7.2. Nodular lymphocyte-predominant Hodgkin's lymphoma (lymph node). The large cells have lobulated nuclei and intermediate-sized nucleoli ("popcorn cells").

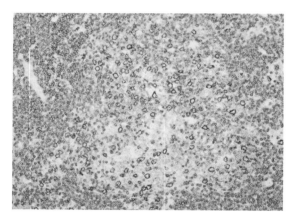

Figure 7.3. Nodular lymphocyte-predominant Hodgkin's lymphoma (lymph node). The "popcorn cells" stain for CD20. They are surrounded by CD20-negative T cells. The remainder of the small lymphocytes in the nodule are small B cells.

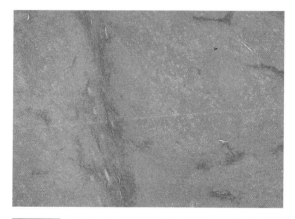

Figure 7.1. Nodular lymphocyte-predominant Hodgkin's lymphoma (lymph node). The lymphoid proliferation has a nodular growth pattern. The nodules consist mainly of small lymphocytes, with scattered large cells and histiocytes.

reactive follicles, some of which may show features of progressive transformation of germinal centers (Fig. 7.1).

The abnormal nodules show a proliferation of small mantle-type cells with round or slightly irregular nuclei and scanty cytoplasm. Histiocytes are usually present, either singly or in small clusters. Within this background is a scattered population of large cells with abundant cytoplasm and large lobulated nuclei with open chromatin and prominent eosinophilic nucleoli. These neoplastic cells are variously termed either L&H cells, after a previous designation of this type of Hodgkin's lymphoma (lymphocytic and histiocytic) in the Lukes and Butler classification, or as popcorn cells, in reference to the complexity of nuclear convolutions (Fig. 7.2). Variable numbers of popcorn cells can be found in the interfollicular zone. Occasionally these interfollicular cells can be strikingly numerous.

Immunophenotypically the popcorn cells express CD45 and the B-cell antigens CD20 (Fig. 7.3) and

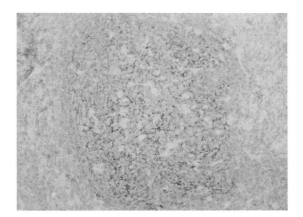

Figure 7.4. Nodular lymphocyte-predominant Hodgkin's lymphoma (lymph node). The nodules are delineated by underlying follicular dendritic cell meshworks stained for CD21, which wrap around the large cells and an attached rim of small lymphocytes.

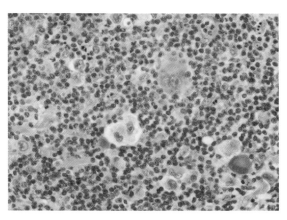

Figure 7.5. Classical Hodgkin's lymphoma. Reed–Sternberg cells are large with abundant cytoplasm. Classical variants have a bilobed nucleus with prominent large inclusion-type nucleoli.

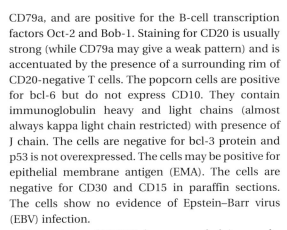

CD79a, and are positive for the B-cell transcription factors Oct-2 and Bob-1. Staining for CD20 is usually strong (while CD79a may give a weak pattern) and is accentuated by the presence of a surrounding rim of CD20-negative T cells. The popcorn cells are positive for bcl-6 but do not express CD10. They contain immunoglobulin heavy and light chains (almost always kappa light chain restricted) with presence of J chain. The cells are negative for bcl-3 protein and p53 is not overexpressed. The cells may be positive for epithelial membrane antigen (EMA). The cells are negative for CD30 and CD15 in paraffin sections. The cells show no evidence of Epstein–Barr virus (EBV) infection.

The nodules of NLPHL have an underlying meshwork of follicular dendritic cells that can be demonstrated by staining for CD21 or CD23 (Fig. 7.4). The small B cells are predominantly IgD-positive, with scattered T cells. The cells around the popcorn cells are CD4-positive, CD57-positive T cells. Residual germinal-center cells may be present either singly or in small clusters. CD30-positive B immunoblastic cells are seen in the interfollicular areas, but these are not part of the neoplastic population.

NLPHL needs to be differentiated from reactive changes in the follicles, particularly progressive transformation of the germinal centers. In the latter condition the classical finding of strongly CD20-positive cells surrounded by rosettes of T cells is not present. Differentiation from classical Hodgkin's

lymphoma (cHL) can be achieved by careful assessment of the immunophenotype of the neoplastic cells. Distinction between NLPHL and diffuse large B-cell lymphoma of T-cell/histiocyte-rich type may be problematic, but NLPHL usually shows at least some residual nodularity or follicular dendritic cell meshwork and there is usually at least a sprinkling of IgD-positive small B cells around the popcorn cells. Residual CD57-positive T cells also favor NLPHL.

Classical Hodgkin's lymphoma (cHL)

The hallmark of classical Hodgkin's lymphoma is the presence of Reed–Sternberg (RS) cells or their variants. These are set in a background that consists of a polymorphous mix of inflammatory cells. The background cellular population, together with other changes, determines the morphological subclassification of cHL (Fig. 7.5).

Reed–Sternberg cells are large with abundant pale eosinophilic cytoplasm. The nuclei of the classical form of RS cells are bilobed and contain large round eosinophilic nucleoli that are surrounded by a thin clear rim. Variants from the classical RS cell include mononuclear forms (sometimes termed Hodgkin cells) and cells with more complex multilobated nuclei. Some RS cells have more deeply staining eosinophilic cytoplasm with pyknotic nuclei (often referred to as mummified cells).

Figure 7.6. Nodular lymphocyte-rich classical Hodgkin's lymphoma (lymph node). The lymphoid population has a nodular/follicular growth pattern. The nodules contain a background of small lymphocytes with scattered large cells.

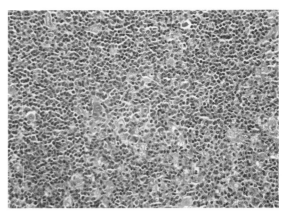

Figure 7.7. Nodular lymphocyte-rich classical Hodgkin's lymphoma (lymph node). The large cells have the morphology of Reed–Sternberg cells rather than popcorn cells, helping to distinguish this from nodular lymphocyte-predominant Hodgkin's lymphoma.

Immunophenotypically the RS cells and variants express CD30. Expression of CD15 is variable and is highly dependent on the sensitivity of the detection method employed, but is probably positive in 75–85%. Positive cases frequently show staining in only a proportion of the neoplastic cell population. Reed–Sternberg cells are now considered to be derived from mature B cells, and they express IRF4/MUM1 and the B-cell-specific transcription factor PAX-5, but they are negative for CD45 and only about 40% express CD20, with a smaller proportion expressing CD79a. Expression of CD20 is frequently heterogeneous in intensity, and in most cases the staining is not seen in all neoplastic cells. Staining for the transcription factor Oct-2 and its co-activator Bob-1 is usually absent, although a small proportion of cases may be positive for one or other of the two. Expression of both together is not seen. The cells are negative for J chain. Reed–Sternberg cells stain with antibodies against fascin but most, although not all, anaplastic large-cell lymphomas (T-cell and null types) also stain with antibodies to this antigen.

The RS cells are usually surrounded by a corona of small reactive T cells, making assessment of T-cell antigen expression difficult. In general RS cells do not express T-cell-related antigens, although aberrant expression of these may be seen in a small number of cases. There is no staining for ALK kinase protein, and RS cells are generally negative for epithelial membrane antigen (EMA).

Expression of Epstein–Barr virus (EBV)-latent membrane protein 1 (LMP-1) is variable and dependent on morphological subtype. Reed–Sternberg cells can overexpress p53 protein. Expression of bcl-2 protein is variable, and both p53 and bcl-2 protein expression may be prognostically important, although this remains controversial. Proliferation in RS cells is high. There is also significant proliferative activity within the background reactive lymphoid population.

Lymphocyte-rich classical Hodgkin's lymphoma (LR-cHL)

In this subtype the background population is predominantly composed of small lymphocytes (Figs. 7.6, 7.7). The growth pattern is usually nodular. The nodules are lymphoid follicles with expanded mantle zones. They may contain residual germinal centers. The RS cells are scattered within the expanded mantle zones. This subtype may therefore mimic the morphological appearance of NLPHL. Eosinophils are scanty or absent. A rare diffuse form also exists.

Immunophenotypically the RS cells show the typical immunophenotype, with expression of CD30 and CD15 (in distinction from the cells of NLPHL) (Figs. 7.8 and 7.9). The RS cells are rimmed by T cells, but the majority of the associated lymphocyte-rich background consists of mantle-type small B cells. The nodules also contain disrupted follicular dendritic cell meshworks (highlighted by staining for CD21 or CD23).

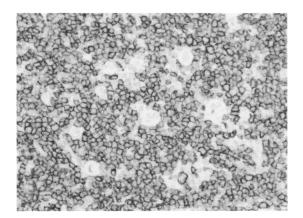

Figure 7.8. Nodular lymphocyte-rich classical Hodgkin's lymphoma (lymph node). The Reed–Sternberg cells are negative for CD20.

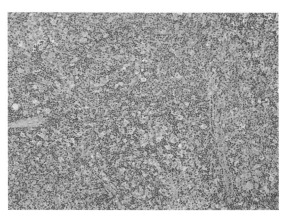

Figure 7.10. Mixed-cellularity Hodgkin's lymphoma. Reed–Sternberg cells are present within a mixed background rich in small lymphocytes, histiocytes, eosinophils and plasma cells. There is no nodule formation and no mature, banded sclerosis.

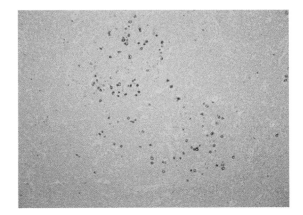

Figure 7.9. Nodular lymphocyte-rich classical Hodgkin's lymphoma (lymph node). Further distinction from lymphocyte-predominant Hodgkin's lymphoma is the strong positive staining of the Reed–Sternberg cells for CD30 (popcorn cells are CD30-negative).

Mixed-cellularity Hodgkin's lymphoma (MC-HL)

In this subtype the nodal architecture is effaced by a polymorphous mixture of cells within which classical RS cells are found. This background contains lymphocytes, histiocytes, plasma cells, eosinophils and neutrophils in proportions that vary from case to case. The nodal capsule is not thickened and there are no well-formed sclerotic fibrous bands formed of mature collagen, although some interstitial fibrosis may be seen. In some cases the nodal architecture is not completely effaced and the infiltrate occupies the interfollicular areas (Fig. 7.10).

Immunophenotypically the RS cells show the typical antigen profile but expression of EBV LMP-1 is frequent.

Nodular sclerosing Hodgkin's lymphoma (NS-HL)

The lymph node usually shows thickening of the capsule. There are fibrosclerotic bands that extend from the capsule into the node pulp with formation of cellular nodules. The degree of nodularity varies between cases and the nodules may contain residual lymphoid follicles. Within the cellular nodules R-S cells are present in variable numbers. There may be confluent sheets of RS cells and there may be areas of necrosis. In formalin-fixed tissue a proportion of the RS cells may show artefactual separation from the surrounding rim of lymphocytes (lacunar cells) (Fig. 7.11).

A grading system has been formulated by the British National Lymphoma Investigation (BNLI) for the assessment of NS-HL, based on the number of RS cells and the background cellular population. In grade 1, 75% of the nodules contain scattered RS cells in a lymphocyte-rich polymorphous infiltrate. In grade 2, at least 25% of the nodules contain sheets of RS cells with a relatively lymphocyte-depleted background. There is frequently associated necrosis in the nodules. Grade 2 lesions have, in the past, been called nodular sclerosis with lymphocyte depletion.

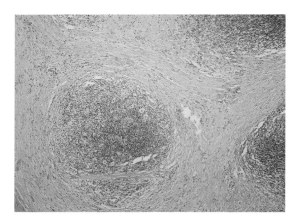

Figure 7.11. Nodular sclerosing Hodgkin's lymphoma (lymph node). The node architecture is effaced. There are cellular nodules that are separated from each other by sclerotic bands. The nodules contain Reed–Sternberg cells in a background of small lymphocytes, histiocytes, eosinophils and plasma cells.

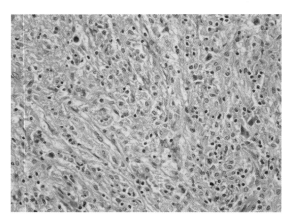

Figure 7.12. Lymphocyte-depleted Hodgkin's lymphoma. A proliferation of pleomorphic cells including occasional Reed–Sternberg cells in a background that shows a paucity of lymphocytes.

Immunophenotypically the RS cells show a typical antigen profile but EBV LMP-1 is less frequently expressed (10–40%).

Lymphocyte-depleted Hodgkin's lymphoma (LD-HL)

The lymph node is effaced by a population that contains a relative predominance of RS cells over background cells. In some cases the RS cells show marked pleomorphism with a sarcomatous appearance. In a proportion of cases there is diffuse fibrosis (without nodule formation) with scattered RS cells (Fig. 7.12).

Immunophenotypically the RS cells show the characteristic antigen profile.

MOLECULAR PATHOLOGY AND CYTOGENETICS

The molecular and genetic analysis of the malignant tumor cells in this lymphoma, the Hodgkin and Reed–Sternberg (HRS) cells, has long been hampered by the paucity of the neoplastic cells (1–2%) in the lymphoma specimen. However, advances in tissue microdissection techniques have enabled a more detailed molecular genetic analysis of HRS cells.

HRS cells in classical Hodgkin's lymphoma (cHL) have a pronounced lineage infidelity concerning the expression of antigen markers and frequently express myeloid (CD15), B-cell (PAX5), plasma cell (MUM1 and syndecan) and activation markers (CD30). The analysis of IgV_H genes, however, demonstrated that the vast majority of HRS cells harbor clonal Ig rearrangements that represent a molecular marker of B-cell derivation. Interestingly, a proportion of these cases (25%) harbors destructive Ig rearrangements with crippling mutations. Since such crippling mutations would result in apoptotic cell death in reactive germinal-center (GC) B cells, it has been postulated that HRS cells might be derived from pre-apoptotic GC B cells. Additional evidence came from the analysis of composite lymphomas consisting of simultaneous HL and non-HL tumors, which demonstrated a clonal relationship between the two lymphomas and a mutational pattern characteristic of GC B cells. Expression of T-cell markers also occurs in a subset of cHL, and a proportion of these cases harbor clonal T-cell receptor rearrangements and germline Ig configuration, pointing to the existence of rare T-cell-derived HL. In contrast to cHL, in nodular lymphocyte-predominant HL (NLPHL), L&H cells show an immunophenotype consistent with B-cell derivation and harbor clonal and somatically mutated IgV_H genes with ongoing mutations. Although derived from B cells, HRS cells usually lack B-cell lineage marker expression. This fact was confirmed in gene expression profiling studies that revealed global downregulation of the B-cell lineage gene repertoire including surface molecules, kinase signaling and B-cell-specific transcription factors (Oct-2, Bob-1 and

Pu.1). Recently, it was demonstrated that the loss of B-cell identity in cHL results from the aberrant expression of the transcription factors ABF-1 and Id2, leading to downregulation of B-cell genes, but also to expression of genes not usually associated with B-cell lineage. A characteristic feature of HRS cells is constitutive NF-κB activity, which is mediated by inactivating mutations of the NF-κB inhibitor IκBα in 30% of the cases, or, to a lesser extent, of IκBε. Additionally, genomic amplification of a component of NF-κB (*c-Rel*) is frequently demonstrated in cHL.

HL cases have been demonstrated to harbor complex clonal chromosomal abnormalities with frequently hyperdiploid karyotypes. Some recurrent chromosomal gains in cHL involve *jak-2* (9p23–24), *REL/BCL-11a* (2p13–16) and *mdm2* (12q14), providing possible explanations for the constitutive NF-κB and STAT member family expression in HL. In a thorough investigation of NLPHL involving microdissection, DOP-PCR and CGH analysis showed that chromosomal regions with a gain included 1p, 1q, 2q, 3p, 3q, 4q, 5q, 6p, 6q, 8, 11q, 12q and X, and losses were demonstrated at 17/17p. Chromosomal translocations occur in a fraction of HL: in NLPHL, *BCL6* rearrangements were identified in up to 48% of cases.

To identify potential transforming events able to rescue HRS cell precursors from apoptosis, candidate genes like *TP53*, *CD95* (*FAS*) and *N-RAS* were investigated, but no mutations were found. HRS cells, nevertheless, are resistant to FAS-mediated apoptosis, but no alterations of downstream effectors of the FAS cascade were found.

Approximately 40% of cHL cases in the Western world are associated with infection by the Epstein–Barr virus (EBV), whereas in some geographic regions, such as Latin America, such involvement can reach up to 90% of cases, depending on age and histological subtype. The transforming capabilities of the viral latent membrane protein 1 (LMP-1) activating NF-κB can be considered a potential transforming event after infection of HRS cell precursors, by rescuing them from apoptosis. It is noteworthy that the viral latent membrane protein 2 (LMP-2) is also expressed in infected HRS cells and is able to mimic B-cell receptor signaling, which is normally defective in HRS cells.

HRS cells in cHL commonly express caspase-3, a component of the extrinsic and intrinsic apoptosis pathways. Functional studies, however, demonstrated that caspase-3 is non-functional in cultured HRS cells.

c-FLIP and X-linked inhibitors of apoptosis molecules, both of which represent NF-κB target genes, inhibit caspase-3 activation, thereby hampering effective apoptosis. In line with these findings, small interfering RNAs directed to c-FLIP were able to reconstitute the apoptosis pathway.

The microenvironment of cHL sets the stage for a cross-talk between clonal and non-clonal elements. A micromilieu is built up in which cytokine and chemokine production promotes survival and escape from immune surveillance. For example, HRS cells produce Th2-related cytokines (IL-4 and IL-13) and Th1 and CD8 inhibitory cytokines (IL-10 and TGFβ), and thus create a favorable milieu for HRS to resist cell-mediated apoptosis. Adding to this scenario, the production of several chemokines including TARC, MDC, IP-10 and eotaxin by infiltrating cells supports the favorable microenvironment for the tumor clone. It is of note that there is an overall higher expression of chemokines in EBV-related cHL cases, possibly reflecting additional mechanisms of hampered immunosurveillance in this cHL subgroup.

STAGING AND RISK STRATIFICATION

Hodgkin's lymphoma patients are usually treated according to stage and risk factors. The histological subtype – except NLPHL – does not influence the treatment decision. The stage of disease is assessed with the Cotswolds classification, a modified version of the Ann Arbor classification that incorporates additional prognostic factors including the number and location of anatomical sites involved, bulky nodal disease, extranodal extension of disease and extent of subdiaphragmatic involvement (Table 7.2).

The clinical staging usually includes chest X-ray, abdominal sonography, CT scans of the neck, thorax, abdomen and pelvis, bone-marrow biopsy and bone-marrow or skeletal radionuclide imaging. In some cases, additional tests such as MRI, PET or a liver biopsy might be indicated. Recently metabolic imaging with PET has attracted increasing attention in the management of lymphoma patients. Based on a higher uptake of the glucose analogue FDG in malignant cells as compared with non-malignant cells, PET imaging might complement CT-scan results at initial diagnosis and at restaging after treatment. PET imaging might also be used to discriminate

Table 7.2. The Cotswolds staging classification for Hodgkin's lymphoma.

Stage I   Involvement of a single lymph-node region or lymphoid structure (e.g. spleen, thymus, Waldeyer's ring) (I); or involvement of a single extralymphatic site (I_E)

Stage II   Involvement of two or more lymph-node regions on the same side of the diaphragm (II); localized contiguous involvement of only one extranodal organ or site and lymph-node region(s) on the same side of the diaphragm (II_E).

The number of anatomic regions involved should be indicated by a subscript (e.g. II_3)

Stage III   Involvement of lymph-node regions on both sides of the diaphragm (III), which may also be accompanied by involvement of the spleen (III_S) or by localized contiguous involvement of only one extranodal organ site (III_E) or both (III_{SE}).

III_1 With or without involvement of splenic, hilar, celiac or portal nodes

III_2 With involvement of para-aortic iliac and mesenteric nodes

Stage IV   Diffuse or disseminated involvement of one or more extranodal organs or tissues, with or without associated lymph-node involvement

Designations applicable to any disease stage

A   No symptoms

B   Fever (temperature $> 38\,°C$), drenching night sweats, unexplained loss of 10% of body weight within the preceding 6 months

X   Bulky disease (a widening of the mediastinum by more than one-third or the presence of a nodal mass with a maximal dimension greater than 10 cm)

E   Involvement of a single extranodal site that is contiguous or proximal to the known nodal site

CS   Clinical stage

PS   Pathological stage (as determined by laparotomy)

---

between active lymphoma and fibronecrotic tissue in those patients with residual tumor masses after treatment. A high negative predictive value of FDG-PET (81–100%) has been reported for this application by some smaller studies, suggesting that patients with a negative PET result after or during treatment might have a better chance for cure. The positive predictive value of PET is more variable (25–100%). However, the exact role of PET imaging for patients with residual masses after therapy has to be determined in prospective randomized trials such as the current HD15 trial of the German Hodgkin Study Group (GHSG). In addition, larger studies are required to confirm the role of PET as a reliable diagnostic tool and prognostic marker in this disease.

Risk stratification

The major prognostic factors used for risk stratification of HL patients are stage, B symptoms and bulky disease (maximum diameter of the largest single tumor mass $> 5–10$ cm). In North America, most centers treat patients according to the traditional classifications of early (CS I–IIA or B) and advanced stages (CS III–IVA or B, CS I–II A or B with bulky disease). European study groups such as EORTC (European Organisation for Research and Treatment of Cancer), GELA (Groupe d'Etudes des Lymphomes de l'Adulte), and GHSG (German Hodgkin Lymphoma Study Group) classify patients into early favorable stages (CS I–II without risk factors) or early unfavorable (intermediate) stages (CS I–II with risk factors) depending on the clinical factors listed in Table 7.3.

In order more precisely to define the risk of patients with advanced disease, the International Prognostic Score (IPS) was developed. The IPS consists of seven factors that are significantly related to an unfavorable prognosis when present at initial diagnosis of HL: serum albumin <40 g/L, hemoglobin <105 g/L, male sex, age >45 years, stage IV disease, leukocytosis $>15 \times 10^9$/L, lymphocytopenia $< 0.6 \times 10^9$/L and/or $<8\%$ of white cells.

Table 7.3. Definition of treatment groups according to EORTC/GELA and GHSG.

Treatment groups	EORTC/GELA	GHSG
Early-stage favorable	CS I–II without risk factors (supradiaphragmatic)	CS I–II without risk factors
Early-stage unfavorable (intermediate)	CS I–II with ≥ 1 risk factors (supradiaphragmatic)	CS I, CSIIA with ≥ 1 risk factors; CS IIB with C/D but without A/B
Advanced stage	CS III–IV	CS IIB with A/B; CS III–IV
Risk factors (RF)	(A) large mediastinal mass	(A) large mediastinal mass
	(B) age ≥ 50 years	(B) extranodal disease
	(C) elevated ESR[a]	(C) elevated ESR[a]
	(D) ≥4 involved regions	(D) ≥3 involved areas

GHSG, German Hodgkin Study Group; EORTC, European Organisation for Research and Treatment of Cancer; GELA, Groupe d'Etude des Lymphomes de l'Adulte

[a] Erythrocyte sedimentation rate (≥ 50 mm/h without or ≥ 30 mm/h with B symptoms)

FIRST-LINE TREATMENT

Early-stage favorable Hodgkin's lymphoma

Until recently, early-stage favorable Hodgkin's lymphoma was treated with extended-field radiation (EF-RT). Due to the high incidence of relapse (25–30%) after EF-RT alone, and fatal long-term effects such as secondary malignancies, cardiac toxicity and pulmonary dysfunction, new treatment strategies have been developed combining involved-field radiotherapy (IF-RT) with short-duration chemotherapy.

The most prominent recently finished or ongoing international studies for early-stage favorable HL are summarized in Table 7.4. The Southwest Oncology Group (SWOG) demonstrated that patients treated with combined modality treatment, consisting of three cycles of doxorubicin and vinblastine followed by subtotal lymphoid irradiation, had a significantly better outcome in terms of freedom from treatment failure (FFTF) than those patients receiving subtotal lymphoid irradiation alone. Studies from Milan and Stanford revealed that subtotal lymphoid irradiation can be effectively replaced by IF-RT after short-duration chemotherapy, such as ABVD (doxorubicin, bleomycin, vinblastine, dacarbazine) or Stanford V (mechlorethamine, doxorubicin, vinblastine, vincristine, bleomycin, etoposide, prednisone), without any change in progression-free and overall survival. The EORTC and GELA trials also demonstrated that combined modality treatment, consisting of either six courses of EBVP (H7F trial) or three cycles of MOPP (mechlorethamine, vincristine, procarbacine, prednisone)/AVB (H8F trial), followed by IF-RT yields a significantly better event-free survival than subtotal nodal radiotherapy alone. A combined modality approach was established in the HD7 trial by the GHSG. In this trial two cycles of ABVD plus EF-RT were shown to be superior to EF-RT alone in terms of FFTF.

Further improvement of treatment, with respect to the excellent long-term survival rates, seems difficult. Thus, strategies to reduce dose and toxicity of treatment while maintaining efficacy are being pursued. In the HD10 trial of the GHSG, a possible reduction of chemotherapy from four to two cycles of ABVD and/or of IF-RT from 30 Gy to 20 Gy was evaluated. After a median observation time of two years, FFTF and overall survival rates were 96.6% and 98.5%, without any significant differences between treatment arms. A longer follow-up is needed to finally answer the question of the best radiation dose, i.e. 20 or 30 Gy. The aim of the ongoing GHSG HD13 study for early stages is to omit the presumably less effective drugs, bleomycin and dacarbazine, from the ABVD regimen. Whether chemotherapy alone is sufficient to control disease has yet to be determined, and is the subject of ongoing trials.

Summary

A combined modality approach consisting of two courses of ABVD followed by 30 Gy IF-RT can be regarded as standard of care for patients with

Table 7.4. Selected trials for early-stage favorable Hodgkin's lymphoma.

Trial	Therapy regimen	Patients (*n*)	Outcome
SWOG #9133	(A) 3 (dox. + vinbl.) + STNI (36–40 Gy)	165	94% FFTF; 98% OS
	(B) STNI (36–40 Gy)	161	81% FFTF; 96% OS (3 years)
Milan 1990–97	(A) 4 ABVD + STNI	65	97% FFP; 93% OS
	(B) 4 ABVD + IF-RT	68	97% FFP; 93% OS (5 years)
Stanford V (C SI–IIA)	8 weeks of Stanford V + modified IF-RT (30 Gy)	65	94.6% FFP; 96.6% OS (16 months; estimated for 3 years)
EORTC/GELA H7F	(A) 6 EBVP + IF-RT (36 Gy)	168	90% RFS; 98% OS
	(B) STNI	165	81% RFS; 95% OS (5 years)
EORTC/GELA H8F	(A) 3 MOPP/ABV + IF-RT (36 Gy)	271	99% RFS; 99% OS
	(B) STNI	272	80% RFS; 95% OS (4 years)
EORTC/GELA H9F	(A) 6 EBVP + IF-RT (36 Gy)	783	87% EFS; 98% OS
	(B) 6 EBVP + IF-RT (20 Gy)		84% EFS; 98% OS (4 years)
	(C) 6 EBVP		C closed because of high relapse rate
GHSG HD7	(A) EF-RT 30 Gy (40 Gy IF)	305	75% FFTF; 94% OS
	(B) 2 ABVD + EF-RT 30 Gy (40 Gy IF)	312	91% FFTF; 94% OS (5 years)
GHSG HD10	(A) 4 ABVD + IF-RT (30 Gy)	847	Interim analysis (2 years) all pts: 96.6% FFTF; 98.5% OS
	(B) 4 ABVD + IF-RT (20 Gy)		
	(C) 2 ABVD + IF-RT (30 Gy)		
	(D) 2 ABVD + IF-RT (20 Gy)		
GHSG HD13	(A) 2 ABVD + IF-RT (30 Gy)		Ongoing trial
	(B) 2 ABV + IF-RT (30 Gy)		
	(C) 2 AVD + IF-RT (30 Gy)		
	(D) 2 AV + IF-RT (30 Gy)		

SWOG, Southwest Oncology Group; EORTC, European Organisation for Research and Treatment of Cancer; GELA, Groupe d'Etude des Lymphomes de l'Adulte; GHSG, German Hodgkin Study Group

EF/IF-RT, extended/involved-field radiotherapy; STNI, subtotal nodal irradiation; FFTF, freedom from treatment failure; RFS, relapse-free survival; FFP, freedom from progression; EFS, event-free suvival; OS, overall survival.

early-stage favorable Hodgkin's lymphoma until a less toxic treatment approach is proven to be equally effective.

Early-stage unfavorable disease

As with early-stage favorable HL, those patients with early-stage unfavorable disease generally receive combined modality treatment. However, the best chemotherapy, the optimal number of cycles and the radiotherapy regimen are not yet clearly defined, and there is an ongoing desire to optimize therapy in this risk group.

Several trials have shown that the reduction of field size to IF radiotherapy does not compromise the efficacy of treatment. A cooperative study comparing

six cycles of MOPP sandwiched around 40 Gy of radiotherapy, applied either in IF or EF, showed no difference in terms of disease-free survival or overall survival (OS). The Milan trial, which compared STNI with IF-RT after four courses of ABVD in patients with early-stage favorable and unfavorable disease (see Table 7.4), also reported a similar treatment outcome in both arms. Other key trials are summarized in Table 7.5. The EORTC randomized patients to six cycles of MOPP/ABV + 36 Gy IF-RT, four cycles of MOPP/ABV + 36 Gy IF-RT and four cycles of MOPP/ABV + STNI. There was no difference between the arms in terms of response rates, failure-free survival or overall survival. The HD8 trial, the largest trial investigating radiotherapy reduction, confirmed these results: patients with early-stage unfavorable disease

Table 7.5. Selected trials for early-stage unfavorable Hodgkin's lymphoma.

Trial	Therapy regimen	Patients (n)	Outcome
EORTC/GELA H8U	(A) 6 MOPP/ABV + IF-RT (36 Gy)	335	94% RFS; 90% OS
	(B) 4 MOPP/ABV + IF-RT (36 Gy)	333	95% RFS; 95% OS
	(C) 4 MOPP/ABV + STNI	327	96% RFS; 93% OS (4 years)
GHSG HD8	(A) 2 COPP + ABVD + EF-RT	532	86% FFTF; 91% OS
	(30 Gy) + bulk (10 Gy)		
	(B) 2 COPP + ABVD + IF-RT (30 Gy) + bulk (10 Gy)	532	84% FFTF; 92% OS (5 years)
SWOG/ECOG #2496	(A) 6 ABVD + IF-RT (36 Gy) to bulk (> 5 cm)		Ongoing trial
	(B) 12 weeks Stanford V + IF-RT (36 Gy) to		
	bulk (>5 cm)		
EORTC/GELA H9U	(A) 6 ABVD + IF-RT	808	94% EFS; 96% OS
	(B) 4 ABVD + IF-RT		89% EFS; 95% OS
	(C) 4 BEACOPP-bas. + IF-RT		91% EFS; 93% OS (4 years)
GHSG HD11	(A) 4 ABVD + IF-RT (30 Gy)	1047	Interim analysis (2 years)
	(B) 4 ABVD + IF-RT (20 Gy)		All pts: 97.4% FFTF; 89.9% OS
	(C) 4 BEACOPP-bas. + IF-RT (30 Gy)		
	(D) 4 BEACOPP-bas. + IF-RT (20 Gy)		
GHSG HD14	(A) 4 ABVD + IF-RT (30 Gy)		Ongoing trial
	(B) 2 BEACOPP-esc. + 2 ABVD + IF-RT (30 Gy)		

ECOG, Eastern Cooperative Oncology Group; Other abbreviations as in Table 7.4.

were randomized to two alternating cycles of COPP (cyclophosphamide, vincristine, procarbacine, prednisone)/ABVD followed by 30 Gy radiotherapy in either EF or IF. Final results at five years showed no significant differences between the two arms in terms of FFTF and overall survival, although more toxicity was reported in the patients who were treated with EF-RT.

Efforts have also been made to improve the efficacy of chemotherapy by altering drugs and schedules as well as the number of cycles. Alternation or hybridization of a MOPP-like regimen with ABVD did not produce better outcomes when compared with ABVD alone.

Despite the excellent initial remission rates obtained with ABVD and radiotherapy, approximately 15% of patients in the early unfavorable stage relapse within five years and about another 5% have primary progressive disease. Because of these disappointing outcome rates, more intensive chemotherapy regimens, originally developed for the treatment of advanced stages, have been evaluated for the treatment of early unfavourable stage (Table 7.5). In their ongoing intergroup trial #2496, the ECOG and SWOG assess whether the

Stanford V regimen (12 weeks) is superior to six cycles of ABVD. In another approach, the HD11 trial (GHSG) and the H9U trial (EORTC-GELA) compared four cycles of ABVD and four cycles of BEACOPP-baseline (bleomycin, etoposide, doxorubicin, cyclophosphamide, vincristine, procarbazine, prednisone). The recently presented H9U trial additionally analyzed whether six cycles of ABVD are more effective than four. After a median follow-up of four years no significant difference was observed between treatment arms in the H9U trial. Interim analysis of the GHSG HD11 trial at two years did not show any significant difference between ABVD and BEACOPP-baseline. The GHSG is evaluating further treatment intensification in the ongoing HD14 trial. Patients are currently being randomized to two cycles of BEACOPP-escalated plus two cycles of ABVD or four cycles of ABVD followed by 30 Gy IF-RT.

Summary

A combined modality treatment consisting of four courses of ABVD followed by 30 Gy IF-RT remains standard treatment for patients with early-stage unfavorable HL until a more efficient chemotherapy regimen is established.

Advanced Hodgkin's lymphoma

Before the introduction of polychemotherapy, only very few patients with advanced HL could be cured. The use of combinations such as MOPP or similar regimens led to long-term remission of approximately 50%. The introduction of ABVD by Bonadonna and colleagues in 1975 resulted in a significant increase of FFTF and OS to 63% and 82% after five years. The hybrid regimen MOPP/ABV and the alternating MOPP/ABVD regimen were demonstrated to be as effective as ABVD but more effective than sequential application of MOPP and ABVD. The application of ABVD alone has been reported to be less toxic than MOPP/ABV in terms of acute toxicity and the incidence of secondary acute leukemia or MDS. Therefore ABVD was accepted as standard chemotherapy in a combined modality strategy. Overall, the prognosis for patients with advanced HL has substantially improved over the last decades (Fig. 7.13).

In order to further improve the results in this group of patients, new regimens have been developed by integrating additional drugs such as etoposide and by increasing dose intensity with the support of colony-stimulating factors and with modern antibiotics. These new approaches include regimens such as Stanford V, BEACOPP-baseline and BEACOPP-escalated (Table 7.6).

Stanford V seemed a promising strategy in a phase II single-center trial, but a randomized comparison of Stanford V with MEC and ABVD showed a clear inferiority of the Stanford V protocol. The FFTF obtained with the MEC protocol was slightly better than the FFTF achieved with ABVD; nevertheless, after a median observation time of three years no significant differences between ABVD and MEC could be detected. To obtain an additional set of data another phase III trial comparing Stanford V with ABVD is being carried out by the BNLI.

In 1992 the GHSG designed the BEACOPP regimen in a baseline and an escalated version, and compared these variants with COPP/ABVD in patients with advanced HL. Radiotherapy was used for bulky disease at diagnosis and for residual disease after eight cycles of chemotherapy. The analysis of this trial, HD9, indicated a significant superiority of BEACOPP-escalated

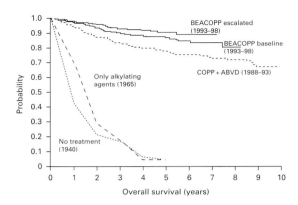

Figure 7.13. Progress made in the treatment of advanced-stage Hodgkin's lymphoma during the past 40 years. (From Diehl and Behringer 2006; data modified from de Vita including data from GHSG trials).

over BEACOPP-baseline and COPP/ABVD: after a median follow-up of seven years FFTF and overall survival rates were 85% and 90% in the BEACOPP-escalated group, 75% and 84% in the BEACOPP-baseline group and 67% and 79% in the COPP/ABVD group. However, the BEACOPP-escalated regimen is associated with more acute and long-term toxicity, and with problems such as secondary leukemias and infertility.

The subsequent GHSG trials, HD12 and HD15, aim to reduce therapy-associated toxicity while maintaining the good results achieved in HD9. This strategy includes modifications of the eight-course BEACOPP-escalated regimen and an attempt to delete consolidative radiotherapy after BEACOPP. Since substantial treatment-associated long-term toxicity can be attributed to radiotherapy, the omission should reduce long-term toxicity. A study conducted by the EORTC and reported by Aleman and colleagues has suggested that only patients with partial remission may benefit from involved-field radiotherapy.

The HD12 trial of the GHSG compares eight courses of BEACOPP-escalated with four courses of BEACOPP-escalated followed by four of BEACOPP-baseline, with or without consolidative radiation to initial bulky and residual disease. In the latest interim analysis, at a median follow-up of 30 months, there has been no significant difference between treatment arms. In the ongoing HD15 trial for advanced stages, patients are randomized between eight courses of BEACOPP-escalated, six courses of BEACOPP-escalated and eight

Table 7.6. Polychemotherapy regimens for Hodgkin's lymphoma.

Regimens of historical interest	Drug combination
MOPP	Mechlorethamine, Oncovin (vincristine), Procarbazine, Prednisone
COPP	Cyclophosphamide, Oncovin (vincristine), Procarbazine, Prednisone
EBVP	Epirubicin, Bleomycin, Vinblastine, Prednisone
MEC	Mechlorethamine, CCNU (Lomustine), Vindesine, Alkeran, Prednisone, Epidoxorubicin, Vincristine, Procarbazine, Vinblastine, Bleomycin

Commonly used regimens	Drug combinations	Dose (mg/m^2)	Route	Schedule (days)
ABVD	Adriamycin (doxorubicin)	25	i.v	1 + 15
(cycle length 28 days)	Bleomycin	10	i.v.	1 + 15
	Vinblastine	6	i.v.	1 + 15
	Dacarbazine	375	i.v.	1 + 15
BEACOPP	Bleomycin	10	i.v.	8
baseline/escalated	Etoposide	100/200	i.v.	1–3
(cycle length 21 days)	Adriamycin	25/35	i.v.	1
	Cyclophosphamide	650/1250	i.v.	1
	Oncovin (vincristine)	1.4 (max. 2 mg)	i.v.	8
	Procarbazine	100	p.o.	1–7
	Prednisone	40	p.o.	1–14
	G-CSF (for escalated regimen)			From day 8
BEACOPP-14	As BEACOPP baseline with a cycle length of only 14 days (prednisone 80 mg/m^2 day 1–7, G-CSF from day 8)			
Stanford	Mechlorethamine	6	i.v.	Wk 1, 5, 9
(12 weeks)	Adriamycin	25	i.v.	Wk 1, 3, 5, 7, 9, 11
	Vinblastine	6	i.v.	Wk 1, 3, 5, 7, 9, 11
	Vincristine	1.4 (max. 2 mg)	i.v.	Wk 2, 4, 6, 8, 10, 12
	Bleomycin	5	i.v.	Wk 2, 4, 6, 8, 10, 12
	Etoposide	60 × 2	i.v.	Wk 3, 7, 11
	Prednisone	40	p.o.	Wk 1–10, every 2d
	G-CSF			After dose reduction or delay

courses of BEACOPP-14. Only those patients with PET-positive residual tumors receive 30 Gy radiotherapy. The BEACOPP-14 regimen is a time-intensified BEACOPP-baseline regimen given in 14-day intervals with the support of G-CSF.

Before worldwide acceptance of BEACOPP-escalated, more data might be needed confirming HD9. The EORTC recently initiated an international trial which directly compares eight courses of ABVD with four courses of BEACOPP-escalated followed by four courses of BEACOPP-baseline with respect to feasibility, toxicity and efficacy.

Summary

Despite the excellent outcome rates achieved with BEACOPP-escalated in the HD9 trial, ABVD is still widely considered the gold standard for the treatment of advanced HL. Because BEACOPP-escalated has been shown to be significantly better than COPP/ABVD in terms of overall survival and freedom from treatment failure in the HD9 trial, the GHSG regards BEACOPP-escalated as standard for patients with advanced HL. Based on the results of the EORTC trial, published in 2003, and on the latest interim analysis of the HD12 trial, only those patients with partial remission after 6–8 cycles of anthracyclin-containing chemotherapy should receive consolidative radiotherapy.

TREATMENT OF PRIMARY PROGRESSIVE AND RELAPSED HODGKIN'S LYMPHOMA

Patients with refractory or relapsed disease after first-line treatment still have the chance of being cured with an adequate salvage therapy. The choice of salvage treatment particularly depends on the first-line treatment.

Relapse after initial radiotherapy

Conventional anthracyclin-containing chemotherapy is the treatment of choice for patients who relapse after initial radiotherapy for early-stage disease. The survival of these patients is comparable to that of patients with advanced-stage disease initially treated with chemotherapy. Age, advanced-stage disease, extranodal involvement and B symptoms at relapse have been described as important prognostic factors for OS and for second relapse (FF2F).

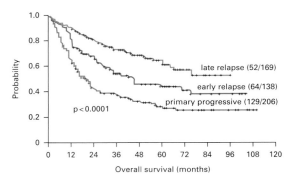

Figure 7.14. Kaplan–Meier analysis showing overall survival in patients with primary progressive, early and late relapsed Hodgkin's lymphoma after first-line polychemotherapy (German Hodgkin Study Group; $n = 513$, total $= 3809$).

Relapse after initial chemotherapy

The therapeutic options for patients with relapse after initial chemotherapy include salvage radiotherapy, conventional salvage chemotherapy, high-dose chemotherapy followed by autologous stem-cell transplantation, or allogeneic stem-cell transplantation in selected cases. As shown in Fig. 7.14, the success of salvage treatment is substantially influenced by the duration of remission after first-line treatment. A relapse within 12 months after initial therapy, stage III or IV disease and a low hemoglobin level (less than 120 g/L for men or less than 105 g/L for women) at relapse are unfavorable prognostic factors according to a risk score developed by the GHSG and published by Josting and colleagues.

Salvage radiotherapy

Salvage radiotherapy alone offers a treatment option for a selected subset of patients with localized relapse in previously non-irradiated areas. In a retrospective analysis of the GHSG the five-year freedom from second failure (FF2F) and overall survival rates were 28% and 51% after salvage radiotherapy alone. Prognostic factors for overall survival were B symptoms and stage at relapse. A retrospective analysis by Campbell and colleagues reported 10-year FF2F and overall survival rates of 33% and 46% for patients with limited-stage recurrent Hodgkin's lymphoma treated with salvage radiotherapy. Adverse prognostic factors for FF2F and overall survival were age over 50 years,

B symptoms and less than complete response to the last chemotherapy regimen. So far, there are no data from controlled trials analyzing the role of salvage radiotherapy in a selected group of patients with relapsed Hodgkin's lymphoma.

High-dose chemotherapy followed by autologous stem-cell transplantation

High-dose chemotherapy (HDCT) followed by autologous stem-cell transplantation (ASCT) has been shown to be superior to conventional chemotherapy in relapsed Hodgkin's lymphoma in two prospective randomized trials. In the BNLI trial, patients with relapsed or refractory HL were treated with conventional-dose mini-BEAM (carmustine, etoposide, cytosine arabinoside, melphalan) or high-dose BEAM and autologous stem-cell transplantation. The three-year event-free survival was significantly better after high-dose chemotherapy (53% vs. 10%). The HDR1 multicenter trial conducted by the GHSG and the EBMT (European Group for Blood and Marrow Transplantation) compared four cycles of Dexa-BEAM with two cycles of Dexa-BEAM followed by BEAM and autologous stem-cell transplantation. The FF2F at three years was significantly better in the transplanted group than in the group receiving conventional salvage chemotherapy (55% vs. 34%). In the subgroup analysis this was true for patients both in early and in late relapse. The overall survival did not differ significantly between the two treatment arms in both trials.

It is not only patients with relapsed Hodgkin's lymphoma, but also those with primary progressive disease, who benefit from HDCT and ASCT. Whereas the results of conventional salvage chemotherapies in primary refractory HL were disappointing (4-year FF2F 0%, 4-year OS 0–8%), a significantly better FF2F and OS (5-year FF2F 32–42%, 5-year OS 36–48%) could be detected in several retrospective analyses for those patients who were treated with HDCT and ASCT. The efficacy of HDCT and ASCT in primary progressive HL was confirmed by a prospective trial run by the Sloan-Kettering Cancer Center. However, a multivariate analysis of this trial showed that chemosensitivity to standard-dose second-line chemotherapy was predictive of a better survival. Moreover, it should be noted that a significant proportion of patients cannot receive HDCT and ASCT because of rapid disease progression, older age, poor performance status or insufficient stem-cell harvest.

Since reduction of tumor volume prior to HDCT and ASCT has been described as an important variable affecting the outcome in relapsed and refractory HL, a cytoreductive chemotherapy seems to be indispensable prior to myeloablative HDCT and ASCT. So far, there is no consensus concerning the strategy of cytoreduction, stem-cell mobilization and transplant conditioning for patients with relapsed or refractory Hodgkin's lymphoma. Some groups employ at least one course of standard-dose second-line chemotherapy, such as ASHAP (doxorubicin, methylprednisolone, cytarabine, cisplatin), ESHAP (etoposide, methylprednisolone, cytarabine, cisplatin) or ICE (ifosphamide, carboplatine, etoposide), prior to HDCT. A more effective cytoreduction might be attained by intensifying salvage induction therapy. One promising approach is the strategy of sequential HDCT prior to autologous stem-cell transplantation. The feasibility and efficacy of sequential high-dose chemotherapy (cyclophosphamide, methotrexate plus vincristine, etoposide) after two cycles of DHAP (dexamethasone, cytosine arabinoside, cisplatin) were demonstrated in a phase II trial conducted by the GHSG. Based on these results, the GHSG initiated a prospective randomized European intergroup trial together with the EORTC and other European groups (HDR2), which compares the efficacy of two courses of DHAP followed by BEAM with the additional sequential strategy in patients with early or late relapse. This approach does not take into account that a considerable number of patients might be over-treated with sequential HDCT and ASCT. Other groups are therefore attempting to develop a risk-adapted therapy for relapsed and refractory Hodgkin's lymphoma.

Allogeneic stem-cell transplantation

Allogeneic stem-cell transplantation following reduced-intensity conditioning might become an appropiate strategy in selected subgroups of young poor-risk patients, such as those in whom autologous transplantation has failed, or for patients with early relapse and additional risk factors. However, to date, the number of patients treated is small, and further clinical studies are required in order to define clear indications for this treatment option.

Summary: primary progressive and relapsed HL

HDCT followed by autologous SCT is the treatment of choice for patients with primary progressive and relapsed Hodgkin's lymphoma after first-line chemotherapy. Alternative treatment approaches have to be developed for those patients with chemotherapy-resistant disease. A selected group of patients with localized relapse in previously non-irradiated areas can be effectively treated with salvage radiotherapy alone. Those patients with relapsed disease after initial radiotherapy should receive an anthracyclin-containing chemotherapy regimen.

TARGETED THERAPY OF HODGKIN'S LYMPHOMA

Based on increasing knowledge of the pathogenesis of HL, new treatment approaches are currently being developed which target cell-surface molecules, modulate the function of certain intracellular proteins via direct interaction ("small molecules") or prevent the expression of the respective protein. An effective targeted therapy, given alone or in combination with chemotherapy, might improve the long-term outcome of relapsed and primary refractory patients. In particular, those patients with chemotherapy-resistant disease might benefit from a targeted therapy. As a component of first-line treatment a biologically based drug might eliminate residual lymphoma cells after chemotherapy. Additionally, combination of chemotherapy with a targeted therapy might help to reduce the amount of cytotoxic drugs needed, resulting in less toxicity than the current regimens.

Monoclonal antibodies

Hodgkin's lymphoma seems an ideal target for antibody-based therapeutic approaches, since HRS cells express the specific surface antigen CD30 and L & H cells strongly express CD20.

Currently, there are two anti-CD30 monoclonal antibodies being developed, the humanized chimeric SGN-30 monoclonal antibody and the fully human 5F11. The efficacy and toxicity of SGN-30 were analyzed in a phase I single-dose trial and in a subsequent phase I/II dose-escalation trial. In the phase II trial, maximal response to SGN-30 was disease stabilization,

reported in 6 of 12 evaluable patients. The fully human IgG1κ monoclonal antibody 5F11 (MDX-60) has been evaluated in a phase I/II dose-escalation study. In the recently finished phase II study, 40 patients with relapsed or refractory HL were treated with 5F11 at 10 or 15 mg/kg without any significant infusion-related reactions; objective responses have been observed in three patients (1 CR, 2 PR). In addition, about one-third of the patients who achieved a stable disease state have survived for two years or more. This preliminary result indicates that 5F11 is clinically active in some patients with relapsed or refractory HL. It remains to be clarified, in the ongoing additional studies, which patients are the best candidates for treatment with this construct.

The efficacy of the anti-CD20 antibody rituximab for patients with NLPHL has been demonstrated in two phase II trials. The multicenter phase II trial performed by the GHSG showed an overall response of 86% (8 CR, 4 PR) in patients with refractory NLPHL after treatment with rituximab at standard dose. With a median follow-up of 12 months, nine patients were still in remission. An overall response rate of 100% was reported in a phase II trial performed at Stanford that included 12 untreated patients and 10 previously treated patients with NLPHL. In contrast to the GHSG trial, nine patients had relapsed at a median follow-up of 13 months.

Radioimmunotherapy

Radiolabeled antibodies for therapeutic use consist of a specific antibody labeled with an α- or β-emitter, such as iodine-131 (^{131}I) or yttrium-90 (^{90}Y). A substantial advantage of radiolabeled antibodies is their ability to kill tumor cells adjacent to cells to which the radio-immunoconjugate is bound. Currently, both non-myeloablative and myeloablative strategies involving radiolabeled antibodies are being pursued. For the treatment of patients with HL, radioimmunotherapeutic approaches using polyclonal antiferritin antibodies labeled with ^{131}I or ^{90}Y and the monoclonal anti-CD30 antibody Ki-4 labeled with ^{131}I have been studied. Low-dose radioimmunotherapy with ^{131}I- or ^{90}Y-labeled polyclonal ferritin-directed antibodies has been evaluated in two trials: tumor response was dose-related and varied from 22% to 86%. After treatment of 90 patients with ^{90}Y-labeled polyclonal antiferritin antibodies, 15 CRs and 29 PRs with a median duration of six months were observed. Toxicity and efficacy of the ^{131}I-labeled

Ki-4 were analyzed in a clinical phase I trial: 22 patients were treated with individual doses of up to 0.35 Gy of ^{131}I-Ki-4, and responses included one CR, five PRs and three minor or mixed responses. The most significant toxicity observed in these studies was hematotoxicity, particularly thrombocytopenia. The support with autologous hematopoietic stem cells after radioimmunotherapy might accelerate hematopoietic recovery. This was shown in a phase I/II trial by the Johns Hopkins Oncology Center in which 29 refractory Hodgkin's patients were treated with different doses of ^{90}Y-labeled polyclonal antiferritin immunoglobulins followed by autologous bone-marrow transplantation. Responses included 9 CRs and 9 PRs; there was no significant difference between 20 mCi and 40 mCi ^{90}Y-labeled antiferritin with respect to overall response. The approach of combining radioimmunotherapy with high-dose chemotherapy followed by autologous bone-marrow transplant was examined in a trial published by Bierman *et al*. A treatment-related mortality of 30% (4/12 patients treated), however, made a revision of the treatment protocol indispensable.

Protein-specific "small molecules"

Several novel drugs have been designed which are supposed to inhibit the anti-apoptotic pathway of HRS cells at the intracellular level. Targets of these small molecules include the IKK-IκBα-NFκB cascade or the anti-apoptotic proteins c-FLIP, XIAP and Bcl-X_L.

One of these small molecules is bortezomib, a reversible inhibitor of the 26S proteasome interfering with degradation of a variety of proteins including IκBα. This drug was recently approved for the treatment of relapsed and refractory multiple myeloma. A phase I trial conducted by the M. D. Anderson Center evaluated the safety and efficacy of bortezomib in patients with relapsed Hodgkin's lymphoma: one of fourteen patients achieved a PR and two had a minor response after treatment with three to six courses of bortezomib.

Summary: targeted therapy

Targeted therapy approaches evaluated for the treatment of Hodgkin's lymphoma include CD30- and CD20-specific monoclonal antibodies, radioimmunoconjugates and so called "small molecules" which directly inhibit the anti-apoptotic pathway of HRS

cells. Preliminary data from a phase I/II trial indicated that the humanized anti-CD30 antibody 5F11 is effective in a small subgroup of patients with relapsed HL. A significantly higher response rate could be achieved in phase I/II trials with ^{90}Y-labeled radioimmunoconjugates such as ^{90}Y-ferritin-directed immunoglobulins; however, a significant hematotoxicity was documented after application of these radioimmunoconjugates. Promising results for the treatment of NLPHL could be obtained with the monoclonal anti-CD20 antibody rituximab. So far there are no clinical data showing the efficacy of "small molecules" in the treatment of Hodgkin's lymphoma.

TREATMENT OF LYMPHOCYTE-PREDOMINANT HODGKIN'S LYMPHOMA (NLPHL)

Most patients with NLPHL are initially diagnosed with limited-stage disease. Despite an excellent response to combined modality treatment, patients with NLPHL tend to relapse continuously over decades. Current treatment strategies should take into account the favorable prognosis of these patients and late toxicity effects after a combined modality treatment. The EORTC and the GHSG currently recommend involved-field radiotherapy (30 Gy) in stage IA/IIA NLPHL. Patients with advanced-stage NLPHL (20–25% of all patients with NLPHL) show a substantially worse overall and tumor-free survival than patients with early-stage NLPHL and are thus treated according to protocols used for cHL.

Experimental approaches for patients with NLPHL focus on the anti-CD20 antibody rituximab, which has given impressive results in relapsed NLPHL. This chimeric antibody is currently being evaluated in a GHSG phase II trial in selected IA NLPHL patients.

TREATMENT OF HODGKIN'S LYMPHOMA IN CHILDREN AND ADOLESCENTS

Biologic features unique to childhood or adolescent HL have not been described; only the relative incidence of histological subtypes varies. Because of similar responsiveness of childhood HL to chemo- and radiotherapy, treatment approaches developed in adults, such as the chemotherapy regimens COPP,

MOPP or ABVD and a consolidative radiotherapy, were initially applied to children suffering from HL. Similarly to treatment of adult HL, children suffering from HL are allocated to three risk groups according to the stage of disease. With risk-adapted, combined modality treatment, an overall survival of 90% in children suffering from HL can be achieved. However, due to the high rate of treatment-induced developmental disturbances and the high risk of developing long-term complications, radiotherapy dose and field have been reduced and new chemotherapy regimens such as OEPA (vincristine, etoposide, prednisone, doxorubicin), COPDIC (cyclophosphamide, vincristine, prednisone, dacarbazine) or ABVE-PC (doxorubicin, bleomycin, vincristine, etoposide, prednisone, cyclophosphamide) have been designed. So far there is no international consensus concerning the optimal chemotherapy regimen and the number of chemotherapy courses required; furthermore, so far the role of consolidative radiotherapy has not been clearly defined.

One promising approach is to individualize therapy by a risk-adapted treatment, reducing treatment intensity in chemosensitive patients, which may maintain excellent results while reducing toxicity. Several trials of the British Paediatric Oncology Group (POG) and the American Children's Oncology Group (COG) have shown that early response to chemotherapy (after six weeks) is of more prognostic importance than end-of-chemotherapy response and is therefore a suitable parameter to determine treatment intensity. Early responders can be treated with fewer courses of chemotherapy than slow responders, and they might be treated without consolidative radiotherapy. Treatment outcome and toxicity of response-adapted therapy will be further evaluated in the EuroNet-PHL-C1 trial initiated by the European Network for Paediatric Hodgkin Lymphoma.

Published data focusing on the treatment of adolescent HL patients (15–19 years old) are scarce. Most of the adult and pediatric trials including adolescents have not performed age-specific survival analyses; those trials performing an age-specific survival analysis did not reveal a significant effect of age on CR or EFS. The DAL-HD-90 trial of the German Paediatric Hodgkin Study Group (GPOH-HD), for example, showed that treatment of adolescent HL patients with a risk-adapted combined modality approach including chemotherapy regimens such as OEPA or OPPA results in event-free survival rates similar to those achieved by protocols for adults. Longer follow-up is needed to confirm the lower long-term toxicity of the pediatric protocol, and a randomized trial is required to establish the optimal treatment regimen for adolescent HL patients.

Summary

Standard of care for childhood HL is chemotherapy combined with low-dose, limited-field radiation. Ongoing pediatric trials aim at further reduction of long-term toxicity and maintenance of high cure rates. A promising approach to the realization of individualized, risk-adapted treatment is early response-adapted therapy. Treatment strategies for adolescent HL patients may be adapted from pediatric protocols; the optimal treatment regimen for adolescents has to be found out in randomized trials.

THERAPY-ASSOCIATED TOXICITY

As a consequence of the impressive long-term remission rates in Hodgkin's lymphoma the reduction of treatment-related complications has become increasingly important.

Short-term toxicity

Acute treatment-associated adverse effects include nausea and vomiting, bone-marrow depression, infections, mucositis and neurological complications such as polyneuropathy. Less frequent acute complications are pulmonary dysfunction or acute cardiac failure. The severity of these therapy-associated complications depends on the chemotherapy regimen and the additional application of radiotherapy. Chemotherapy with BEACOPP-escalated results in a significantly higher incidence of grade 3 and 4 leukopenia, thrombocytopenia and anemia than treatment with BEACOPP-baseline, COPP-ABVD or ABVD alone. The pronounced myelosuppressive effect of BEACOPP-escalated translates into a significantly higher incidence of severe infections and severe mucositis.

Bleomycin-based chemotherapy regimens, such as ABVD or BEACOPP, as well as mediastinal irradiation, may induce acute pneumonitis followed by lung fibrosis. Clinical symptoms of therapy-associated pneumonitis such as dyspnea and cough usually appear 3–4 months after treatment; fatal courses of pulmonary toxicity typically occur in the peri-treatment period. Clinical symptoms of acute pneumonitis and progression resulting in lung fibrosis might be influenced by application of steroids.

Acute cardiac toxicity as a result of mediastinal radiotherapy or an anthracycline-containing chemotherapy regimen is rather rare. It most frequently presents with coronary heart disease or acute cardiac failure due to therapy-induced cardiomyopathy.

Long-term toxicity

As with short-term treatment-related toxicity, long-term complications vary in frequency and severity depending on the chemotherapy regimen and the additional application of radiotherapy. Chemotherapy-associated long-term toxicity is particularly dependent on the cumulative dose of certain chemotherapeutic agents.

The most serious long-term treatment-associated complications are secondary neoplasia and cardiovascular disease. Further late effects contributing to morbidity and/or mortality of long-term survivors of HL are pulmonary dysfunction, infectious complications, hypothyroidism, infertility and fatigue.

The most frequent subtypes of secondary malignancy are solid tumors, particularly breast cancer and lung cancer. Leukemia and non-Hodgkin's lymphoma account for only 20–25% of the observed secondary cancers. While the risk of developing secondary leukemia is predominantly confined to the first 10 years of follow-up, the incidence of secondary solid tumors continuously increases up to a cumulative risk of 23% at a follow-up of 25 years. Treatment with alkylating chemotherapy substances has been described as the most important risk factor for the development of secondary leukemia. Radiotherapy, chemotherapy with alkylating agents and smoking are the most relevant risk factors for the pathogenesis of secondary lung cancer. One important strategy to reduce the incidence of secondary malignancies is the reduction of treatment intensity, for example by abbreviation of chemotherapy regimens or by reduction of radiation field size and radiation dose. Further prevention strategies include smoking cessation programs and counseling on sun-safety practice. Since early detection through screening tests can reduce mortality in many cancer types,

several screening tests have been evaluated in patients surviving Hodgkin's lymphoma. As a result of one of these screening trials yearly screening mammography is recommended, beginning eight years after mediastinal radiotherapy or at the age of 40. Whether lung-cancer screening with annual chest CT scans is of benefit to survivors of HL is still a point of discussion.

Treatment-related long-term cardiac toxicity comprises a wide spectrum of cardiac disease such as coronary artery disease, cardiomyopathy, pericardial disease, valvular disease, arrhythmia and autonomic dysfunction. Among these cardiac abnormalities, coronary artery disease accounts for 66% of all cases of fatal cardiac events in HL survivors. Since mediastinal irradiation is the most important risk factor for developing cardiopulmonary complications, strategies to reduce treatment-associated cardiac disease focus on improvement of radiation therapy techniques and on further dose and field size reduction. In order to detect subclinical cardiac abnormalities non-invasive cardiac screening tests such as resting and stress echocardiogram should be performed; a standardized screening strategy is yet to be defined.

Sterility is a long-term treatment-related complication with serious impact on the quality of life of young HL patients. A high incidence of primary ovarian insufficiency or oligo/azoospermia has been documented after treatment with alkylating agents such as cyclophosphamide or procarbazine or after radiotherapy to the pelvis or the testes. Chemotherapy regimens such as BEACOPP and MOPP are therefore reported to be more gonadotoxic than ABVD. Advanced-stage HL and age over 30 are further risk factors for female infertility. A lower incidence of therapy-induced amenorrhea may be achieved by administration of oral contraceptives or gonadotropin-releasing hormone agonists. Cryopreservation prior to therapy is another approach to preserve fertility. While cryopreservation of semen is a standardized procedure, ovarian cryopreservation is still experimental.

Summary: therapy-associated toxicity

The most relevant acute treatment-related adverse effects are mucositis, bone-marrow suppression, infections, polyneuropathy and less frequently acute pneumonitis and acute cardiac toxicity. Delayed treatment-associated complications include the development of secondary malignancy, cardiac disease,

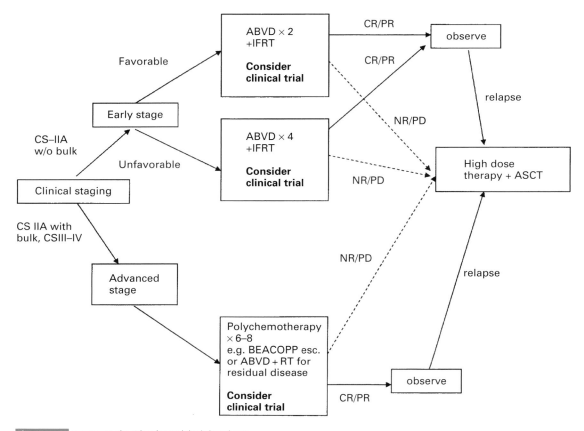

Figure 7.15. Treatment algorithm for Hodgkin's lymphoma.

pulmonary dysfunction, infections, infertility, hypothyroidism and fatigue. In particular, secondary malignancy and cardiovascular disease represent the leading causes of excess mortality of long-term HL survivors. In order to reduce treatment-related toxicity ongoing trials are evaluating the efficacy and toxicity of less intensive chemotherapy protocols and of reduced radiation field size and dose. Regular cardiac screening tests might also contribute to reducing the mortality amongst HL survivors.

SUMMARY

Classical Hodgkin's lymphoma is a B-cell lymphoma characterized by the presence of HRS cells which derive from germinal-center B cells. L&H cells are pathognomonic for the less frequent NLPHL. Both variants share common features, i.e. the neoplastic cells are

surrounded by reactive nonclonal hematopoietic cells and represent less than 2% of the total tumor load.

While the initial transformation process is still unclear, it has become evident that the constitutive activation of the NF-κB pathway is an important survival signal for HRS cells. It has also been demonstrated that cytokines and chemokines secreted by HRS cells or "bystander cells" contribute to the anti-apoptotic phenotype of HRS cells, or may stimulate their proliferation.

Treatment strategies for patients with Hodgkin's lymphoma (Fig. 7.15) are based on an individual risk-factor assessment. The major prognostic factors used for risk stratification include stage of disease, bulky disease and B symptoms. According to the risk stratification applied by most European groups, including the GHSG and the EORTC, patients are assigned to early-stage favorable, early-stage unfavorable or advanced-stage risk groups. The recommended treatment for patients with

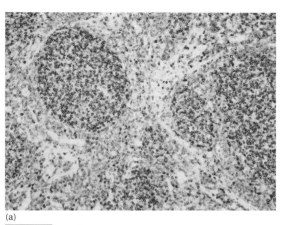
(a)

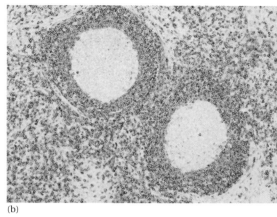
(b)

Figure 8.5. Follicular lymphoma stained for bcl-2 protein (lymph node). The cells of follicular lymphoma show strong staining for bcl-2 protein (a) in distinction to the cells of reactive germinal centers, which are (with the exception of the intrafollicular T cells) bcl-2 negative (b).

lymphoma the areas of diffuse growth composed of sheets of cells with centroblast morphology are considered to represent diffuse large B-cell lymphoma.

Other histological variants have been described which take into account an unusual growth pattern (floral variant), morphological characteristics (monocytoid differentiation, plasma cell differentiation, signet ring cell morphology, immunoglobulin inclusions) or presence of stromal changes (sclerosis, PAS-positive extracellular material).

Immunophenotypically the cells of follicular lymphoma are CD20- and CD79a-positive B cells that have surface immunoglobulin (sIg). In the majority of cases they have a germinal center cell phenotype with expression of CD10 and bcl-6 protein. A proportion of cases show loss of CD10. There is no staining for Mum1. In contrast to reactive germinal centers the cells of follicular lymphoma express bcl-2 protein in the majority (about 85%) of cases. This is more frequently the case in grade 1 lymphoma (almost 100%) but is found in only 75% of grade 3 follicular lymphomas. A proportion of cases express CD23 but the cells are negative for CD5 and cyclin D1. The neoplastic follicles contain an FDC meshwork that is highlighted by staining for CD21 or CD23 and contain a component of reactive T cells (Fig. 8.5).

MOLECULAR PATHOLOGY AND CYTOGENETICS

The cytogenetic hallmark of follicular lymphoma, the t(14;18)(q32;q21) chromosome translocation, is present in roughly 85% of grade 1 and 2 tumors. By this translocation, easily detectable by fluorescence *in-situ* hybridization (FISH) techniques, the *BCL-2* proto-oncogene is juxtaposed to enhancer sequences of the IgH gene promoter region, leading to bcl-2 deregulation and overexpression in the neoplastic follicles. This rearrangement occurs during the recombination of variable (V), diversity (D) and joining (J) regions in precursor B cells. In reactive follicles, the bcl-2 protein is not expressed, thus enabling the removal of B cells with non-functional B-cell receptors via apoptosis. The constitutive activation of the anti-apoptotic bcl-2 via the t(14;18) bypasses this physiological mechanism, and hence FL may be viewed as a disease of programmed cell death deregulation. An exciting new finding is the presence of the translocation in FL samples not only in the neoplastic lymphoid cells but also in microvascular endothelial cells within the tumor. However, according to data obtained from mouse models the introduction of a t(14;18) in a lymphoid cell may not be sufficient to cause a lymphoma on its own. Instead, this event may rather constitute a prerequisite for the acquisition of secondary chromosomal aberrations by prolonging the life span of a germinal center B cell.

Secondary chromosome aberrations are well defined in follicular lymphoma. In particular, (partial) trisomies of chromosomes 1q, 7, 12, 18 and X, as well as deletions in the short arm of chromosome 1 (1p) and the long arm of chromosome 6 (6q), have been reported. The acquisition of these secondary chromosomal alterations appears to be non-random, and certain aberration cascades may be determined by genetic alterations in the early steps of progression. In a large cohort of FL cases, the concept of varied cytogenetic pathways central to pathogenesis has emerged from the analysis of secondary chromosomal alterations defined by the acquisition of aberrations like 6q−, +7 or der(18)t(14;18). The presence of a deletion in the long arm of chromosome 6 (6q−) has been associated with inferior outcome in FL. Follicular lymphoma frequently progresses to DLBCL, and this event seems to be associated with certain recurring chromosome aberrations. Transformed follicular lymphomas frequently acquire deletions in the short arms of chromosomes 9 and 17, the sites of the $p16^{INK4A}$ and *TP53* tumor suppressor genes. The additional introduction of a t(8;14)(q24;q32)/MYC rearrangement in FL leads to a highly aggressive "Burkitt-like" neoplasia, sometimes with a precursor B-cell phenotype. Follicular lymphoma grade 3a, in accordance to its morphological and immunophenotypical similarities to FL grades 1 and 2, is also frequently t(14;18)-positive, although to a slightly lesser extent than its grade 1 and 2 counterparts. In contrast, FL 3b and especially those tumors with a DLBCL component frequently harbor *BCL-6* rearrangements, while *BCL-2* translocations are rarely present.

Recently, gene expression profiling emerged as a powerful tool to identify robust prognostic subgroups in FL. The analysis of a large cohort of FL resulted in the definition of two gene expression signatures with highly predictive potential. One of these signatures, termed "immune response 1 signature," was associated with a favorable clinical course, while the "immune response 2 signature" conferred inferior survival times. As suggested by their names, these signatures do not appear to be derived from the malignant B cells, but instead from reactive tumor-infiltrating cells. In particular, the immune response 1 signature may primarily be derived from certain T-cell subsets and the immune response 2 signature from macrophages and dendritic cells. A mathematical model combining these two signatures predicts that the relative levels of subsets of these cells in the lymphoma specimen are crucial for survival times in FL, arguing for a prominent role of immunologic cross-talk between the malignant B cells and infiltrating bystander cells.

STAGING INVESTIGATIONS

Treatment decisions critically depend upon the distinction between early-stage disease and advanced disease. Staging investigations should therefore include whole-body CT scanning, full blood count, biochemical assessment including lactate dehydrogenase (LDH) and bone-marrow biopsy. Marrow involvement by follicular lymphoma is typically patchy and may not be identified by a bone marrow aspirate alone. It is more readily detected as a paratrabecular infiltrate on the trephine biopsy. The incidence of CNS involvement by follicular lymphoma is rare and routine examination of the cerebrospinal fluid unnecessary.

The role of FDG-PET scanning in the staging of follicular lymphoma is currently under investigation. Its use may lead to the upstaging of many cases of apparent early-stage disease.

PROGNOSTIC FACTORS

This topic is covered in greater detail in Chapter 4.

The International Prognostic Index, developed for use in high-grade lymphoma treated with anthracycline-based chemotherapy, has been applied to follicular lymphoma. However, its use is limited by the fact that in follicular lymphoma extranodal disease is rare and elevation of the LDH is uncommon. As such only a small minority of patients are classified as high risk and the index does not effectively identify those cases of FL at high risk. More recently the Follicular Lymphoma International Prognostic Index (FLIPI) has been developed from multivariate analysis of 4167 cases of follicular lymphoma. The index includes age, stage, hemoglobin level, LDH and number of nodal sites involved, and distinguishes three roughly equal-sized risk groups – low, intermediate and high – based on scores of 0–1, 2, ≥3 respectively. The five-year overall survivals for low, intermediate and high-risk groups respectively are 91, 78 and 52%, and the ten-year survivals are 71, 51 and 36%. Notably there is no plateau in the survival curve of any risk group.

More recently cDNA microarray has identified two separate gene expression signatures associated with the immune response to the tumor. Immune response 1 is associated with overexpression of T-lymphocyte genes and confers a favorable prognosis.

Immune response 2 is associated instead with macrophage and dendritic-cell gene expression and confers an unfavorable prognosis independent of the FLIPI.

Whilst cDNA microarray technology is not routinely available in clinical practice the immune response patterns described above can also be partially distinguished by simple immunohistochemistry and CD68 staining of macrophages. A heavy infiltration of macrophages (>15 per high-power field) correlates with immune response 2 and a poorer survival.

It is important to note that all these prognostic models were derived from studies of patients prior to the widespread use of rituximab. Current studies are under way to establish whether these models still apply in patients who receive immunochemotherapy.

TREATMENT OF EARLY-STAGE DISEASE

Follicular lymphoma is exquisitely sensitive to radiation, and in the minority (15–20%) of patients who present with stage I or II and small-volume disease radiotherapy alone has the potential to be curative. Numerous studies confirm long-term disease-free survival in a proportion of patients treated with involved field radiotherapy alone. Relapses, when they occur, do so at sites outside the original field of radiation and usually do so within the first 15 years. Beyond this time relapses are extremely rare.

In a series of 460 patients with stage I/II FL treated with involved field radiation (IF-RT), disease-free survival (DFS) rates were 56% at 5 years and 41% at 10 years. Beyond 15 years only 2% of patients relapsed. As expected, most relapses occurred outside the original field of radiation. Similar results were seen in a series of 80 patients from M. D. Anderson treated with IF-RT alone. Progression-free survival (PFS) at 15 years was 66% for stage I patients and 26% for stage II. Beyond 17 years no relapses were seen. There is no randomized study comparing radiotherapy with observation alone.

In an attempt to improve long-term PFS, the role of adjuvant chemotherapy has been examined in single-arm studies. Seymour reported a 10-year time to treatment failure (TTF) of 72% in stage I–III FL patients treated with 10 cycles of CVP-bleo (cyclophosphamide, vincristine, prednisolone and bleomycin) and IF-RT. Whilst these results are superior to historical controls treated with IF-RT there was a significant increase in secondary malignancy. No randomized trial compares IF-RT with combined modality treatment. A randomized phase III study to address this question is currently under way in Australia, examining IF-RT with and without six cycles of CVP. Clearly any improvement in disease control must be balanced against immediate and late toxicity of this approach, and in particular the risk of secondary malignancy.

Partly because of concerns over late toxicity, other researchers have examined the approach of "no initial therapy" in early-stage disease. Advani reported the outcome of 11 stage I and 32 stage II FL patients who received no initial therapy. More than half remained untreated at 6 years, and 10-year survival was comparable to reports of patients treated up-front with IF-RT.

There is little evidence to guide therapy in completely excised stage I disease.

Summary

At present IF-RT (30–40 Gy) remains the standard of care for small-volume stage I and II follicular lymphoma. In around 40% of such patients this approach will be curative. In completely excised stage I disease the toxicity of treatment may outweigh the potential reduction in risk of recurrence.

TREATMENT OF ADVANCED DISEASE IN ASYMPTOMATIC PATIENTS

The majority of patients with FL present with advanced disease, and many of these are asymptomatic at diagnosis. In contrast to early-stage FL, conventional treatment is not curative and the aim of treatment is to control the disease sufficiently to avoid symptoms. Three randomized trials, conducted by the NCI, GELA and BNLI, have confirmed that early treatment with chemotherapy offers no survival advantage in asymptomatic patients with follicular lymphoma. In 1988 Young reported on a randomized study of 99 patients with indolent NHL, comparing watchful waiting versus aggressive combined modality treatment with ProMACE–MOPP (prednisone, methotrexate, doxorubicin, cyclophosphamide, etoposide plus mechlorethamine, vincristine, procarbazine and prednisone) followed by total nodal irradiation. No survival difference was detected between the two arms. In 1997 Brice and colleagues reported on a study of 193 patients with low tumor volume FL randomized to receive watchful waiting, prednimustine or interferon (IFN), and detected no survival difference between the three arms at 5 years. In the largest trial run by the BNLI 309 patients with asymptomatic FL were randomized to "watchful waiting" or immediate chlorambucil. Although the chance of complete remission was increased by immediate treatment (63% vs. 27%), no difference in overall survival or lymphoma-related death was observed between the two arms. The mean time to treatment in the observation arm was 2.6 years. Furthermore, in the observation arm 19% of patients had required no treatment by 10 years. Elderly patients (over 70 years) had an even greater chance of requiring no therapy, with 40% untreated at 10 years after diagnosis.

Whilst there is no role for conventional chemotherapy in asymptomatic FL, it is possible that newer less toxic agents such as rituximab may prolong the time to disease progression and requirement for chemotherapy. Currently open trials are investigating the role of immediate rituximab and rituximab maintenance in patients with newly diagnosed asymptomatic FL.

Summary

Watchful waiting remains an appropriate management for asymptomatic patients with advanced follicular lymphoma. Data from trials of monoclonal antibodies and radioimmunotherapy may lead to a change in practice in the future.

FIRST-LINE TREATMENT OF ADVANCED DISEASE IN SYMPTOMATIC PATIENTS

The indications to initiate treatment in follicular lymphoma are generally considered to be overt progression of bulky disease, compromise of a vital organ, bone-marrow failure and B symptoms. Patients are treated with the expectation that the disease will pursue a relapsing and remitting course and that patients may require several lines of treatment during the course of their disease. The usual strategy is to treat to remission or best response and then manage with regular surveillance until progression. At this time restaging and repeat biopsy (to exclude high-grade transformation) should be performed to guide

subsequent therapy. For many years standard first-line treatment has been alkylator-based therapy, frequently in combinations including vinca alkaloids, corticosteroids and anthracyclines. No single alkylator-based regimen shows superiority in terms of overall survival over any other. Recently the addition of rituximab to alkylator-based regimens has been shown to improve TTF (time to treatment failure) in several randomized trials, including two which demonstrate an improvement in overall survival.

Conventional chemotherapy

Single-agent chlorambucil or cyclophosphamide induces response rates up to 80%, although few complete responses are seen. The addition of corticosteroid and vincristine may increase the rates of complete remission but does not affect overall survival. Attempts to increase the intensity of chemotherapy by addition of an anthracycline have similarly failed to show a survival advantage. In 1994 Kimby and colleagues reported a study of 259 patients with untreated, symptomatic low-grade NHL randomized between ChP (chlorambucil and prednisone) and CHOP (cyclophosphamide, doxorubicin, vincristine and prednisone). Although the response rate was greater in the CHOP-treated patients (60% vs. 36%), 5-year overall survival was equivalent (54% vs. 59%). Most recently Peterson randomized 228 patients with previously untreated FL to receive either daily oral cyclophosphamide or CHOP–bleomycin. Responses were seen in 91% of patients, but there were no significant differences in complete response (CR) (66% vs. 60%), 10-year TTF (25% vs. 33%) or overall survival (OS) (44% vs. 46%). Although a number of other studies have suggested response rates are improved by the addition of an anthracycline, no study has identified a survival advantage. Any improvement in response with anthracycline-containing combinations must be balanced against the inevitable increase in toxicity, and against the preclusion of anthracycline, due to cumulative dose-related cardiotoxicity, as a therapeutic agent in the event of subsequent transformation to high-grade disease. Table 8.2 summarizes the results of some recent studies of first-line treatment of symptomatic FL.

The purine analogue fludarabine has been shown to have considerable activity against follicular lymphoma as first-line treatment when used both as a single agent

Table 8.2. Studies of first-line treatment of follicular lymphoma.

Study	Treatment	n	ORR (%)	CR (%)	TTP (months)
Kimby (1994)	Chlorambucil/Prednisone	132	36%	5%	41% (5 yr OS)
	CHOP	127	60%	18%	44% (5 yr OS)
Solal-Céligny (1998)	CHVP	119	58%	13%	18 mo
	CHVP + IFN	123	76%	20%	34 mo (PFS)
Hagenbeek (1998)	CVP	315	79%	45%	20 mo
	CVP + IFN	120	n/a	n/a	30 mo
Hagenbeek (2001)	CVP	187	51%	15%	15 mo
	Fludarabine	194	68%	38%	21 mo
Fisher (2000)	ProMACE–MOPP ProMACE–MOPP + IFN	500	83%	47%	36 mo
		144	n/a	n/a	48 mo

ORR, overall response rate
CR, complete response
TTP, time to progression
OS, overall survival
PFS, progression-free survival

and in combination with either cyclophosphamide or mitoxantrone. High rates of response including complete remissions and molecular remissions are seen. But prolonged PFS is not consistently observed and no trial has identified a survival advantage. Furthermore, the first-line use of fludarabine may have a detrimental effect on any subsequent attempt to mobilize hematopoietic stem cells for autologous transplantation. It carries an increased risk of opportunistic infection and it may be associated with an increased risk of secondary acute myeloid leukemia or myelodysplasia.

Combined immunochemotherapy

The anti-CD20 chimeric antibody rituximab was originally shown to have activity against FL when used as a single agent in the treatment of relapsed or refractory FL. Four recent phase III trials have now confirmed the efficacy of rituximab in combination with an alkylator-containing regimen, both with and without the inclusion of anthracycline (Table 8.3).

Marcus *et al.* randomized 321 patients with previously untreated advanced FL to eight cycles of CVP (cyclophosphamide, vincristine and prednisolone) chemotherapy with or without rituximab. At a median follow-up of 30 months patients treated with

rituximab had significantly superior outcomes: TTF (27 vs. 7 months), TTP (32 vs. 15 months), ORR (81% vs. 57%) and CR (41% vs. 10%). Notably the improvement in TTP (time to progression) was seen across all prognostic groups. Although a survival benefit was not detected at the time of original publication, an update of the data has since revealed a survival benefit in the rituximab treated patients.

On behalf of the GLSG Hiddeman and colleagues reported a study of 428 patients with untreated advanced-stage FL who were randomized to receive 6–8 cycles of CHOP chemotherapy with or without rituximab. A significantly improved ORR (96% vs. 90%) and PFS were seen in the rituximab arm. In addition, rituximab led to an improvement in survival, with 6 deaths vs. 17 deaths in the first three years. Although the numbers were small this achieved statistical significance. Survival advantage for immunochemotherapy over chemotherapy alone was confirmed in another phase III study conducted by the OSHO group and reported by Herold in 2004. They randomized 358 patients with previously untreated advanced indolent NHL to receive eight cycles of MCP (mitoxantrone, cyclophosphamide and prednisolone) with or without rituximab. Although the trial included mantle cell lymphoma and

Table 8.3. First-line treatment of follicular lymphoma: immunochemotherapy phase III trials.

Study	Treatment	n	ORR	CR	Response duration
Marcus (2005)	CVP	159	57%	41%	15 mo TTP
	R-CVP	162	81%	10%	34 mo TTP
Hiddemann (2005)	CHOP	205	90%	17%	31 mo TTF
	R-CHOP	223	96%	20%	Not reached
Herold (2004) (abstract)	MCP	96	75%	n/a	43% (2 yr EFS)
	R-MCP	105	92%	n/a	83% (2 yr EFS)
Salles (2004) (abstract)	CHVP + IFN	175	85%	49%	62% (2.5 yr EFS)
	R-CHVP + IFN	184	94%	76%	78% (2.5 yr EFS)

ORR, overall response rate

CR, complete response

TTP, time to progression

TTF, time to treatment failure

EFS, event-free survival

lymphoplasmacytic lymphoma, 201 patients had follicular lymphoma. The ORR and CR were 85.5% and 42% in the R-MCP arm and 65.5% and 20% in the MCP arm ($p < 0.0001$). The results were even more striking in the FL subgroup, with an ORR of 92.4% vs. 75% and a CR of 49.5% vs. 25% ($p < 0.0001$). Within the FL subgroup 30-month PFS was 80% vs. 52% ($p < 0.0001$). Most notably, the addition of rituximab to MCP in patients with FL was associated with a significantly improved overall survival at 30 months (89% vs. 75%, $p = 0.007$).

Finally, in the FL-200 study conducted by GELA and reported by Salles, 359 patients with previously untreated FL and high tumor burden were randomized to 12 cycles of CHVP/interferon (cyclophosphamide, doxorubicin, etoposide, prednisolone and alpha-interferon) or six cycles of CHVP/interferon with six doses of rituximab. Patients receiving rituximab had a significantly higher response rate at 6 months (ORR 94% vs. 85%; CR/CRu 76% vs. 49%). An update of this trial has shown a survival advantage in the rituximab-treated arm in both FLIPI low- and high-risk patients (FLIPI 0–2 3-year OS 72% vs. 55%, $p = 0.019$; FLIPI 3–5 3-year OS 61% vs. 38%, $p = 0.0005$).

The survival benefit of combined immunochemotherapy as first-line treatment of FL has been confirmed by a recent Cochrane meta-analysis, which combined survival data from the above randomized trials, although it was composed prior to the updated survival data from the GELA and Marcus trials.

This analysis favored immunochemotherapy, with a hazard ratio (HR) of 0.57 (95% CI 0.43 – 0.77).

Further support for a survival advantage from immunochemotherapy over chemotherapy alone comes from a retrospective review by Fisher *et al.* of patients treated by the Southwest Oncology Group (SWOG) over the last 30 years using three sequential regimens – CHOP, ProMACE–MOPP and CHOP+MoAb. Although the MoAb cohort included some patients treated with radioimmunotherapy the majority received rituximab. The four-year estimated survival for each group is 69% for CHOP regimens, 79% for ProMACE–MOPP regimens and 91% for the CHOP + MoAb regimens ($p < 0.001$). This suggests that overall survival of patients with FL has indeed improved over the last decade, and that the use of immunochemotherapy may be at least partly responsible for this improvement.

Summary

In patients who require treatment the combination of chemotherapy with rituximab is now the standard of care for first-line treatment of stage III and IV follicular lymphoma.

Rituximab maintenance

The efficacy of rituximab maintenance after conventional first-line chemotherapy has been demonstrated in a prospective phase III randomized trial undertaken by ECOG. Previously untreated patients with FL received up to eight cycles of CVP chemotherapy. Importantly, these patients did not receive rituximab as part of induction therapy. Responding patients were then randomized to either rituximab maintenance (four once-weekly infusions every 6 months for 2 years) or observation only. The estimated PFS at 4 years was 56% in the maintenance arm and 33% in the observation arm (HR = 0.39, $p < 0.0001$). Differences in PFS were most significant for patients with high initial tumor burden and minimal residual disease after CVP. A survival benefit was also observed in the rituximab maintenance arm at 4 years (88% vs. 72%, HR = 0.51, $p = 0.03$).

The benefit of maintenance rituximab in patients who have already received rituximab as part of induction therapy is less clear, and at the time of writing no trial has yet answered this question. The value of rituximab maintenance after rituximab-based reinduction has, however, been confirmed in the setting of relapsed FL (see below). Interestingly these results appear to contrast with the data in diffuse large B-cell lymphoma treated with R-CHOP, where subsequent maintenance rituximab has not been shown to be of clinical benefit.

Interferon maintenance

A large number of trials have examined the role of IFN (interferon-alpha) either as an adjunct to induction therapy or as maintenance. The results of 10 such phase III trials, including 1922 newly diagnosed patients with FL, have been incorporated into a meta-analysis by Rohatiner *et al.* Although the addition of IFN to induction chemotherapy did not significantly improve response rates, an improved overall survival and remission duration was seen in patients treated with IFN. However, this survival benefit was limited to those receiving IFN concurrent with (but not after) intensive remission induction, at a dose of > 5 million units and at a cumulative dose of > 36 million units per month. It is important to note that this analysis was based upon studies performed prior to the use of rituximab immunochemotherapy, and the benefit of IFN in this setting is currently unknown.

Autologous stem-cell transplantation (ASCT) in first remission

Autologous stem-cell transplantation has been shown to be effective in relapsed FL. In an attempt

to prolong remission a number of groups have investigated its role as consolidation in first remission. The three most important studies have generated conflicting results.

The GLSG (Lenz and colleagues) carried out a study in which patients with FL in first remission were randomized to receive IFN or autologous SCT as maintenance therapy. Induction treatment consisted of either CHOP or MCP. Although autografting was associated with a prolonged PFS at 5 years (64.7% vs. 33.3%, $p < 0.0001$), this failed to translate into an improved overall survival, partly due to an excess of secondary malignancy. GOELAMS randomized 172 patients with advanced, previously untreated FL to either anthracycline-based chemotherapy and autograft or anthracycline-based chemotherapy and IFN. The conditioning used was total body irradiation (TBI) and cyclophosphamide, and stem cells were purged ex-vivo. Although an improved event-free survival (EFS) was seen (most pronounced in FLIPI high-risk patients), in the autograft arm this was balanced by an excess of fatal secondary malignancy (8.5%), and no survival advantage was seen in any group. The GELA group randomized 401 patients to receive standard therapy (CHVP × 12 followed by IFN) or CHOP × 4 followed by autologous stem-cell transplantation (TBI, cyclophosphamide, etoposide conditioning). At a median follow-up of 7 years no significant difference in EFS (28% vs. 38%, $p = 0.11$) or OS (71% vs. 76%, $p = 0.53$) was detected. Interestingly, no excess of secondary malignancy was observed in this trial. These results, and data from the GLSG trial, suggest that the risk of secondary malignancy may depend at least partly on initial chemotherapy rather than solely on the transplant conditioning used.

Summary

The results of these studies are conflicting and provide insufficient evidence to justify routine autografting in first remission. The high risk of secondary malignancy seen in some trials is a serious concern. Furthermore, all these studies were conducted prior to the use of monoclonal antibody therapy. Our own view is that the improvements in EFS and OS seen with the use of rituximab may now mean that autografting in first remission after immunochemotherapy may add little more than toxicity.

Radioimmunotherapy

Radioimmunotherapy has been demonstrated to be effective in the treatment of relapsed FL. Recently a phase II trial by Kaminski and colleagues has examined the role of ^{131}I-tositumomab in the treatment of previously untreated FL. Seventy-six patients with stage III/IV FL received a single one-week course of ^{131}I-tositumomab. The ORR was 95% and CR was 75%. Molecular responses were seen in 80% of patients achieving a complete response. At a median follow-up of 5.1 years the PFS was 59% and median PFS was 6.1 years. Patients tolerated the treatment without problem and no case of treatment-related myelodysplasia (t-MDS) was seen. Whilst the ORR and PFS quoted are extremely impressive, the study included patients with a very favorable profile: the median age was 49 years and less than 50% of patients had bulky disease. The SWOG studied the use of ^{131}I-tositumomab as consolidation after CHOP chemotherapy in 90 previously untreated patients with FL, as reported by Press. Treatment was well tolerated and myelosuppression was more severe with the CHOP than with the radioimmunotherapy. The ORR was 90%, including 67% complete response. Of the patients who failed to achieve a CR with CHOP, 57% converted to CR after radioimmunotherapy. The two-year PFS was estimated to be 81%. On the basis of this study a phase III trial is currently under way to compare R-CHOP with CHOP ^{131}I-tositumomab in previously untreated FL.

Summary

Despite the ease of administration, tolerability and impressive response rates, solid evidence of the clinical benefit of radioimmunotherapy in previously untreated FL is awaited.

Summary: first-line treatment of advanced follicular lymphoma

Asymptomatic patients with advanced follicular lymphoma should be managed with observation alone, and do not benefit from early intervention. Those patients who do require treatment should receive an alkylator-based regimen in combination with rituximab. The inclusion of an anthracycline may improve response rate but does not improve overall survival. Furthermore, if an anthracycline is used as first-line

therapy the cumulative risk of cardiotoxicity may then preclude its future use in the event of high-grade transformation. The role of maintenance rituximab after immunochemotherapy is currently unclear. In patients who have received rituximab-based induction therapy there is no evidence to justify either maintenance interferon or autologous stem-cell transplantation in first remission. Phase III trials are currently under way to establish the role of radioimmunotherapy in first-line treatment of FL.

MANAGEMENT OF RELAPSED FOLLICULAR LYMPHOMA

The management of patients with relapsed disease is influenced by the tempo, nature and timing of the relapse. Similar to the situation in patients with FL at presentation, provided the patient remains asymptomatic and the disease quiescent no treatment may be required at relapse. The risk of transformation to high-grade lymphoma is approximately 20% at 5 years. It is therefore important to rule out transformation by biopsy at each recurrence before considering therapeutic approaches. Restaging of the disease is also recommended at each relapse to establish the extent of the lymphoma and to provide a baseline from which to define response to therapy.

There are a number of treatment options available to clinicians in the management of symptomatic relapsed follicular lymphoma, but the heterogeneity of the patient population, specifically the nature of previous treatments and the duration of previous remissions, combined with a lack of good-quality randomized controlled trial data, means that treatment at relapse is far from standardized.

Chemotherapy

There has been no direct comparison of single-agent alkylating agents with combinations such as CVP or CHOP carried out in the context of relapsed disease and in the context of patients who have had durable remissions to first-line therapies.

The superiority of combination therapies over single-agent alkylators in terms of overall survival cannot be assumed.

Other approaches include the use of purine analogues such as fludarabine. This is a highly effective agent in patients who relapse following first-line alkylator-based therapy. The majority of studies have used intravenous fludarabine (25 mg/m^2 per day for 3–5 days), but oral fludarabine (40 mg/m^2 per day for 5 days) appears to show equal efficacy. Fludarabine showed improved progression-free survival (PFS), treatment-free survival (TFS) and social function scores in comparison with CVP but did not significantly improve response rate or overall survival. In patients with refractory and relapsed FL response rates appear to be improved by combining fludarabine with an anthracycline (fludarabine/mitoxantrone, ORR 94%) or an alkylating agent (fludarabine/cyclophosphamide, ORR 72%) or both (fludarabine/cyclophosphamide/mitoxantrone, RR 88%). However, no direct comparison was made to alkylator therapy alone, and superiority in terms of OS has not been demonstrated.

Fludarabine treatment is also associated with significantly greater toxicity than alkylator- or anthracycline-based regimens: infection (including opportunistic organisms) occurred in up to 12% and 44% of patients in the above studies. As discussed earlier, fludarabine also reduces the subsequent likelihood of successful stem cell mobilization. Finally, t-MDS has been found to occur at a crude incidence of 4%, one to five years after fludarabine/anthracycline-based chemotherapy. Therefore the benefits of fludarabine as second-line treatment must be weighed against the risks of infection, stem cell toxicity and t-MDS.

Rituximab

Early experience with rituximab demonstrated that approximately 50% of patients with relapsed FL (who had not previously received antibody therapy) treated with monthly rituximab 375 mg/m^2 showed a response, with a median time to treatment failure of 13 months. Single-agent rituximab also appears to be active in patients with FL who have previously responded to rituximab therapy, with a response rate in this group of 40% and a median time to progression estimated at 18 months.

The addition of rituximab to a combination of fludarabine, cyclophosphamide, mitoxantrone (FCM) significantly increases response rates and prolongs survival as compared with FCM alone in patients with relapsed and refractory FL. Response rates after four courses of treatment were 94% and 70% in the R-FCM and FCM groups respectively. Progression-

free survival was not reached at 3 years in the R-FCM group and was estimated at 21 months in the FCM-treated cases. Furthermore, in patients with relapsed FL who have objective response or stable disease with single-agent rituximab therapy, duration of rituximab benefit is substantially prolonged with either scheduled maintenance treatment or rituximab re-treatment at the time of progression. Progression-free survival was 31 versus 7 months in the maintenance and re-treatment groups respectively, but duration of rituximab benefit was similar in both groups at approximately 31 months, suggesting the two approaches were equally effective. In a single study of patients with relapsed or refractory FL the addition of rituximab to CHOP at first randomization in the remission induction schedule has been shown to improve PFS, and in a second randomization rituximab maintenance was demonstrated to improve PFS and OS. Median PFS from first randomization was 20.2 months after CHOP versus 33.1 months after R-CHOP. Subsequently rituximab maintenance treatment resulted in a median PFS of 51.5 months versus 14.9 months in the observation arm. Intriguingly, on further analysis this improvement of PFS was found to occur after both induction with CHOP (42 months versus observation 12 months) and R-CHOP (rituximab maintenance 52 months versus observation 23 months). A significant benefit was also demonstrated for overall survival in the entire group: 85% at 3 years in the rituximab maintenance arm versus 77% in the observation arm.

Summary of immunochemotherapy as second-line treatment

Alkylating agents, anthracyclines and fludarabine are all effective in a proportion of patients with relapsed FL. Response rates appear to be higher when these drugs are used in combination, although at the cost of greater short- and long-term toxicity. Rituximab should be used in patients who have previously responded well to rituximab (>2 year remission) and in those who are rituximab-naive. Rituximab may also be considered as maintenance in patients who respond to second-line therapy. It remains unclear which are the optimal drugs to use in combination with rituximab. Patients who have achieved durable remissions from previous therapies may be considered for a regimen containing the same agents at relapse. Chemotherapy or antibodies that have previously failed or have induced only short remissions should be avoided. Patients with clinically aggressive or advanced disease at relapse should be considered for more intensive combination regimens.

High-dose therapy and autologous stem-cell transplantation (ASCT)

Only one randomized controlled trial to date (Schouten *et al.*) has compared chemotherapy and ASCT in relapsed FL. Between 1993 and 1997, 89 patients with relapsed or refractory FL who had achieved a CR or PR following induction therapy (the majority of patients treated with CHOP), and who had a WHO performance status of 0–2 and limited bone-marrow infiltration (defined as < 20% B cells in the marrow aspirate), were randomized to receive three further chemotherapy courses, an unpurged ASCT or a purged ASCT. As the numbers in the three groups were small the two transplant groups (unpurged and purged) were combined and compared with chemotherapy and an overall survival benefit for ASCT was reported (HR = 0.40 [range 0.18–0.89], $p = 0.026$) with an OS at 2 years of 71% in the ASCT group and 46% in the chemotherapy group.

Several retrospective case series have evaluated the role of ASCT in relapsed follicular lymphoma. Durable responses are reported in this patient group, with median disease-free survival of about 4 years, which compares well to historical data on chemotherapy alone. There is a suggestion that fewer previous courses of chemotherapy, TBI-based conditioning regimens and complete remission at the time of transplant are associated with the best outcomes. These data offer support for the idea of ASCT in relapsed FL, but importantly these studies do not compare ASCT with rituximab-based chemotherapy regimens.

Summary
Currently the precise role for ASCT in relapsed FL remains unclear. The morbidity and mortality of the procedure must be considered. It is currently difficult to recommend ASCT for patients with relapsed FL who may otherwise respond well to antibody-based therapy (i.e. rituximab-naive patients and those with a previous good remission following rituximab-based therapy). ASCT is best reserved for patients with early relapse, those with aggressive disease and those who

have failed antibody treatment. The exact role for ASCT in the antibody era remains to be defined in randomized clinical trials.

Allogeneic stem-cell transplantation (allo-SCT)

The potential to exploit a graft-versus-lymphoma effect makes allogeneic stem-cell transplantation (allo-SCT) a potentially attractive proposition, particularly in a selected group of younger patients with relapsed aggressive FL. However, in contrast to other hematological malignancies, where relapsed disease is often untreatable, relapsed FL may still be amenable to treatment with many lines of therapy including novel agents. This fact must be weighed against the considerable morbidity and mortality attached to allogeneic transplantation.

There are limited data available to guide patient selection and the optimum timing of transplantation in the natural history of disease. In an IBMTR report by van Besien and colleagues of 176 patients with FL who underwent allo-SCT, the reported treatment-related mortality (TRM) was 24% at 1 year and 30% at 5 years, with a recurrence rate of 19% at 1 year and very few relapses thereafter. Disappointingly, despite the low relapse rate, the high TRM resulted in overall survival of 51% at 5 years. This was not significantly different from that following ASCT at a similar time point.

Reduced-intensity conditioned allogeneic stem-cell transplantation (RIC-allo-SCT) aims to improve survival by exploiting the low relapse rates that have been observed following allo-SCT whilst reducing the TRM. Case series and registry data of RIC-allo-SCT suggest that this approach may be effective in patients with low-grade lymphoproliferative disorders, with reported 2-year TRM rates of 11%, 16% and 31% and OS rates of 74% at 2 years, 74% at 3 years and 65% at 2 years. No study has yet directly compared allo-SCT with RIC-allo-SCT in relapsed FL.

Summary
Allogeneic stem-cell transplantation should be considered for younger patients with aggressive disease who have relapsed or progressed despite conventional treatments (chemotherapy, antibody therapy and ASCT) and who are considered otherwise fit enough for the procedure. The high TRM means that

allogeneic transplantation will be an option for only a minority of patients. The optimum conditioning regimen is unclear but it is suggested that the youngest and fittest patients receive full allo-SCT conditioning whilst the remainder receive reduced-intensity conditioning. Allogeneic transplantation remains an experimental therapy and patients should be treated where possible within the context of a clinical trial.

Radiolabeled monoclonal antibodies

Both ^{131}I-tositumomab and ^{90}Y-ibritumomab have shown clinical benefit in relapsed and refractory FL. In a randomized comparison with rituximab, patients who received ^{90}Y-ibritumomab were shown to have a superior ORR (80% vs. 56%). Although the study was not powered to detect differences in time-to-event variables, the results trend toward longer median TTP (15 vs. 10.2 months), response duration (16.7 vs. 11.2 months) and time to next therapy (21.1 vs. 13.8 months). Furthermore, in patients with rituximab-refractory FL, treatment with ^{90}Y-ibritumomab has been shown by Witzig *et al.* to induce a response in 54% of patients, with a median duration of 6 months.

[131]I-tositumomab has also been found to be effective in patients with relapsed FL. In patients who had not responded or progressed within 6 months after their last qualifying chemotherapy (LQC) the ORR was 65% after ^{131}I-tositumomab, in comparison to 28% after the LQC. The median duration of response was 6.5 months after ^{131}I-tositumomab, compared with 3.4 months after the LQC. In a separate study ^{131}I-tositumomab myeloablation followed by ASCT in 27 patients with relapsed FL led to an estimated 5-year OS and PFS of 67% and 48% respectively and 100-day treatment-related mortality of 3.7%.

Summary

The data available suggest that radioimmunotherapy is effective in relapsed FL and demands urgent further study to define the appropriate context in which it should be used.

High-grade transformation of FL

Transformation of FL to high-grade lymphoma appears to be an early event in the course of the disease and is mainly observed in patients with known adverse prognostic factors or those who do not achieve CR after initial treatment. Furthermore, transformed FL carries a poor prognosis despite treatment with aggressive chemotherapy. In a retrospective analysis of 220 patients over 15 years Bastion and colleagues reported a probability of transformation of 22% at 5 years and 31% at 10 years and observed a plateau after 6 years. Predictive factors for transformation were non-achievement of CR after initial therapy, low serum albumin level (< 35 g/L) and beta 2-microglobulin level greater than 3 mg/L at diagnosis. Transformation accounted for 44% of deaths and was associated with a poor outcome, with a median survival time of 7 months.

Data are limited as to the most appropriate course of treatment in transformed FL. Anthracycline-based combinations (e.g. CHOP or FMD) should be used to induce remission induction. Intuitively it seems reasonable to add rituximab to the remission induction regimen although data are lacking. In the event of an inadequate response or progressive disease, therapeutic options include salvage chemotherapy (e.g. ESHAP) to establish disease response and subsequent ASCT in those with responsive disease. In patients treated this way 5-year survival is approximately 30%. Radioimmunotherapy and allo-SCT are more experimental strategies but may also be effective in selected individuals. The management of high-grade lymphoma is described in more detail in Chapter 12.

Summary: relapsed follicular lymphoma

Presently, relapsed FL remains an incurable disease for the majority of patients. While the increasing number of treatment options at relapse provides optimism the appropriate timing of the various therapies available has yet to be clearly defined. Intervention is generally recommended only in the context of symptomatic or progressive disease. Re-biopsy and restaging of the lymphoma is recommended at each relapse. The choice of therapy will be dictated principally by the tempo of disease, the response to previous therapies and the patient's general medical condition. Chemotherapy or antibody combinations that have provided a previous remission of 2 years or more should be considered again. Rituximab-naive patients should receive rituximab-based immuno-chemotherapy. Rituximab may also be considered as maintenance. Patients with aggressive disease and those who relapse early after immunochemotherapy

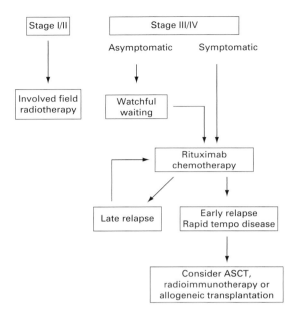

Figure 8.6. Proposed treatment algorithm for follicular lymphoma.

should be considered for radioimmunotherapy or ASCT. Younger patients who relapse despite the above should be considered for an allogeneic transplant. Where possible, patients should be managed in the context of a clinical trial.

FURTHER READING

Advani, R., Rosenberg, S. A. and Horning, S. J. Stage I and II follicular non-Hodgkin's lymphoma: long-term follow-up of no initial therapy. *J. Clin. Oncol.* **22** (2004), 1454–1459.

Ardeshna, K. M., Smith, P., Norton, A. *et al.* Long-term effect of a watch and wait policy versus immediate systemic treatment for asymptomatic advanced-stage non-Hodgkin lymphoma: a randomised controlled trial. *Lancet* **362** (2003), 516–522.

Bastion, Y., Sebban, C., Berger, F. *et al.* Incidence, predictive factors, and outcome of lymphoma transformation in follicular lymphoma patients. *J. Clin. Oncol.* **15** (1997), 1587–1594.

Fisher, R. I., LeBlanc, M., Press, O. W., Maloney, D. G., Unger, J. M. and Miller, T. P. New treatment options have changed the survival of patients with follicular lymphoma. *J. Clin. Oncol.* **23** (2005), 8447–8452.

Ganguly, S., Divine, C. L., Deauna-Limayo, D. *et al.* Autologous transplantation in patients with relapsed or high-grade follicular lymphoma provides long term disease-free survival and best median duration of response. *Ann. Hematol.* **84** (2005), 526–531.

Gopal, A. K., Gooley, T. A., Maloney, D. G. *et al.* High-dose radioimmunotherapy versus conventional high-dose therapy and autologous hematopoietic stem-cell transplantation for relapsed follicular non-Hodgkin lymphoma: a multivariable cohort analysis. *Blood* **102** (2003), 2351–2357.

Hainsworth, J. D., Litchy, S., Shaffer, D. W., Lackey, V. L., Grimaldi, M. and Greco, F. A. Maximizing therapeutic benefit of rituximab: maintenance therapy versus re-treatment at progression in patients with indolent non-Hodgkin's lymphoma. A randomized phase II trial of the Minnie Pearl Cancer Research Network. *J. Clin. Oncol.* **23** (2005), 1088–1095.

Hiddemann, W., Kneba, M., Dreyling, M. *et al.* Frontline therapy with rituximab added to the combination of cyclophosphamide, doxorubicin, vincristine, and prednisone (CHOP) significantly improves the outcome for patients with advanced-stage follicular lymphoma compared with therapy with CHOP alone: results of a prospective randomized study of the German Low-Grade Lymphoma Study Group. *Blood* **106** (2005), 3725–3732.

Kaminski, M. S., Tuck, M., Estes, J. *et al.* ^{131}I-tositumomab therapy as initial treatment for follicular lymphoma. *N. Engl. J. Med.* **352** (2005), 441–449.

Kimby, E., Bjorkholm, M., Gahrton, G. *et al.* Chlorambucil/prednisone vs. CHOP in symptomatic low-grade non-Hodgkin's lymphomas: a randomized trial from the Lymphoma Group of Central Sweden. *Ann. Oncol.* **5** Suppl 2 (1994), 67–71.

Klasa, R. J., Meyer, R. M., Shustik, C. *et al.* Randomized phase III study of fludarabine phosphate versus cyclophosphamide, vincristine, and prednisone in patients with recurrent low-grade non-Hodgkin's lymphoma previously treated with an alkylating agent or alkylator-containing regimen. *J. Clin. Oncol.* **20** (2002), 4649–4654.

Lenz, G., Dreyling, M., Schiegnitz, E. *et al.* Myeloablative radiochemotherapy followed by autologous stem-cell transplantation in first remission prolongs progression-free survival in follicular lymphoma: results of a prospective, randomized trial of the German Low-Grade Lymphoma Study Group. *Blood* **104** (2004), 2667–2674.

Mann, R. B. and Berard, C. W. Criteria for the cytologic subclassification of follicular lymphomas: a proposed alternative method. *Hematol. Oncol.* **1** (1983), 187–192.

Marcus, R., Imrie, K., Belch, A. *et al.* CVP chemotherapy plus rituximab compared with CVP as first-line treatment for advanced follicular lymphoma. *Blood* **105** (2005), 1417–1423.

McLaughlin, P., Grillo-Lopez, A. J., Link, B. K. *et al.* Rituximab chimeric anti-CD20 monoclonal antibody therapy for relapsed indolent lymphoma: half of patients respond to a four-dose treatment program. *J. Clin. Oncol.* **16** (1998), 2825–2833.

McLaughlin, P., Hagemeister, F. B., Romaguera, J. E. *et al.* Fludarabine, mitoxantrone, and dexamethasone: an effective new regimen for indolent lymphoma. *J. Clin. Oncol.* **14** (1996), 1262–1268.

Morris, E., Thomson, K., Craddock, C. *et al.* Outcomes after alemtuzumab-containing reduced-intensity allogeneic transplantation regimen for relapsed and refractory non-Hodgkin lymphoma. *Blood* **104** (2004), 3865–3871.

Peterson, B. A., Petroni, G. R., Frizzera, G. *et al.* Prolonged single-agent versus combination chemotherapy in indolent follicular lymphomas: a study of the cancer and leukemia group B. *J. Clin. Oncol.* **21** (2003), 5–15.

Press, O. W., Unger, J. M., Braziel, R. M. *et al.* A phase 2 trial of CHOP chemotherapy followed by tositumomab/iodine I 131 tositumomab for previously untreated follicular non-Hodgkin lymphoma: Southwest Oncology Group Protocol S9911. *Blood* **102** (2003), 1606–1612.

Rohatiner, A. Z., Gregory, W. M., Peterson, B. *et al.* Meta-analysis to evaluate the role of interferon in follicular lymphoma. *J. Clin. Oncol.* **23** (2005), 2215–2223.

Schouten, H. C., Qian, W., Kvaloy, S. *et al.* High-dose therapy improves progression-free survival and survival in relapsed follicular non-Hodgkin's lymphoma: results from the randomized European CUP trial. *J. Clin. Oncol.* **21** (2003), 3918–3927.

Sebban, C., Mounier, N., Brousse, N. *et al.* Standard chemotherapy with interferon compared to CHOP followed by high-dose therapy with autologous stem-cell transplantation in untreated patients with advanced follicular lymphoma: the GELF-94 randomized study from the GELA. *Blood* **108** (2006), 2540–2544.

van Besien, K., Loberiza, F. R. Jr., Bajorunaite, R. *et al.* Comparison of autologous and allogeneic hematopoietic stem-cell transplantation for follicular lymphoma. *Blood*, **102** (2003), 3521–3529.

van Oers, M. H., Klasa, R., Marcus, R. E. *et al.* Rituximab maintenance improves clinical outcome of relapsed/resistant follicular non-Hodgkin's lymphoma, both in patients with and without rituximab during induction: results of a prospective randomized phase III intergroup trial. *Blood* **108** (2006), 3295–3301.

Wilder, R. B., Jones, D., Tucker, S. L. *et al.* Long-term results with radiotherapy for Stage I–II follicular lymphomas. *Int. J. Radiat. Oncol. Biol. Phys.* **51** (2001), 1219–1227.

Witzig, T. E., Gordon, L. I., Cabanillas, F. *et al.* Randomized controlled trial of yttrium-90-labeled ibritumomab tiuxetan radioimmunotherapy versus rituximab immunotherapy for patients with relapsed or refractory low-grade, follicular, or transformed B-cell non-Hodgkin's lymphoma. *J. Clin. Oncol.* **20** (2002), 2453–2463.

MALT LYMPHOMA AND OTHER MARGINAL ZONE LYMPHOMAS

Emanuele Zucca and Francesco Bertoni

Pathology: Andrew Wotherspoon
Molecular cytogenetics: Andreas Rosenwald and German Ott

EXTRANODAL MARGINAL ZONE B-CELL LYMPHOMA (MALT LYMPHOMA): CLINICAL FEATURES

Lymphoma of the mucosa-associated lymphoid tissue (MALT lymphoma) comprises about 7–8% of all non-Hodgkin's lymphomas. It is a neoplasm of adults with a median age at presentation of about 60 years and with a slightly higher proportion of females than males. The presenting symptoms are essentially related to the primary location. Few patients present with elevated lactate dehydrogenase (LDH) or β_2 microglobulin levels. Constitutional B symptoms are extremely uncommon. MALT lymphoma usually remains localized for a prolonged period within the tissue of origin, but dissemination to multiple sites is not uncommon and has been reported in up to one-quarter of cases, with either synchronous or metachronous involvement of multiple mucosal sites or non-mucosal sites such as bone marrow, spleen or liver. Regional lymph nodes can also be involved. Bone-marrow involvement is reported in up to 20% of cases. The stomach is the commonest localization, representing about one-third of the cases. Other typical presentation sites include the salivary glands, the orbit, the thyroid and the lung; the frequency at different organs is shown in Table 9.1.

Within the stomach, MALT lymphoma is often multifocal, possibly explaining the reports of relapses in the gastric stump after surgical excision. Gastric MALT lymphoma can often disseminate to the small intestine and to the splenic marginal zone. Concomitant GI and non-GI involvement can be detected in approximately 10% of cases. Disseminated disease appears to be more common in non-GI MALT lymphomas. It has been postulated that dissemination of

MALT lymphoma may be due to specific expression of special homing receptors or adhesion molecules on the surface of most B cells of mucosa-associated lymphoid tissue, whether normal or transformed.

MALT lymphoma usually has a favorable outcome, with overall survival at five years higher than 85% in most series. Patients at high risk according to the International Prognostic Index (IPI) were found to have a worse prognosis in one retrospective study, whilst other series have reported that those with lymph-node or bone-marrow involvement at presentation, but not those with involvement of multiple mucosal sites, may have a worse prognosis. If initially localized, the disease is generally slow to disseminate. Recurrences may involve either extranodal or nodal sites. The median time to progression has been reported to be better for the GI than for the non-GI lymphomas, but with no significant differences in overall survival between the groups. Localization may have prognostic relevance because of organ-specific clinical problems that determine particular management strategies, but also because of specific local pathogenetic mechanisms, as suggested by the reports of different frequency of different chromosomal translocations at distinct anatomic locations.

In a radiotherapy study from Toronto, gastric and thyroid MALT lymphomas had the best outcome, whereas distant recurrences were more common for other sites. In a multicenter series from the International Extranodal Lymphoma Study Group (IELSG) patients with the disease initially presenting in the upper airways appeared to have a slightly poorer outcome (Table 9.1), but their small number prevents a definitive conclusion. In general, despite

Lymphoma: Pathology, Diagnosis and Treatment, ed. Robert Marcus, John W. Sweetenham and Michael E. Williams. Published by Cambridge University Press. © Cambridge University Press 2007.

Table 9.1. Main clinical features and survival of MALT lymphomas at different presentation sites.

Extranodal site	Frequency	Stage I	Elevated LDH	Nodal involvement	Bone-marrow involvement	Overall survival at 5 years (95% CI)
GI localization						
Stomach	33%	88%	2%	4%	8%	82% (67–91)
Intestine	3–9%	56%	11%	44%	0	100%
Non-GI localization						
Skin	8–10%	82%	9%	0	9%	100%
Ocular adnexa[a]	10–12%	84%	26%	10%	13%	94% (77–98)
Salivary glands	16%	83%	17%	11%	9%	97% (81–100)
Lung	6–10%	60%	27%	27%	7%	100%
Upper airways	5–10%	50%	42%	33%	33%	46% (7–80)
Breast	2–3%	100%	33%	0	0	100%
Thyroid	4%	60%	10%	40%	0	100%
Multiple mucosal sites[b]	9–11%	Not applicable	26	45	33%	77% (43–93)

Derived from Pinotti *et al.* 1997, Thieblemont *et al.* 2000, Zucca *et al.* 2003.

[a] recalculated from the published split data on orbital and conjunctival cases (Zucca *et al.* 2003)

[b] with or without nodal and/or bone marrow involvement

frequent relapses, MALT lymphomas most often have an indolent course. Histologic transformation to large-cell lymphoma is reported in about 10% of the cases, usually late during the course of the disease and independently from dissemination. It is not known whether the incidence of transformation is different at different anatomic sites.

MALT LYMPHOMA: PATHOLOGY

In early cases the neoplastic cells infiltrate around the periphery of lymphoid follicles outside the mantle zone in the region that would normally be occupied by marginal zone B cells (such as are found in the Peyer's patches of the terminal ileum). As the disease progresses the lymphoma may overrun the lymphoid follicles, and residual germinal centers may be difficult to identify, although the lymphoma usually retains at least a focal nodular growth pattern. Even in those cases with preserved lymphoid follicles, colonization of the reactive germinal centers is frequently encountered (Fig. 9.1).

The morphology of the cells is variable, and this cellular variation can be seen within a single lesion. Classically the cells are described as having moderate amounts of cytoplasm with small irregular nuclei, fine chromatin and indistinct nucleoli that resemble the centrocyte of the germinal center. However, the cells may have less abundant cytoplasm and round nuclei resembling small lymphocytes, or may have more abundant cytoplasm with crisp cytoplasmic borders and round nuclei, giving the cell a monocytoid appearance. Plasma cell differentiation is frequent and may be so pronounced as to raise the possibility of a plasma cell neoplasm (Fig. 9.2). Scattered large cells with abundant cytoplasm, vesicular nuclei and prominent nucleoli are present within the infiltrate.

In cells associated with epithelial structures the infiltrate lies between the follicle and the epithelium, and neoplastic cells infiltrate and destroy the epithelial structures to form lymphoepithelial lesions (Fig. 9.3). The disruption of the epithelial structures is associated with morphological changes in the epithelial cells, imparting an eosinophilic appearance to their cytoplasm.

Involved lymph nodes show either a perifollicular infiltrate or, in more advanced cases, a nodular proliferation of similar cells. These cases may mimic nodal MZL.

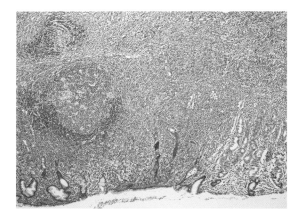

Figure 9.1. Extranodal marginal zone B-cell (MALT) lymphoma (stomach). There is a perifollicular infiltrate of small lymphoid cells with irregular nuclei. Glands are infiltrated and destroyed to form lymphoepithelial lesions.

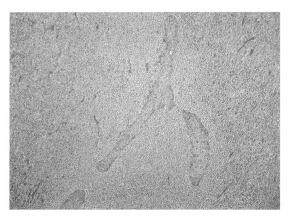

Figure 9.3. Extranodal marginal zone B-cell (MALT) lymphoma (salivary gland). MALT lymphomas at all sites share the common morphological appearance. The cells infiltrate associated epithelial structures to form lymphoepithelial lesions.

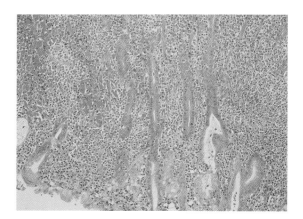

Figure 9.2. Extranodal marginal zone B-cell (MALT) lymphoma (stomach). Some cases show prominent plasma cell differentiation. In this case the plasma cells are distended by accumulated immunoglobulin.

Immunophenotypically these lymphomas express Ig (usually IgM, less often IgA or IgG). The special type of MALT lymphoma occurring in the small intestine (immunoproliferative small intestinal disease, IPSID) shows IgA expression without production of light chain. The lymphocytes express CD20 and CD79a and are usually negative for CD5, CD23, CD10 and cyclin D1. There is expression of bcl-2 protein. A small percentage of cases show expression of CD5, and these may be associated with a more aggressive presentation including a leukemic phase.

MALT lymphomas need to be distinguished from other low-grade lymphomas including follicular lymphoma, mantle cell lymphoma and small lymphocytic lymphoma/B-CLL. This can usually be done by morphological examination and immunophenotypic studies. Distinction from underlying reactive conditions that are known to be precursor lesions to the development of MALT lymphoma (e.g. Hashimoto's thyroiditis in the thyroid and Sjögren's syndrome in the salivary glands) is essential.

MALT LYMPHOMA: MOLECULAR PATHOLOGY AND CYTOGENETICS

The molecular genetic and cytogenetic features of these extranodal lymphomas are in keeping with their marked heterogeneity with respect to morphology, immunophenotype, clinical presentation and clinical outcome.

Extranodal marginal zone B-cell lymphomas of MALT type represent mature B-cell lymphomas with productively rearranged IgH genes. Interestingly, the V_H4, V_H3 and V_H1 family genes known to be involved in autoantibody formation are preferentially used, suggesting a possible derivation from autoreactive B-cell clones. The rearranged IgV_H genes are usually mutated and occasionally show a mutation pattern indicative of selective antigen pressure. Recent studies provide evidence that MALT lymphomas from specific localizations (gastric and salivary gland), in contrast to any other lymphoma subtype, frequently express B-cell receptors with strong homology to the rheumatoid factor (RF). This finding underscores the strong link between chronic antigenic stimulation, autoimmunity and development of MALT lymphomas.

Recurrent genetic aberrations in MALT lymphomas include trisomies of chromosomes 3, 7, 12 and 18, structural abnormalities at 1q21 and 1p34 and translocations t(1;14)(p22;q32), t(11;18)(q21;q21), t(14;18)(q32;q21), t(3;14)(q27;q32) and t(3;14)(p13;q32). In addition, extranodal MALT lymphomas lack translocations common in other low-grade B-cell lymphomas, e.g. t(11;14)(q13;q32), or t(14;18)(q32;q21) affecting *BCL-2*. In some MALT lymphomas, disease progression and high-grade transformation is associated with *MYC* rearrangements and inactivation/deletion of the *TP53* and *$p16^{INK4a}$* genes.

Three translocations, t(1;14)(p22;q32), t(11;18) (q21;q21) and t(14;18)(q32;q21), are of particular interest, since they appear to be specific for this subtype of B-cell lymphoma. In addition, they target a common oncogenic pathway, resulting in nuclear factor kappa B (NF-κB) activation. The translocation t(11;18)(q21;q21) generates a chimeric fusion between the *API2* and *MALT1* genes, whereas translocations t(1;14)(p22;q32) and t(14;18)(q32;q21) result in deregulated expression of *BCL-10* and *MALT1*, respectively, by juxtaposing them to regulatory sequences of the IgH gene cluster. The translocation t(11;18)(q21;q21) is specifically associated with MALT lymphoma and has not been detected in any other lymphoma subtype or in uncomplicated *Helicobacter pylori*-associated gastritis. Cytogenetically, t(11;18) is almost always the sole chromosomal aberration, in contrast to t(11;18)-negative tumors, which often show other alterations such as trisomies 3, 12 and 18 and allelic imbalances. Importantly, gastric MALT lymphomas with t(11;18) do not respond to *Helicobacter pylori* eradication therapy and also rarely undergo high-grade transformation. These data suggest that lymphomas carrying the t(11;18)(q21;q21) may constitute a distinct subgroup of MALT lymphoma that may require specific treatment strategies. On the molecular level, the API2–MALT1 fusion product consists of three BIR (Baculovirus Inhibitor of apoptosis protein Repeat) domains present in the N-terminus of the API2 protein and a variable part of the MALT1 protein, which always contains the caspase-like p20 domain. The chimeric protein API2–MALT1 effectively activates the NF-κB survival pathway in vitro, and it has been proposed that constituents of the BIR domain may mediate the oligomerisation of the API2–MALT1 fusion protein, thereby conferring its ability to activate NF-κB.

The translocations t(1;14)(p22;q32) and t(1;2) (p22;p12) occur in less than 4% of MALT lymphomas. *BCL-10*, the target gene of these translocations, specifically links antigen receptor signaling to the NF-κB pathway. Wild-type bcl-10 protein is expressed in the cytoplasm in normal germinal-center and marginal-zone B cells. MALT lymphomas with translocations t(1;14)(p22;q32) and t(1;2)(p22;p12) show strong nuclear bcl-10 labeling, as is also the case in t(11;18) positive tumors. This suggests that nuclear bcl-10 expression may confer oncogenic activity.

In addition to the t(11;18)(q21;q21), *MALT1* is also targeted by the translocation t(14;18)(q32;q21) and by genomic amplifications. *MALT1* alone is not able to activate NF-κB, but acts synergistically with *BCL-10*. Upon antigen receptor stimulation, a member of the membrane associated guanylate kinase (MAGUK) family of scaffolding proteins such as CARMA1 is recruited to the receptor complex. CARMA1 subsequently recruits bcl-10 and induces its oligomerisation. This is followed by bcl-10-mediated MALT1 oligomerisation, which activates the IκB kinase complex and, through a cascade of events, results in NF-κB activation. Interestingly, t(14;18)(q32;q21)-positive MALT lymphomas co-express bcl-10 and MALT1 protein in the cytoplasm, with perinuclear accumulation of bcl-10. Recently, a novel recurrent translocation, t(3;14)(p13;q32), was reported in MALT lymphomas from different localizations, resulting in the deregulated expression of the *Forkhead Box P1* (*FOXP1*) gene by juxtaposing it to the IgH regulatory elements. In subsequent studies, *FOXP1* translocations were also identified in cases of diffuse large B-cell lymphomas (DLBCL), suggesting that this genetic event may not be confined to MALT lymphomas alone. Interestingly, the frequencies of the translocations t(11;18), t(14;18), t(1;14) and t(3;14), and also the number of cases with numerical aberrations, are clearly differing between tumors arising at different localizations, pointing to the possible importance of local factors influencing the transformation pathways.

Table 9.2. Staging systems for GI-tract lymphoma.

Ann Arbor (Carbone 1971)	Musshof (Musshoff 1977)	Lugano (Rohatiner 1994)	TNM modifications in the Paris system (Ruskone-Fourmestraux 2003)	Lymphoma extension
I_E	I_{E1}	I = confined to GI tract (single primary or	T1m N0 M0	mucosa
I_E	I_{E2}	multiple, non-contiguous)	T1sm N0 M0	submucosa
I_E			T2 N0 M0	muscolaris propria
			T3 N0 M0	serosa
II_E	II_{E1}	II = extending into abdomen	T1-3 N1 M0	perigastric lymph nodes
II_E	II_{E2}	II_1 = local nodal involvement	T1-3 N2 M0	more distant regional nodes
		II_2 = distant nodal involvement	T1-3 N3 M0	extra-abdominal lymph nodes
I_E	I_E	II_E = penetration of serosa to involve adjacent organs or tissues	T4 N0 M0	invasion of adjacent structures
III_E	III_E	IV = disseminated extranodal involvement	T1-4 N3 M0	lymph nodes on both sides of
IV_E	IV_E	or concomitant supradiaphragmatic	T1-4 N0-3 M1	the diaphragm, and/or additional extranodal sites with non-continuous involvement of separate GI site
		nodal involvement		
			T1-4 N0-3 M2	or non-continuous involvement of non-GI sites
			T1-4 N0-3 M0-2 BX	bone marrow not assessed
			T1-4 N0-3 M0-2 B0	bone marrow not involved
			T1-4 N0-3 M2 B1	bone marrow involvement

MALT LYMPHOMA: STAGING

Since patients presenting with lymphoma disseminated at multiple mucosal sites may have a favorable outcome similar to the patients with localized disease, the traditional Ann Arbor staging system, which is mainly based on the extension of nodal areas, is not optimal. Alternative staging systems (Table 9.2) for extranodal lymphomas were proposed in the 1970s, but a general consensus has not yet been achieved.

The main problem in staging patients with MALT lymphoma is the number of extranodal sites to be explored at diagnosis. The finding at pathologic investigations of asymptomatic dissemination in patients with apparently localized disease, and the relatively high proportion of patients with early dissemination, suggests the need for extensive staging procedures in all patients with MALT lymphoma. However, patients with disseminated disease seem to have the same long-term outcome as those with localized disease.

Outside clinical trials, aggressive staging procedures should be tailored to the individual patient according to the clinical conditions (presenting localization, age, intended treatment, performance status, symptoms). Staging procedures should always comprise a complete clinical history and physical examination with a careful evaluation of all lymph-node regions, inspection of the upper airway and tonsils, thyroid examination and clinical evaluation of the size of liver and spleen. Standard chest radiographs and a CT scan of thorax, abdomen and pelvis should be performed. Bone-marrow biopsy must be performed at diagnosis. Laboratory tests should include complete blood counts with cytological examination, LDH and β_2 microglobulin levels, evaluation of renal and liver function, HCV and HIV serology. Then, depending upon the particular

Table 9.3. Site-specific investigations that may be useful for the staging of extranodal lymphomas of MALT type.

Stomach	Gastroduodenal endoscopy with multiple gastric biopsies from all the visible lesions and the non-involved areas with a complete mapping
	Histological and histochemical examination for *H. pylori* (Genta stain or Warthin–Starry stain of antral biopsy specimen) and serology studies if histology results are negative
	FISH for the t(11;18) translocation
	Endoscopic ultrasound
Small intestine (IPSID)	Endoscopy
	Small bowel double-contrast X-ray
	Campylobacter jejuni search in the tumor biopsy by PCR, immunohistochemistry or *in-situ* hybridization
Large intestine	Colonoscopy
	Endoscopic ultrasound
Ocular adnexa	MRI (or CT scan) and ophthalmologic examination
	Chlamydophila psittaci in the tumor biopsy and blood mononuclear cells by PCR
Lung	Bronchoscopy with bronchoalveolar lavage
Salivary gland, tonsils, parotid	ENT examination and ultrasound
Thyroid	Ultrasound ± CT scan of the neck and thyroid function tests
Breast	Mammography and MRI
Skin	*Borrelia burgdorferi* in the tumor biopsy by PCR

FISH, fluorescent in-situ hybridization; PCR, polymerase chain reaction; ENT, ear, nose and throat; CT, computed tomography; MRI, magnetic resonance imaging.

clinical presentation, the investigations should focus on the specific organs suspected of being involved (Table 9.3). We now focus mainly on the diagnosis, staging, and treatment of gastric MALT lymphoma, since the stomach is the commonest and best-known site.

Diagnosis and staging of gastric MALT lymphoma

The most common presenting symptoms of gastric MALT lymphoma are non-specific upper GI complaints (dyspepsia, epigastric pain, nausea and chronic manifestations of gastrointestinal bleeding such as anemia), often leading to an endoscopy that usually reveals non-specific gastritis or peptic ulcer, with mass lesions being unusual. Diagnosis is based on the histopathologic evaluation of the gastric biopsies.

In addition to routine histology and immunohistochemistry, FISH analysis for detection of t(11;18) may be useful for identifying cases that are unlikely to respond to antibiotics.

The best staging system is still controversial. The Ann Arbor staging system, routinely used for non-Hodgkin's lymphoma, was developed for Hodgkin's disease and is not adequate for the specific problems posed by GI-tract lymphomas. A variety of alternative systems have therefore been proposed, and these are summarized in Table 9.2. We have largely used the modification of the Blackledge system known as the "Lugano" staging system. However, this system was proposed before the wide use of endosonography and does not accurately describe the depth of infiltration in the gastric wall, a parameter that is highly predictive for the MALT lymphoma response to anti-*Helicobacter* therapy. There is a general consensus that initial staging procedures should include a gastroduodenal endoscopy, with multiple biopsies from each region of the stomach, duodenum and gastroesophageal junction, as well as from any abnormal-appearing site. Fresh biopsy and washings material should be available for cytogenetic studies in addition to routine histology and immunohistochemistry. The presence of active *H. pylori* infection must be

Table 9.4. Response rate and time needed to document a complete response after antibiotic therapy for Stage I gastric MALT lymphoma.

Author	No. of patients	Staging procedure	CR (%)	Months to CR	No. of relapses
Wotherspoon, 1993	6	US	83	—	—
Savio, 1996	12	CT	84	2–4	0
Pinotti, 1997	45	CT	67	3–18	2
Neubauer, 1997	50	CT ± EUS	80	1–9	5
Nobre Leitao, 1998	17	CT + EUS	100	1–12	1
Steinbach, 1999	23	CT ± EUS	56	3–45	0
Montalban, 2001	19	CT ± EUS	95	2–19	0
Ruskone-Formestraux, 2001	24	CT + EUS	79	2–18	2
Bertoni, 2002	189	CT	56	3–24	15

CR, complete response; US, ultrasound; CT, computed tomography; EUS, endoscopic ultrasound.

determined by histochemistry and breath test; serology studies are recommended when the results of histology are negative. Endoscopic ultrasound is recommended in the initial follow-up for evaluation of depth of infiltration and presence of perigastric lymph nodes. Deep infiltration of the gastric wall is associated with a higher risk of lymph-node involvement, and a lower response rate with antibiotic therapy. Presentation with multiple MALT localizations is more frequent in patients with non-gastrointestinal lymphoma. Staging should include complete blood counts, basic biochemical studies (see above), CT of the chest, abdomen and pelvis, and a bone-marrow biopsy. Although the disease usually remains localized in the stomach, systemic dissemination and bone-marrow involvement should be excluded at presentation, since prognosis is worse with advanced-stage disease or with unfavorable IPI score. Utility of PET scan is controversial.

Staging procedures in non-gastric MALT lymphoma

Significantly more patients with extragastric than with gastric MALT lymphoma present with dissemination to another MALT organ, and a careful initial staging is therefore important. Staging should include basic laboratory studies (see above), total-body CT scans and a bone-marrow biopsy. In addition, the different anatomic sites may require specific procedures, as summarized in Table 9.3.

MALT LYMPHOMA: MANAGEMENT AND FOLLOW-UP

H. pylori eradication in gastric MALT lymphoma

A major change in the management of gastric lymphoma occurred following the identification of *Helicobacter pylori* as the etiologic agent for gastric MALT lymphoma. The therapeutic strategies in primary extranodal low-grade lymphoma used to be based on surgical excision. Surgical resection, often followed by postoperative radiotherapy or chemotherapy, was standard. Eradication of *H. pylori* with antibiotics as the sole initial treatment of localized (i.e. confined to the gastric wall) MALT lymphoma has now become the best-studied therapeutic approach, with more than 20 reported non-randomized studies (Table 9.4). The regression of gastric MALT lymphoma after antibiotic eradication of *H. pylori* was first reported in 1993 by Wotherspoon and colleagues, who described histologic regression following anti-*Helicobacter* therapy in five of six patients with superficially invasive gastric MALT lymphoma. The long-term follow-up of these six patients confirmed the achievement of prolonged lymphoma remissions and also described the occurrence of transient histological and molecular relapses, suggesting that the neoplastic clone can re-expand, but that without the growth stimulus from *H. pylori* this may remain a self-limiting event.

Several groups thereafter confirmed the achievement of durable lymphoma remissions in 60–100% of patients with localized *H. pylori*-positive gastric MALT lymphoma treated with antibiotics. The histologic remission can usually be documented within six months from the *H. pylori* eradication, but sometimes the period required is more prolonged and the therapeutic response may be delayed up to more than one year. Several effective anti-*H. pylori* programs are available. The choice should be based on the epidemiology of the infection in the different countries, taking into account the locally expected antibiotic resistance. The most commonly used regimen is triple therapy with a proton pump inhibitor (e.g. omeprazole, lansoprazole, pantoprazole or esomeprazole) in association with amoxicillin and clarithromycin. Metronidazole can substitute for amoxicillin in penicillin-allergic individuals. Other regimens that include bismuth or H2-receptor antagonists with antibiotics are also effective.

Anti-*Helicobacter* therapy in gastric diffuse large B-cell lymphoma

Anti-*Helicobacter* therapy may be of benefit also in some cases of diffuse large B-cell lymphoma (DLBCL) of the stomach, since in the subset of cases that may have been derived from a MALT lymphoma antibiotics may eliminate a residual or relapsed low-grade component that can be responsible for tumor recurrence following antigen stimulation. Cases of regression of high-grade lesions after anti-*H. pylori* therapy have been reported, suggesting that high-grade transformation is not necessarily associated with the loss of *H. pylori* dependence. However, relying solely on antibiotic therapy for gastric large-cell lymphomas cannot be advised outside clinical trials until large-scale prospective studies have validated its use as first-line therapy, and at present we recommend treating them as localized DLBCL.

Post-treatment histologic evaluation

The interpretation of residual lymphoid infiltrate in post-treatment gastric biopsies can be very difficult,

and there are no uniform criteria in the literature for the definition of histologic remission.

The Wotherspoon score shown in Table 9.5 can be very useful to express the degree of confidence in the MALT lymphoma diagnosis on small gastric biopsies but it is difficult to apply in the evaluation of the response to therapy, and other criteria have been proposed. The lack of standard reproducible criteria can affect the comparison of the results of the different clinical trials. Copie-Bergmann and colleagues have proposed a new (GELA) histological grading system with the aim of providing relevant information to the clinician. This system, which is also summarized in Table 9.5, may become a useful tool if its reproducibility can be confirmed in larger series.

Factors predicting the lymphoma response to *H. pylori* eradication

Endoscopic ultrasound can be useful to predict the lymphoma response to *H. pylori* eradication. There is a significant difference between the response rates of lymphomas restricted to the gastric mucosa and those with less superficial lesions. The response rate is highest for the mucosa-confined lymphomas (approximately 70–90%) and then decreases markedly and progressively for the tumors infiltrating the submucosa, the muscularis propria and the serosa. In cases with documented nodal involvement the response is highly unlikely. Nearly all gastric lymphomas with the t(11;18) translocation will not respond to *Helicobacter pylori* eradication therapy, and presence of the t(11;18) translocation can therefore predict the therapeutic response of gastric MALT lymphoma to antibiotics, although not necessarily to other therapeutic approaches such as chemotherapy or immunotherapy. Moreover, the cases carrying this translocation rarely undergo high-grade transformation and have been reported to have a significantly longer relapse-free survival irrespective of treatment modality. There are no large-scale studies to suggest the utility of any specific treatment strategy in this subgroup. *Helicobacter pylori* eradication may have some benefit on symptoms, but is usually unable to induce a lymphoma regression. The treatment of antibiotic-resistant gastric MALT lymphoma, as discussed later, is a controversial issue, with no evidence to suggest that one therapeutic approach is better than another.

Table 9.5. The Wotherspoon and GELA systems for the histological evaluation of gastric MALT lymphoma endoscopic biopsies.

Wotherspoon's score (for diagnosis and post-treatment evaluation)

0	Normal	Scattered plasma cells in LP
1	Chronic active gastritis	Small clusters of lymphocytes in LP, no lymphoid follicles, no LEL
2	Chronic active gastritis with lymphoid follicles	Prominent lymphoid follicles with surrounding mantle zone and plasma cells, no LEL
3	Suspicious lymphoid infiltrate, probably reactive	Lymphoid follicles surrounded by small lymphocytes that infiltrate diffusely in LP and occasionally into epithelium
4	Suspicious lymphoid infiltrate, probably lymphoma	Lymphoid follicles surrounded by centrocyte-like cells that infiltrate diffusely in LP and into epithelium in small groups
5	Low-grade MALT lymphoma	Dense diffuse infiltrate of centrocyte-like cells in LP with prominent LEL

GELA grading score (for post-treatment evaluation)

CR	Complete histological remission	Normal or empty LP and/or fibrosis with absent or scattered plasma cells and small lymphoid cells in the LP, no LEL
pMRD	Probable minimal residual disease	Empty LP and/or fibrosis with aggregates of lymphoid cells or lymphoid nodules in the LP/MM and/or SM, no LEL
rRD	Responding residual disease	Focal empty LP and/or fibrosis with dense, diffuse or nodular lymphoid infiltrate, extending around glands in the LP, focal or absent LEL
NC	No change	Dense, diffuse or nodular lymphoid infiltrate, LEL usually present

LEL, lymphoepithelial lesions; Lp, lamina propria; MM, muscolaris mucosa; SM, submucosa.

Clinical and molecular follow-up

A number of molecular follow-up studies have shown that post-antibiotic histological and endoscopic remission does not necessarily mean a cure. The long-term persistence of monoclonal B cells after histologic regression of the lymphoma has been reported in about half of the cases, suggesting that *H. pylori* eradication suppresses but does not eradicate the lymphoma clones. Transient histological and molecular relapses have been reported during long-term follow-up of antibiotic-treated patients, but without the stimulus from *H. pylori* this usually remains a self-limiting event and does not imply a frank clinical progression. The clinical relevance of the detection of monoclonal B cells by molecular methods remains unclear. In the long-term follow-up of some cases with minimal residual disease neither lymphoma clinical growth nor histological transformation was documented despite persistent clonality, suggesting that a watch-and-wait policy could be feasible and safe, and these patients do not necessarily require additional treatment. On the other hand, cases of lymphoma recurrence following *H. pylori* reinfection have been reported, suggesting that residual dormant tumor cells can be present despite histological remission. Relapses have also been documented in the absence of *H. pylori* reinfection, indicating the presence of lymphoma clones that may have escaped the antigenic drive. Histological transformation into DLBCL has also been described in some cases. Regular follow-up is strongly advised, and histological evaluation of repeated biopsies continues to be the fundamental follow-up procedure. We perform a breath test two months after treatment to document *H. pylori* eradication and repeat post-treatment endoscopies with multiple biopsies every six months for two years, then yearly to monitor the histological regression of the lymphoma.

Management of *H. pylori*-negative or antibiotic-resistant cases

No definite guidelines exist for the management of the subset of *H. pylori*-negative cases, and for the patients who fail antibiotic therapy. There are no published randomized studies to help the treatment choice. In two retrospective series of patients with gastric low-grade MALT lymphoma, no statistically significant difference was apparent in survival between patients who received different initial treatments (including chemotherapy alone, surgery alone, surgery with additional chemotherapy or radiation therapy, or antibiotics against *H. pylori*).

A modest dose of involved-field radiotherapy (30 Gy given in four weeks to the stomach and perigastric nodes) gives excellent disease control and it might be the treatment of choice for patients with stage I–II MALT lymphoma of the stomach without evidence of *H. pylori* infection, or with persistent lymphoma after antibiotics.

Surgery has been widely and successfully used in the past. It leads to excellent long-term local control, but its role should be redefined in view of the promising results of the conservative approach. Whether stage I patients treated with radical gastrectomy need further treatment is unclear, but a wait-and-see policy is most often appropriate.

Patients with systemic disease should be considered for systemic treatment (i.e. chemotherapy and/or immunotherapy with anti-CD20 monoclonal antibodies). In the presence of disseminated or advanced disease, chemotherapy is an obvious choice, but only a few compounds and regimens have been tested specifically in MALT lymphomas. Oral alkylating agents (either cyclophosphamide or chlorambucil, with median treatment duration of one year) can result in a high rate of disease control. Phase II studies have demonstrated some anti-tumor activity of the purine analogs fludarabine and cladribine, which might however be associated with an increased risk of secondary MDS, and of a combination regimen of chlorambucil/mitoxantrone/prednisone. Aggressive anthracycline-containing chemotherapy should be reserved for patients with high tumor burden (bulky masses, high IPI score). The activity of the anti-CD20 monoclonal antibody rituximab has also been demonstrated in a phase II study (with a response rate of about 70%), and this may represent an additional option for the treatment of systemic disease. The efficacy of the combination of rituximab with chemotherapy is being explored in a randomized study of the IELSG.

Similar considerations may apply to the treatment of patients relapsing after an initial lymphoma response to antibiotics. Local relapses may benefit from involved-field radiotherapy, while systemic relapses may require systemic treatment.

Management of non-gastric localizations

MALT lymphomas have been described in various non-gastrointestinal sites, such as salivary glands, thyroid, skin, conjunctiva, orbit, larynx, lung, breast, kidney, liver, prostate and even the intracranial dura. In general, MALT lymphoma arises in mucosal sites where lymphocytes are not normally present and where a MALT is acquired in response either to autoimmune processes such as Hashimoto's thyroiditis and Sjögren's syndrome or to chronic infectious conditions. *Helicobacter pylori* gastritis is the best-studied condition, but other infectious agents have more recently been implicated in the pathogenesis of MALT lymphomas arising in the skin (*Borrelia burgdorferi*), in the ocular adnexa (*Chlamydophila psittaci*) and in the small intestine (*Campylobacter jejuni*). Among viruses, the involvement of HCV infection in the development of some marginal zone lymphomas (especially the splenic type) has been recently proposed.

Non-gastric MALT lymphomas have been difficult to characterize because these tumors are distributed so widely throughout the body that it is difficult to assemble adequate series of any given site. One-quarter of non-gastrointestinal MALT lymphomas have been reported to present with involvement of multiple mucosal sites or non-mucosal sites such as bone marrow. Non-gastrointestinal MALT lymphomas, despite presenting with stage IV disease more often than the gastric variant, frequently have a quite indolent course regardless of treatment type, but they are significantly more prone to relapse than the primary gastric cases (most often at other mucosal sites). A multicenter retrospective survey of 180 non-gastric cases showed no evidence of a clear advantage for any type of therapy and, despite the high proportion of cases with disseminated disease, which should require systemic therapy, no clear advantage was associated with any chemotherapy program.

In general, the treatment of non-gastric MALT lymphoma can be approached in the same way as that of the *H. pylori*-negative cases described above. The sole use of moderate-dose radiotherapy for the patients with localized disease results in a high rate of local

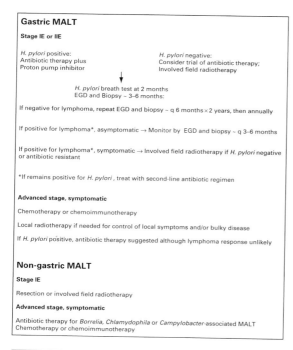

Gastric MALT

Stage IE or IIE

H. pylori positive:
Antibiotic therapy plus
Proton pump inhibitor

H. pylori negative:
Consider trial of antibiotic therapy;
Involved field radiotherapy

H. pylori breath test at 2 months
EGD and Biopsy ~ 3–6 months:

If negative for lymphoma, repeat EGD and biopsy ~ q 6 months×2 years, then annually

If positive for lymphoma*, asymptomatic → Monitor by EGD and biopsy ~ q 3–6 months

If positive for lymphoma*, symptomatic → Involved field radiotherapy if H. pylori negative
or antibiotic resistant

*If remains positive for H. pylori , treat with second-line antibiotic regimen

Advanced stage, symptomatic

Chemotherapy or chemoimmunotherapy

Local radiotherapy if needed for control of local symptoms and/or bulky disease

If H. pylori positive, antibiotic therapy suggested although lymphoma response unlikely

Non-gastric MALT

Stage IE

Resection or involved field radiotherapy

Advanced stage, symptomatic

Antibiotic therapy for Borrelia, Chlamydophila or Campylobacter-associated MALT
Chemotherapy or chemoimmunotherapy

Figure 9.4. Treatment algorithm for MALT lymphoma.

control and often cure. Effective radiotherapy is frequently possible for both common and rare presentations of the disease. Side effects of RT are mild and reversible. For patients with localized non-gastric MALT lymphoma, given the unique biologic behavior with a tendency to relapse in MALT tissues and an indolent course, RT is often the first-line treatment of choice. The emerging literature on localized MALT lymphomas confirms a high rate of local control in MALT lymphoma, with a high proportion of patients likely to be cured of the disease. The moderate doses of radiation required for cure (25–35 Gy) are generally associated with a minimal risk of long-term toxicity, although special considerations are needed for particular localizations such as the eye or the lung.

For some patients with stage III or IV disease, radiotherapy can also be an effective therapy in providing local disease control, but the optimal management of disseminated MALT lymphomas is less clearly defined. Because no curative treatment exists, expectant observation can be an adequate initial policy in most patients. In general, the treatment should be "patient-tailored," taking into account the site, the stage and the clinical characteristics of the individual patient. Systemic antibiotic treatment should be

tried first in patients with *B. burgdorferi*-associated cutaneous lymphomas. Similarly, the finding that *C. psittaci* is associated with MALT lymphoma of the ocular adnexa may provide the rationale for the antibiotic treatment of localized lesions, and preliminary encouraging results have been reported, but this approach remains investigational and will need to be confirmed by larger clinical studies.

A treatment algorithm for MALT lymphoma is shown in Fig. 9.4.

IMMUNOPROLIFERATIVE SMALL INTESTINAL DISEASE (IPSID)

This condition, known in the past as alpha-heavy-chain disease or Mediterranean lymphoma, is nowadays considered a special subtype of MALT lymphoma. The distinguishing feature of IPSID is the synthesis of alpha heavy chain that is secreted and detectable in the serum, urine, saliva and duodenal fluid in approximately two-thirds of cases; in the remainder, the protein is demonstrable by immuno-histochemistry but not secreted. Most of the cases have been described in the Middle East, especially in the Mediterranean area, where the disease is endemic, affecting young adults of both sexes, but predominantly males. A few cases have been reported from industrialized Western countries, usually among immigrants from the endemic area. The natural course of IPSID is usually prolonged, often over many years, including a potentially reversible early phase, with the disease usually confined to the abdomen. If untreated it degenerates, with high-grade transformation, into large B-cell lymphoma. Since the histology of mucosal lesions and mesenteric lymph nodes can be discordant, with a higher grade in the latter, staging laparotomy can be useful in the evaluation of the mesenteric nodal involvement, but surgery has no therapeutic role due to a generally diffuse intestinal involvement. It has been known since the 1970s that early IPSID phases could achieve durable remissions with sustained antibiotic treatment (such as tetracycline or metronidazole and ampicillin for at least six months). Recently, the presence of *Campylobacter jejuni* has been demonstrated in IPSID tumor sections. At an early stage, antibiotic treatment directed against *C. jejuni* may lead to lymphoma regression, but there is no clear evidence that antibiotics alone are of benefit in the advanced phases. Although the early studies reported that aggressive chemotherapy is not well tolerated by patients with advanced disease and severe malabsorption, anthracycline-containing regimens, combined with nutritional support plus antibiotics to control diarrhea and malabsorption, may offer the best chance of cure, with five-year survival rates up to 70 percent.

PRIMARY SPLENIC MARGINAL ZONE LYMPHOMA

Clinical features

Splenic marginal zone lymphoma (splenic MZL) is a very rare disorder, comprising less than 1% of all lymphomas. Up to two-thirds of the patients with splenic MZL have circulating villous lymphocytes with characteristic fine short cytoplasm polar projections. When these are more than 20% of the lymphocyte count, the term "splenic lymphoma with villous lymphocytes" is commonly used. Despite relevant geographical variations, hepatitis C virus (HCV) seems to be involved in lymphomagenesis of a portion of cases. An association with malaria and with EBV infection has been shown in tropical Africa, and the tropical cases are characterized by a high percentage of circulating villous lymphocytes.

Most patients with primary splenic MZL are over 50, with a similar incidence in males and females. The disease usually presents with massive splenomegaly, which produces abdominal discomfort and pain. Diagnosis is often made at splenectomy, performed to establish the cause of unexplained splenic enlargement. B symptoms are not uncommon: anemia, thrombocytopenia or leukocytosis are reported in one-quarter of cases. Autoimmune hemolytic anemia can be found in up to 15% of patients. Involvement of the splenic hilar lymph nodes and/or the liver is reported in 25–30% of cases.

According to the WHO classification peripheral lymph-node involvement is typically absent. However, patients with disseminated marginal zone lymphomas can be seen and a precise diagnosis can be very difficult in cases presenting with concomitant splenic, extranodal and nodal involvement. In a retrospective French series of 124 patients with non-MALT-type marginal zone lymphoma four clinical subtypes were observed: splenic (48% of cases), nodal (30%), disseminated (splenic and nodal, 16%) and leukemic (neither splenic nor nodal, 6%). Even when the disease is restricted to cases presenting with splenomegaly, nearly all patients have bone-marrow involvement, often accompanied by involvement of peripheral blood (defined as the presence of absolute lymphocytosis of more than 5%). Serum paraproteinemia is observed in about 10–25% of cases and is most frequently of IgM type, posing the problem of differential diagnosis with lymphoplasmacytic lymphoma/Waldenström's macroglobulinemia. The two diseases often present with similar clinical features (splenomegaly, bone-marrow lymphoplasmacytic infiltration, anemia), but marked hyperviscosity and hypergammaglobulinemia are uncommon in splenic MZL. The clinical course is most usually indolent with five-year overall survival ranging from 65% to 80%. Histological transformation is rare, often associated with B symptoms, disease dissemination and poorer outcome. A prognostic model for clinical use was recently proposed, based on the results of a large cooperative retrospective study of 309 patients from Italy. Using three readily available parameters, hemoglobin less than 120 g/L, LDH higher than normal and serum albumin less than 35 g/L, three prognostic groups can be identified: low-risk patients (five-year cause-specific survival 88%) with no adverse factors, intermediate-risk patients (five-year cause-specific survival 73%) with one adverse factor and high-risk patients (five-year cause-specific survival 50%) with two or three adverse factors.

Pathology

Splenic MZL usually presents with splenomegaly and absent peripheral nodal involvement. In the spleen the disease is predominantly within the white pulp, with a less pronounced nodular and interstitial infiltration of the red pulp. The white pulp is partially or completely effaced by the neoplastic cells. These areas show an inner zone of small lymphocytes resembling mantle cells that either surround residual germinal centers or, more commonly, replace them. Around this small cell layer there is a further zone composed of slightly larger cells that have more abundant cytoplasm. Large transformed cells with more abundant cytoplasm and vesicular nuclei that contain nucleoli are scattered within the outer layer. Plasma cell differentiation may occur. The red-pulp nodules are frequently composed of cells resembling those of the inner zone of the white pulp (Fig. 9.5).

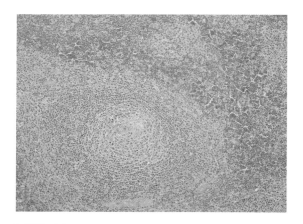

Figure 9.5. Splenic marginal zone B-cell lymphoma (spleen). The white pulp shows infiltration by a population of lymphoid cells that surround residual reactive germinal centers with a biphasic pattern. There is an inner rim of cells with scanty cytoplasm and an outer rim of cells with larger nuclei and more abundant cytoplasm. Scattered larger cells are seen in the outer layer. The red pulp contains small nodular aggregates of lymphoma cells.

Spread to the lymph nodes of the spleen hilum is frequent. These nodes may show a nodular pattern based on pre-existing follicles or may show a zoned appearance similar to that seen in the splenic white pulp.

The bone marrow shows interstitial infiltration by small lymphocytes, usually with a nodular component. In the interstitium cells can frequently be seen within sinusoids, although this pattern is not specific to splenic MZL.

The cells show sIg, usually IgM and IgD. They express CD20 and CD79a and are usually negative for CD5, CD23, CD10 and cyclin D1. There is expression of bcl-2 protein. Proliferation shows a characteristic pattern, with infrequent cells staining for Ki67/MIB1 in the inner, small-cell zone and scattered cells positive in the outer zone.

Splenic marginal zone lymphomas have to be distinguished from other small B-cell lymphomas, almost all of which can adopt an organizational pattern that mimics that of splenic MZL. This can usually be accomplished by immunocytochemical studies.

Molecular pathology and cytogenetics

Splenic marginal zone B-cell lymphoma is a relatively newly recognized lymphoma entity, whose precise molecular pathogenesis is largely unknown. Recent studies indicate that these tumors may harbor unmutated or mutated IgV$_H$ genes, thus being derived from naive or antigen-experienced B cells. The pattern of IgV$_H$ gene usage (biased usage of V$_H$1–2 gene family) and the finding of somatic hypermutations in some cases suggest an antigen-driven lymphomagenesis. In line with these findings, a possible relationship between HCV infection and splenic MZL has recently been established. Cytogenetic and molecular genetic studies have demonstrated that approximately 45% of splenic MZLs harbor allelic losses in the 7q32–q33 chromosome region, and these cases are possibly more aggressive clinically. Other cytogenetic alterations include trisomies 3, 5 and 18, +9q, +12q, +20q, and translocations t(10;14)(q24;q32), t(6;14)(p12;q32) and t(2;7)(p12;q22) with deregulation of Cyclin D3 and CDK6. Recent gene expression profiling studies have confirmed the homogeneity of this disease entity at the molecular level and point to different pathways that may be involved in lymphomagenesis. The molecular signature of splenic ZML includes upregulation of several genes involved in NF-κB activation, B-cell receptor and tumor necrosis factor (TNF) signaling, and of genes associated with the splenic microenvironment (*SELL*, *LPXN*). Genes located in the 7q31–7q32 deletion region have been reported to be downregulated.

Management

The reported largest series show that most patients can initially be managed with a wait-and-see policy, and they do not seem to have a worse outcome. When treatment is needed this is usually because of large symptomatic splenomegaly or cytopenia. Splenectomy appears to be the treatment of choice: it allows a reduction/disappearance of circulating tumor lymphocytes and recovery of the lymphoma-associated cytopenia. The benefit of splenectomy often persists for several years and time to next treatment can be longer than five years. Adjuvant chemotherapy after splenectomy may result in a higher rate of complete response, but there is no evidence of a survival benefit.

Chemotherapy alone may be considered for patients who require treatment but have contraindications to splenectomy, and for the patient with clinical progression after spleen removal. Alkylating agents (chlorambucil or cyclophosphamide) have been reported to be active and can be used as single agents or in combination (as in the CVP and CHOP regimens). Among the purine analogues, fludarabine has been shown to be effective but, curiously, cladribine seems not to be active. Rituximab, alone or in combination with chemotherapy, induces good responses in cases refractory to standard chemotherapy. Very interesting is the observation from one study that some patients with splenic lymphoma with villous lymphocytes and HCV infection obtained a complete response after treatment with interferon alpha, alone or in combination with ribavirine. Interferon treatment had no anti-tumor effect on HCV-negative splenic lymphomas. Analogous to *H. pylori* infection in gastric MZL, it appears that HCV may be responsible for an antigen-driven stimulation of the lymphoma clone. This report suggests that all the cases should be tested for HCV infection, and antiviral therapy should be considered in the positive cases before any decision is reached about more aggressive therapeutic approaches.

NODAL MARGINAL ZONE LYMPHOMA

Clinical features

In contrast with mucosa-based extranodal MALT lymphoma, nodal marginal zone (previously known as monocytoid lymphoma) lymphoma is typically lymph-node-based. This type of lymphoma is exceedingly rare, accounting for less than 10% of all marginal zone lymphomas and less than 1% of all non-Hodgkin's lymphomas. It also has been associated with HCV infection in some epidemiologic studies. The clinical data are sparse and have been largely drawn from pathologic series rather than clinical ones. Nodal MZL is a disease of older people, with the median age at presentation in the sixth decade, and affects both sexes, with a slight female predominance.

The commonest presenting feature is a localized – most often in the neck – or sometimes a generalized adenopathy. Bone marrow is involved at presentation in less than half of the cases. Transformation to high-grade lymphoma has been described in some cases.

Pathology and genetics

The histologic pattern of lymph-node involvement by primary nodal MZL is often indistinguishable from that of extranodal MZL of MALT type, and this lymphoma has previously been thought to be a nodal variety of MALT lymphoma. The tumor cell morphology is heterogeneous and is similar to the lymph-node involvement of extranodal MZL and splenic MZL. Sometimes the tumor cells resemble monocytes; indeed, the term monocytoid lymphoma was used in the past to indicate this type of lymphoma.

Analysis of the IgH genes suggests a prevalence of cases with mutated IgH genes, but, similarly to splenic MZL, unmutated cases do exist. No specific genomic aberration is known to occur in nodal MZL. The most common alterations, such as gain of 3q, are also present in extranodal MZL and splenic MZL.

Management

Because no curative treatment exists, most patients can be initially managed with expectant observation. There is at present no consensus about the best treatment, individual cases being managed differently according to site and stage. Treatment options may include single-agent chlorambucil or fludarabine or combination chemotherapy regimens (such as CVP or CHOP). Rituximab may also have some efficacy and can be combined with chemotherapy. Anti-HCV treatment may induce lymphoma regression in some HCV-infected patients. Autologous stem-cell transplantation has been used in younger patients with adverse prognostic factors or with increased large-cell numbers.

FURTHER READING

Arcaini, L., Lazzarino, M., Colombo, N. *et al.* Splenic marginal zone lymphoma: a prognostic model for clinical use. *Blood* **107** (2006), 4643–4649.

Berger, F., Felman, P., Thieblemont, C. *et al.* Non-MALT marginal zone B-cell lymphomas: a description of clinical presentation and outcome in 124 patients. *Blood* **95** (2000), 1950–1956.

Bertoni, F. and Zucca, E. State-of-the-art therapeutics: marginal-zone lymphoma. *J. Clin. Oncol.* **23** (2005), 6415–6420.

Bertoni, F., Conconi, A., Capella, C. *et al.* Molecular follow-up in gastric mucosa-associated lymphoid tissue lymphomas: early analysis of the LY03 cooperative trial. *Blood* **99** (2002), 2541–2544.

Chen, L. T., Lin, J. T., Tai, J. J. *et al.* Long-term results of anti-*Helicobacter pylori* therapy in early-stage gastric high-grade transformed MALT lymphoma. *J. Natl. Cancer Inst.* **97** (2005), 1345–1353.

Conconi, A., Cavalli, F. and Zucca, E. MALT lymphomas: the role of chemotherapy. In *MALT Lymphomas*, ed. E. Zucca and F. Bertoni (Georgetown, TX: Landes/Kluwer, 2004) pp. 99–103.

Copie-Bergman, C., Gaulard, P., Lavergne-Slove, A. *et al.* Proposal for a new histological grading system for post-treatment evaluation of gastric MALT lymphoma. *Gut* **52** (2003), 1656.

Lecuit, M., Abachin, E., Martin, A. *et al.* Immunoproliferative small intestinal disease associated with *Campylobacter jejuni*. *N. Engl. J. Med.* **350** (2004), 239–248.

Martinelli, G., Laszlo, D., Ferreri, A. J. *et al.* Clinical activity of rituximab in gastric marginal zone non-Hodgkin's lymphoma resistant to or not eligible for anti-*Helicobacter pylori* therapy. *J. Clin. Oncol.* **23** (2005), 1979–1983.

Mollejo, M., Camacho, F. I., Algara, P., Ruiz-Ballesteros, E., Garcia, J. F. and Piris, M. A. Nodal and splenic marginal zone B cell lymphomas. *Hematol. Oncol.* **23** (2005), 108–118.

Pinotti, G., Zucca, E., Roggero, E. *et al.* Clinical features, treatment and outcome in a series of 93 patients with low-grade gastric MALT lymphoma. *Leuk. Lymphoma* **26** (1997), 527–537.

Ruskone-Fourmestraux, A., Dragosics, B., Morgner, A., Wotherspoon, A. and De Jong, D. Paris staging system for primary gastrointestinal lymphomas. *Gut* **52** (2003), 912–913.

Thieblemont, C. and Coiffier, B. MALT lymphoma: sites of presentations, clinical features and staging procedures. In *MALT Lymphomas*, ed. E. Zucca and F. Bertoni (Georgetown, TX: Landes/Kluwer, 2004) pp. 60–80.

Thieblemont, C., Berger, F., Dumontet, C. *et al.* Mucosa-associated lymphoid tissue lymphoma is a disseminated disease in one third of 158 patients analyzed. *Blood* **95** (2000), 802–806.

Thieblemont, C., Felman, P., Callet-Bauchu, E. *et al.* Splenic marginal-zone lymphoma: a distinct clinical and pathological entity. *Lancet Oncol.* **4** (2003), 95–103.

Tsang, R. W. and Gospodarowicz, M. K. Radiation therapy for localized low-grade non-Hodgkin's lymphomas. *Hematol. Oncol.* **23** (2005), 10–17.

Wenzel, C., Dieckmann, K., Fiebeger, W., Mannhalter, C., Chott, A. and Raderer, M. CD5 expression in a lymphoma of the mucosa-associated lymphoid tissue (MALT)-type as a marker for early dissemination and aggressive clinical behaviour. *Leuk. Lymphoma* **42** (2001), 823–829.

Wotherspoon, A. C. and Savio, A. Molecular follow-up in gastric MALT lymphomas. In *MALT Lymphomas*, ed E. Zucca and F. Bertoni (Georgetown, TX: Landes/Kluwer, 2004) pp. 91–98.

Zucca, E. and Cavalli, F. Are antibiotics the treatment of choice for gastric lymphoma? *Curr. Hematol. Rep.* **3** (2004), 11–16.

Zucca, E., Bertoni, F., Roggero, E. and Cavalli, F. The gastric marginal zone B-cell lymphoma of MALT type. *Blood* **96** (2000), 410–419.

Zucca, E., Conconi, A., Pedrinis, E. *et al.* Nongastric marginal zone B-cell lymphoma of mucosa-associated lymphoid tissue. *Blood* **101** (2003), 2489–2495.

10 SMALL LYMPHOCYTIC LYMPHOMA AND ITS VARIANTS

Peter Hillmen

Pathology: Andrew Wotherspoon
Molecular cytogenetics: Andreas Rosenwald and German Ott

INTRODUCTION

Small lymphocytic lymphoma (SLL) and chronic lymphocytic leukemia (CLL) are in the midst of a period of huge change due to advances on several fronts. One important development is the appreciation that SLL and CLL are two manifestations of the same disorder. Throughout this review, therefore, it should be assumed that SLL is managed in a similar manner to CLL, though the studies drawn upon and recommendations made will be based mainly on publications on the diagnosis and therapy for CLL.

There have been major advances in our understanding both of the pathophysiology of CLL/SLL and of the mechanism by which the disease becomes resistant to conventional therapies. This has coincided with the application of novel approaches to define remissions including the use of modern imaging techniques, which have never previously been applied in CLL, and the development of techniques to detect minimal residual disease, particularly by multi-parameter flow cytometry. To some extent a major driver of these changes has been the development of novel therapeutic approaches which yield higher proportions of complete remissions. We have now moved from standard therapies which achieve complete responses in less than 10% of patients to novel approaches which result in greater than 70% complete responses. There is now the prospect of achieving response rates which for other hematopoietic malignancies are associated with a prolongation in survival – and even cures! Treatment paradigms are evolving rapidly towards risk stratification by molecular prognostic factors and tailoring therapy to an individual patient's disease. These changes have largely happened over the last five years, and this rapidity

of movement results in two principal problems: firstly, randomized clinical trials cannot be performed rapidly enough to address the wide variety of relevant questions, and secondly, the application of these modern tests is not straightforward, neither in their availability in most health economies nor in their application to clinical practice. It is not unreasonable to believe, however, that considering a curative intent for more than just a small minority of patients is now a realistic prospect. The current and future management of patients with CLL will require treatment stratification by individual patient risk, the application of techniques to detect minimal residual disease and the intelligent use of the variety of novel therapies that are currently being developed. In this chapter I will review the recent changes in our understanding of CLL as they impact on treatment and the results of recent trials which define the gold-standard therapeutic approach, as well as the questions that are being addressed in the current series of clinical studies.

PATHOLOGY

B-cell small lymphocytic lymphoma/ chronic lymphocytic leukemia

The lymph-node architecture is effaced by a diffuse proliferation of small lymphocytes that have scanty cytoplasm and round nuclei with minimal nuclear irregularity (Figs. 10.1, 10.2). The chromatin is clumped and nucleoli are not seen. Within the small-cell population are scattered larger cells which are frequently clustered into discrete areas that appear pale when the node is examined at low power. These are termed proliferation centers or pseudofollicles and contain a mixture of intermediate-sized

Lymphoma: Pathology, Diagnosis and Treatment, ed. Robert Marcus, John W. Sweetenham and Michael E. Williams. Published by Cambridge University Press. © Cambridge University Press 2007.

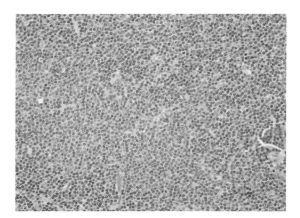

Figure 10.1. B-cell small lymphocytic lymphoma/chronic lymphocytic leukemia (lymph node). The nodal architecture is effaced by a diffuse proliferation of small cells with scanty cytoplasm and round nuclei. Occasional larger cells are present singly and in small groups (proliferation centres/pseudofollicles).

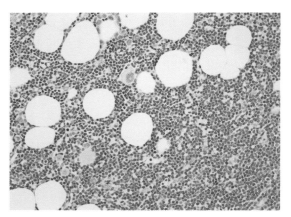

Figure 10.2. B-cell small lymphocytic lymphoma/chronic lymphocytic leukemia (bone marrow). There is an infiltrate of small lymphocytes in the bone marrow with a nodular and interstitial growth pattern.

cells with round nuclei and central eosinophilic nucleoli (prolymphocytes) and large cells with a moderate amount of pale cytoplasm, oval nuclei and large central eosinophilic nucleoli (paraimmunoblasts). In some cases residual normal germinal centers may be seen entrapped within the diffuse lymphomatous proliferation. A proportion of cases may show plasmacytic differentiation.

Immunophenotypically the cells show sIg of IgM type, usually with co-expression of IgD. The cells are positive for CD20 (although this can be weak) and CD79a. The majority of cases show expression of CD5, CD43 and CD23 but without staining for cyclin D1 or CD10. A proportion of cases may lack CD23 or, rarely, CD5. Staining for bcl-2 protein is invariably positive. Proliferation is low and, where present, is usually most prominent in the proliferation centers.

Lymphoplasmacytic lymphoma

In the early stages the lymphoma has an interfollicular growth pattern with sparing of the sinuses, but this may efface the underlying nodal architecture to become diffuse. This lymphoma is composed of a polymorphous mixture of cells including small lymphocytes, cells with plasmacytoid features, classical plasma cells and scattered large cells with abundant cytoplasm and large nuclei that contain nucleoli. Scattered small lymphocytes or plasma cells may

contain intranuclear eosinophilic (usually PAS+) pseudo-inclusions (Dütcher bodies).

These lymphomas are distinguished from other B-cell lymphomas that can show plasma cell differentiation by the lack of neoplastic follicles, proliferation centers and monocytoid/marginal zone cells.

Immunophenotypically the cells have sIg with a proportion of cells containing Ig in the cytoplasm – usually IgM. They are positive for CD20 and CD79a and lack CD5, CD23, CD10 and cyclin D1. They usually express bcl-2 protein.

B-cell prolymphocytic leukemia (B-PLL)

Lymph nodes are not usually enlarged in this lymphoproliferation, and the histopathology usually relates to the appearances within the spleen and bone marrow. In the bone marrow there is infiltration of the interstitium with a non-paratrabecular distribution. In the spleen the red and white pulp is effaced by a diffuse population of cells that are larger than normal lymphocytes. There is moderately abundant cytoplasm, and the nuclei contain single central eosinophilic nucleoli.

Immunophenotypically the cells are positive for CD20 and CD79a. There is variable expression of CD5, and CD23 is usually negative. The cells do not express CD10. Distinction between true B-PLL and a nucleolated version of mantle cell lymphoma that presents in leukemic phase is important. True B-PLL is negative for cyclin D1, while this protein is expressed in the nuclei of nucleolated mantle cell lymphoma.

MOLECULAR PATHOLOGY AND CYTOGENETICS

Chronic lymphocytic leukemia of B-cell lineage (B-CLL) does not seem to constitute a homogeneous genetic entity. In particular, recent molecular studies investigating the occurrence of somatic hypermutations in the variable regions of the immunoglobulin heavy chain (IgV$_H$) genes provide evidence that B-CLL may consist of at least two important subgroups. In roughly 50% of cases, the tumor cells do not display somatic mutations and, hence, are derived from B cells that have not undergone a germinal-center reaction. In the remaining cases somatic mutations are present, indicating a germinal-center passage of the tumor cells. The IgV$_H$-mutated form of B-CLL clearly is associated with a better prognosis. In contrast to many other B-cell non-Hodgkin's lymphomas, reciprocal chromosome translocations are not a frequent feature in B-CLL, although the t(1;6)(p35;p25) has recently been identified as a recurrent translocation in rare cases. While translocations appear to be uncommon in B-CLL, chromosomal imbalances at several loci characterize this leukemia on the genetic level. In particular, frequent aberrations include deletions in chromosomal band 13q14, detected in up to 40% of cases, trisomy 12, and deletions in 17p13 and 11q22–23. Deletions in 17p frequently target the *TP53* gene and 11q deletions commonly result in the loss of one copy of the *ATM (ataxia-telangiectasia mutated)* gene. Both aberrations have been shown to be of prognostic significance in defining patient subgroups with inferior prognosis and are commonly found in the IgV$_H$-unmutated B-CLL variant.

Despite the presence of IgV$_H$-mutated and IgV$_H$-unmutated B-CLL subsets, there is evidence from DNA microarray studies that the two B-CLL subgroups share a homogeneous gene expression profile. B-CLL, therefore, can be viewed as a single entity with a distinct transcriptional profile distinguishing it from other low-grade lymphomas. One major new finding derived from gene expression profiling that may have important implications for the clinical management of B-CLL patients is the identification of the tyrosine kinase ZAP-70 as a powerful surrogate marker for the identification of IgV$_H$-unmutated B-CLL.

Lymphoplasmacytic lymphoma (LPL) constitutes an entity that still lacks a thorough (cyto-) genetic definition. This may, at least in part, be due to difficulties in the definition of the disease on morphological and clinical grounds. A recurring chromosomal translocation, t(9;14)(p13;q32), had been demonstrated in the large majority of small B-cell lymphomas with plasmacytoid differentiation in one study, and this was later shown to juxtapose the *PAX5* (*Paired-Homeobox-5*) and *IgH* genes, resulting in *PAX5* deregulation. Several more recent studies, however, which also included cases of Waldenström's macroglobulinemia (WM), have considered the t(9;14) an infrequent genetic event in LPL.

Similar problems are encountered in B-cell prolymphocytic leukemia (B-PLL). In contrast to both B-CLL and mantle cell lymphoma, IgV$_H$ genes in B-PLL are generally mutated. According to older reports, the most prevalent cytogenetic marker is a rearranged chromosome 14 with 14q32 breaks. Other genetic aberrations in B-PLL include trisomy 12 and structural rearrangements of 1p32 and 6q21. Previously, a t(11;14)(q13;q23) translocation was considered to be a recurring aberration in this tumor, but a critical review of these cases points to a significant overlap with a more refined classification of these tumors as mantle cell lymphoma.

THERAPY

Treatment of CLL by risk stratification

Conventional prognostic variables, such as clinical stage (either Rai or Binet staging; Tables 10.1, 10.2) or lymphocyte doubling time, have been used to predict the proportion of patients who will progress to treatment or who will respond well to therapy. These variables are useful for predicting the outcomes of groups of patients, for example when assessing the merits of different trials, but are not useful for predicting the outcome of individual patients or for stratifying patients to specific therapies. In contrast, the more recently described prognostic factors can more accurately predict the outcome for individual patients, and these have now been validated by large prospective studies. These newer biological variables, which are now being used to stratify treatment in current clinical studies, fall into four principal types:

Table 10.1. Rai staging system for CLL.

Stage	Risk	Clinical features	Median survival
0	Low	Lymphocytes $> 5 \times 10^9$/L and $> 40\%$ lymphocytes in the marrow	>10 years
I	Intermediate	Stage 0 plus enlarged lymph nodes	7 years
II		Stages 0 or I with an enlarged liver or spleen	
III	High	Stages 0, I or II with hemoglobin < 100 g/L	1.5 to 4 years
IV		Stages 0, I, II or III with platelets $< 100 \times 10^9$/L	

Table 10.2. Binet staging system for CLL.

Stage	Clinical features	Median survival
A	< 3 areas of lymphadenopathy and no anemia or thrombocytopenia	12 years
B	3 or more areas of lymphadenopathy and no anemia or thrombocytopenia	7 years
C	Hemoglobin < 100 g/L and/or platelets $< 100 \times 10^9$/L	2–4 years

(1) those that are inherent to the individual patient's disease and which will not alter during the course of their illness – such as somatic mutation of the immunoglobulin gene

(2) genetic abnormalities that develop during the disease course and which are indicative of genetic evolution, and in some cases therapeutic resistance, of disease – such as deletion of the short arm of chromosome 17, studied by FISH

(3) prognostic factors that may vary during a patient's disease or even in response to infections or similar acute events – such as CD38

(4) those that are related to tumor bulk – such as LDH, β_2 microglobulin or thymidine kinase

The factors that are most appropriately used for stratification into different treatment intentions are those that are inherent to a patient's CLL (group 1), as they predict whether or not a patient will eventually develop treatment resistance. In contrast, genetic abnormalities (group 2) that explain chemotherapy resistance, for example disruption of the p53 pathway, are probably most appropriate to tailor an individual patient's treatment, for example by using therapies that are independent of the p53 pathway.

Therefore the two most extensively studied and robust prognostic markers are the presence or absence of somatic mutations in the immunoglobulin gene of the CLL cell and chromosomal abnormalities detected by fluorescence *in-situ* hybridization (FISH). Mutational status and FISH can be used to predict the course of a patient's disease, and are now being evaluated to determine whether patients with poor-risk disease should have therapy initiated before disease progression, as is currently recommended, or whether different therapeutic approaches should be applied to different risk groups. Patients with CLL cells that have no or few ($> 98\%$ homology with germ-line sequence) somatic mutations in the immunoglobulin disease (V_H unmutated) have similar response rates to therapy compared with patients with mutated CLL but remain in remission for a shorter period with a poorer overall survival. In addition, it appears that when patients with unmutated CLL relapse after initial therapy there are frequently abnormalities of the p53 pathway (deletion of either 17p or 11q), leading to a poorer response to conventional therapy and subsequently a poorer survival (Fig. 10.3). It is not clear whether the treatment itself creates abnormalities in the p53 pathway or simply

Table 10.3. Criteria for NCI-WG complete response.

B symptoms	Absent
Lymph nodes	Not palpable[a]
Liver/spleen	Not palpable[a]
Peripheral blood lymphocytes	$\leq 4 \times 10^9$/L
Peripheral blood neutrophils	$\geq 1.5 \times 10^9$/L
Hemoglobin	> 110 g/L
Bone-marrow aspirate	$< 30\%$ lymphocytes[b]
Bone-marrow trephine	No nodules[c]

[a] No requirement for imaging

[b] No requirement for immunophenotyping

[c] This can equate to up to 2% CLL cells

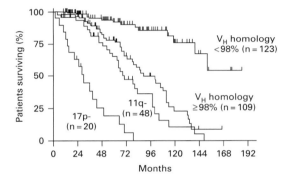

Figure 10.3. Survival of patients with CLL according to cytogenetics (from Doehner *et al.* 2000).

selects for a pre-existing subclone which was present at a low level prior to starting the initial therapy. In contrast, when mutated CLL progresses after therapy, these poor-risk chromosomal abnormalities appear to occur only rarely. When patients either present with or develop a dysfunctional p53 pathway (either 17p or 11q deleted) they are inherently resistant to therapies that damage DNA or interfere with its repair, such as alkylating agents or purine analogues. These patients have a very low response rate to conventional therapy, and this may explain the mechanism of resistance in most, if not all, patients who fail to respond to fludarabine-based combination therapies. In these cases it is logical to use treatments that do not depend upon an intact p53 pathway for their activity, such as high-dose steroids or monoclonal antibodies.

It is logical to treat unmutated CLL intensively, with the aim of achieving more profound remissions, and then to consolidate remissions with therapies that are not dependent upon an intact p53 pathway for their function. In contrast, for good-risk mutated CLL it is logical to de-escalate therapy in order to reduce toxicity, because when patients relapse they are more likely to respond to second-line therapy. For example, the LRF CLL4 trial in the United Kingdom demonstrated that CLL can be divided into three different risk groups by the molecular characteristics of the leukemic cells:

(1) "Good risk" CLL can be defined by the presence of somatic mutations in the immunoglobulin gene of the CLL cell, excluding those cases utilizing the V_H segment V_H3–21, and comprises approximately 30% of patients requiring therapy.

(2) Standard-risk patients can be defined as those cases with unmutated immunoglobulin genes or utilizing V_H3–21, or 11q deletion, comprising approximately 65% of patients.

(3) Poor-risk patients are those with greater than 20% CLL cells which have loss of the short arm of chromosome 17 (17p−) on FISH, comprising about 5% of patients.

Minimal residual disease

The NCI Working Group response criteria in CLL define a complete response on purely clinical examination, blood counts and morphological examination of the bone marrow. This was because when the criteria were published in 1996 there were limited effective therapies available for CLL – this was prior to the advent of purine analogues, monoclonal antibodies and stem-cell transplantation as conventional therapies in CLL, or the development of sensitive tests that can detect minimal residual disease (MRD). A complete response was defined as a patient in whom the clinical examination was normal with an almost normal blood count and a morphologically normal bone marrow (Table 10.3). These criteria have proved to be extremely useful to allow comparison between the results of trials from the various collaborative groups. However, there can be as many as 2% CLL cells in the marrow of a patient who is in an NCI complete remission.

The advent of therapies that result in profound reductions in levels of CLL has necessitated the development of techniques that can detect extremely low levels of CLL. The two most important approaches are molecular techniques, such allele-specific oligonucleotide polymerase chain reaction

Table 10.4. Comparison of methods of residual-disease monitoring in CLL.

	MRD flow cytometry	Allele-specific oligonucleotide PCR
Applicable patients	>95%	85% to 95%
Sensitivity limit	0.01%	0.001%
Quantitative range	0.1% to 0.01%	0.01%
Cost and complexity	Moderate	Initially high, follow-up low
Pre-treatment material required	Preferable	Essential
Turn-round time	Hours	Weeks

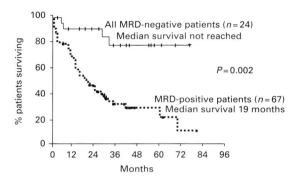

Figure 10.4. Impact of minimal residual disease on overall survival in CLL. Ninety-one patients with relapsed or refractory CLL were treated with alemtuzumab in an attempt to eradicate detectable CLL using a highly sensitive MRD flow cytometric assay. Twenty-four patients achieved MRD negativity: 18 with alemtuzumab monotherapy, 4 following autologous stem-cell transplantation after alemtuzumab and the remaining 2 patients following combined alemtuzumab and fludarabine. The overall survival of patients achieving MRD negativity was significantly better than those remaining MRD-positive.

(ASO-PCR) directed against the immunoglobulin gene of the CLL clone, or multi-parameter, four-color flow cytometry (MRD flow). Both of these techniques will detect as low as a single CLL cell in 10 000 leukocytes or more. ASO-PCR is slightly more sensitive than MRD flow but has several disadvantages (Table 10.4), which means that MRD flow is likely to become the standard approach used in routine practice if and when CLL patients are routinely tested for MRD. In all reports of MRD in CLL, patients who achieve an MRD-negative response have a better progression-free and overall survival than patients who remain MRD-positive, regardless of the therapy used to achieve such a profound response, including combination chemotherapy, immunochemotherapy, monoclonal-antibody-based therapy or stem-cell transplantation (Fig. 10.4).

However, in all of these series the aim of therapy was to eradicate MRD and therefore they do not prove beyond doubt that MRD eradication is critical (the patients achieving MRD negativity may have been biologically better-risk and therefore could have had a better survival regardless of therapy compared to their more resistant counterparts). The next series of clinical trials will therefore address in a randomized fashion whether attempting to eradicate MRD is an important endpoint of therapy.

Chemotherapeutic approach

The time to initiate therapy in CLL is defined by the NCI-WG criteria of 1996 (Table 10.5). Effectively patients require therapy if they are symptomatic from their CLL, or if they have cytopenias due to marrow replacement or rarely a rapidly evolving disease due to refractory immune cytopenias. The absolute level of lymphocytosis in the absence of any other features indicating active disease should not be used to justify initiation of therapy.

There is no proven benefit for the initiation of therapy with asymptomatic Binet stage A CLL, although the randomized trials only tested relatively ineffective therapies, namely alkylating-agent-based therapy, against no therapy in unselected early-stage patients. The advent of better prognostic markers and more effective therapy raises the question whether a subset of poor-risk patients may benefit from early intervention. This question is currently being addressed by collaborative CLL trials groups in Europe.

Alkylating agents in CLL

Randomized controlled trials in the 1990s demonstrated that alkylating agents used as monotherapy

Table 10.5. Indications for therapy in chronic lymphocytic leukemia.

(1) Any one of the following symptoms:
  (a) weight loss > 10% body weight over 6 months
  (b) extreme fatigue (WHO performance status 2 or worse)
  (c) fevers of over 39 °C for over 2 weeks without evidence of infection
  (d) night sweats without evidence of infection
(2) Evidence of progressive bone-marrow failure with either progressive anemia (unless there is another cause) or thrombocytopenia (platelets < 100×10^9/L). If the cytopenia is stable then treatment may not be immediately required.
(3) Autoimmune anemia and/or thrombocytopenia poorly responsive to corticosteroids.
(4) Massive (i.e. > 6 cm below the costal margin) or progressive splenomegaly.
(5) Massive lymphadenopathy (i.e. > 10 cm in longest diameter) or progressive lymphadenopathy.
(6) Progressive lymphocytosis with an increase of > 50% over a 2-month period, or anticipated doubling time of less than 6 months.
(7) Marked hypogammaglobulinemia or the development of a monoclonal pattern, in the absence of any of the above criteria for active disease, is not sufficient for protocol therapy.

were equally effective when compared to combinations of alkylating agents with steroids and vinca alkaloids (CVP) or with the inclusion of an anthracycline (CHOP). Randomized trials comparing purine analogues with alkylating agents have all demonstrated a significantly higher response rate (in the region of 15% complete response for fludarabine monotherapy, compared to less than 5% for chlorambucil) and improved progression-free survival for purine analogues (mainly fludarabine) but no improvement in overall survival (median progression-free survival for fludarabine monotherapy in the range of 18–24 months). It appears that this lack of improvement in overall survival is largely due to the crossover from chlorambucil to fludarabine. Therefore until recently chlorambucil remained the therapy most commonly used as the initial therapy in CLL.

Combination chemotherapy (FC, FCM)

Purine analogues, and in particular fludarabine, are the most active chemotherapeutic agents in CLL and are an essential component for most of the effective combination therapies. There is no convincing evidence that any of the three widely available purine analogues, fludarabine, cladrabine or deoxycoformycin, is more effective than the others. Three recently reported large trials have randomized a total of over 900 patients between fludarabine and fludarabine plus cyclophosphamide (FC). All three showed a

significant improvement in complete responses for FC, over double that for fludarabine monotherapy. In addition, FC resulted in a doubling of PFS compared to fludarabine monotherapy, which was the primary endpoint of the trials and again was statistically significant (Table 10.6). In the LRF CLL4 trial there was no upper age limit and 30% of the patients recruited were over 70 years of age. It is very likely that these older patients were selected, in that they were unlikely to have other significant comorbidity, but it was still somewhat surprising that they had no significant increase in treatment-related toxicity or mortality. In addition, the benefit in response rates for combined fludarabine plus cyclophosphamide was seen across all age groups. There was, however, no improvement in overall survival, which is probably due to a crossover from fludarabine to FC at progression. However, in the LRF CLL4 trial there was extensive quality-of-life assessment, which showed that patients who achieved a complete or nodular partial remission had a significantly better quality of life over the next two years. Therefore the combination of fludarabine plus cyclophosphamide can now be considered the "gold standard" for the initial treatment of CLL, including for elderly patients without significant comorbidities.

Recently Bosch and colleagues have reported the addition of mitoxantrone to fludarabine and cyclophosphamide (FCM) in relapsed, refractory and untreated patients. FCM yields high overall response

Table 10.6. Randomized controlled trials comparing fludarabine monotherapy with fludarabine plus cyclophosphamide.

		Fludarabine monotherapy	Fludarabine plus cyclophosphamide	*p*-value
Eichhorst *et al.* (German CLL Study Group)	No. evaluable	151	148	
	ORR	84.1%	95.3%	0.002
	CR	8.6%	20.3%	0.004
	Median PFS (mo)	21.0	46.7	0.003
Catovsky *et al.* (LRF CLL4)	No. evaluable	176	176	
	ORR	81%	94%	
	CR	15%	39%	
	% PFS at 3 yr	31%	59%	< 0.0005
Flinn *et al.* (Intergroup Trial E2997)	No. evaluable	121	125	
	ORR	49.6%	70.4%	0.001
	CR	5.8%	22.4%	0.0002
	Median PFS (mo)	17.7	41.0	< 0.001

ORR, overall response rate; CR, complete response; PFS, progression-free survival.

rates, with 78% previously treated patients achieving a complete or partial response. FCM also appears effective in previously untreated patients with CLL, with 55% achieving a complete response and a significant minority of patients with CLL below the level of detection by highly sensitive techniques. In fact the only patients who were refractory to FCM were the eight patients with deletion of the short arm of chromosome 17 (p53 deleted). The median duration of response in previously untreated patients receiving FCM was 36 months. The hematological toxicity was acceptable, with only 8% grade 3 or 4 neutropenia. There were two patients who experienced reactivation of hepatitis B, one of which was fatal. This combination now needs to be tested for efficacy and tolerability in randomized phase III trials.

Monoclonal antibody therapy in CLL

The only monoclonal antibody that is approved for use in CLL is alemtuzumab (Campath or MabCampath), which is approved for fludarabine-refractory CLL. Rituximab (Rituxan or MabThera) has also been used in large numbers of patients with CLL, both alone and in combination. Rituximab as a single agent used at the conventional dose of 375 mg/m^2 weekly for 4 weeks has little efficacy in relapsed or

refractory CLL, with only partial remissions observed in a minority of patients, and these remissions only persist for a few months. The partial-response rate increases with higher doses of rituximab but still complete responses were not achieved and the doses used were extremely high (up to 2250 mg/m^2). The use of "conventional" doses of rituximab has also been reported in untreated CLL, with higher response rates (up to 50% of patients), but still very few complete responses, and these are not durable. Rituximab therefore appears to have no role as monotherapy in CLL, but it will probably find a place in combination with chemotherapy as the initial therapy for CLL at least in a proportion of patients (see below).

In contrast, alemtuzumab does have efficacy as a single agent in refractory and untreated CLL. The response rates to single-agent alemtuzumab in relapsed, refractory CLL range between 33% and 50% with up to 25% of patients achieving a complete response. The most important predictor of response to alemtuzumab is the presence or absence of significant lymphadenopathy. Patients with massive lymphadenopathy (single lymph nodes greater than 5 cm in diameter) have a very low response rate. In these patients a more effective strategy is to control the lymphadenopathy with an alternative therapy, such as high-dose methylprednisolone or CHOP chemotherapy, prior to alemtuzumab therapy. Two recently reported phase II trials of subcutaneous alemtuzumab in fludarabine-refractory CLL suggest a similar efficacy to when the drug is given intravenously but with a much improved toxicity profile.

A phase II trial of subcutaneous alemtuzumab in previously untreated CLL was reported on by Lundin and colleagues in 2002. The response rates were in excess of 80%, with a reasonable toxicity profile. This led to the CAM307 trial, in which 297 previously untreated patients with CLL were randomized between chlorambucil and intravenous alemtuzumab. Somewhat surprisingly, the toxicity to alemtuzumab was not significantly higher and the only treatment-related death occurred in the chlorambucil arm of the trial. The response rates of this trial have recently been reported, and show a significantly higher overall and complete response rate for alemtuzumab compared to chlorambucil (ORR 83.2% vs. 56.1%; CR 24.2% vs. 2.0%, $p < 0.0001$). Alemtuzumab monotherapy may well be most useful in the consolidation of response to chemotherapy in an attempt to eradicate minimal residual disease, particularly for patients who have poor-risk disease.

Chemoimmunotherapy

Although the activity of single-agent rituximab in CLL is limited, there is a dose–response relationship when the drug is used at doses up to 2250 mg/m^2. Thus there is some activity in CLL which has encouraged the use of rituximab in combination with other therapies. The logical approach is to combine rituximab with the most effective front-line therapy for CLL, namely FC. Extremely high response rates have been reported for the combination of R-FC in a group of 300 previously untreated patients, with an overall response rate of 95% and 72% of patients achieving a complete remission by NCI response criteria. In addition, in this series, patients who had no detectable disease by a sensitive PCR-based assay at the end of therapy had a very small chance ($< 10\%$) of progression at five-year follow-up. The combination of R-FC is currently the subject of at least two large international studies to address whether or not it is more effective than FC; these studies should complete recruitment within the next year, with results eagerly anticipated.

Since alemtuzumab is the most effective monoclonal antibody when used as a single agent in CLL, then it would appear sensible to combine this with conventional chemotherapy. However, the major concern is that since both alemtuzumab and purine analogues result in T-cell suppression, combining these classes of drugs may lead to immunosuppression and a potential increase in infections. In one trial, alemtuzumab at the standard dosing of 30 mg intravenously three times a week was combined with fludarabine (25 mg/m^2 per day) for 3 days every 28 days, and it was found that patients who were refractory to both fludarabine and alemtuzumab as single agents could respond to the two agents combined. In fact, in a subsequent update of these data, eight of eleven refractory patients responded better to the combination than to either fludarabine or alemtuzumab alone, with two patients having eradication of detectable minimal residual disease. In another trial, an alternative combination of alemtuzumab and fludarabine, in which patients received both fludarabine and alemtuzumab for 3 days every 28 days, resulted in a high overall response rate of 83%, with 30% of patients achieving a complete remission in a group of relapsed or refractory patients. This combination is now being studied in a randomized phase III trial for relapsed CLL.

Alemtuzumab consolidation therapy

It is almost inevitable that patients who achieve an NCI complete remission will eventually relapse, but it appears that patients who achieve MRD-negative remissions have a prolongation of their disease-free period. This suggests that consolidating patients into deeper remissions after conventional therapy might be an effective strategy. In addition, since alemtuzumab is relatively ineffective in the presence of bulky nodal disease, it is likely to be most effective in the consolidation setting. There has been one randomized trial of alemtuzumab consolidation following fludarabine-based initial therapy. This was the GCLLSG CLL4B trial reported on by Wendtner and colleagues, in which patients received intravenous alemtuzumab consolidation at a dose of 30 mg three times a week, given two months after completing initial therapy of a fludarabine-based regimen. This randomized trial against no consolidation showed a significant prolongation in progression-free survival for alemtuzumab consolidation. However, this trial was stopped prematurely as there was a high inci-dence of infections during alemtuzumab therapy. Why was this? Probably because the alemtuzumab was given a median of two months post-fludarabine, which is possibly not sufficient time to allow recovery from the initial therapy. Three other studies of alemtuzumab as consolidation therapy have been reported, and these all had a longer interval between completing the "induction" chemotherapy and alem-tuzumab therapy, and/or the alemtuzumab was given subcutaneously. Each of these studies has shown a degree of activity with an acceptable toxicity profile. Therefore it appears that the strategy of using alem-tuzumab to consolidate remissions following con-ventional therapy is very likely to be effective, if an appropriate schedule and dose can be identified. There are a variety of trials ongoing investigating the optimal schedule for alemtuzumab as consolidation therapy.

Autologous stem-cell transplantation

Autologous stem-cell transplantation has been stu-died in CLL over the last decade or more. There are inherent problems both with transplantation and with analyzing the results of phase II studies resulting from the fact that CLL is predominantly a marrow-based disorder and the therapies employed to achieve responses prior to harvesting very rarely eradicate detectable disease. It is therefore difficult to find an appropriate comparative group as all patients under-going autologous transplantation will have to have achieved a complete or very good partial remission prior to stem-cell harvesting. In addition, almost all autologous stem-cell harvests will contain a con-siderable number of residual CLL cells which are re-infused into the patient. Therefore it is not surprising that there is no evidence of a plateau in either the progression-free or overall survival curves following autologous transplants. In addition, there have been reports of up to 12% of patients experiencing therapy-related myelodysplastic syndrome, with some pro-gressing to acute myeloid leukemia. Such procedures cannot be generally recommended in CLL, and at present there is a phase III randomized trial recruiting in Europe under the auspices of the EBMT which will formally address the role of autologous transplanta-tion in CLL.

Allogeneic stem-cell transplantation

There is convincing evidence of graft-versus-CLL effect in the setting of both conventional myelo-ablative and reduced-intensity conditioning stem-cell transplantation. Gribben and colleagues have reported a six-year overall survival for patients receiving T-cell-depleted HLA-matched sibling bone-marrow trans-plants of 55% with a transplant-related mortality of 24%. It is apparent that patients with MRD detectable post-transplant can frequently become MRD-negative during follow-up or post donor-lymphocyte infusions. This reversion to MRD negativity has not been reported after the completion of other therapies, strongly supporting the significance of graft-versus-CLL as an important biological phenomenon. The major problem at present is to define which patients will benefit from allogeneic transplantation. The cur-rent consensus suggests that patients who are fit enough to withstand an allogeneic transplant with relapsed poor-risk disease or refractory disease should be considered for transplantation.

Novel therapies

There are a number of novel agents that are now being developed in CLL. These include flavopiridol, which, although the initial clinical studies had dis-appointing results, appears to be potentially very effective with a modified dosing schedule. Recently both thalidomide and lenalidomide have been reported to have activity in CLL and are being devel-oped in the disease. Bcl-2 is upregulated in the vast majority of patients with CLL, and this has led to the use of bcl-2 antisense in initial studies in CLL. A variety of new monoclonal antibodies to pre-existing and novel targets are now being studied in CLL.

Recommended therapeutic approaches in CLL

As a general rule, patients should be offered entry into well-designed clinical trials if available and if the patient is eligible. In the absence of such studies, a summary of the evidence presented above with recom-mendations for therapy at the various time points in a patient's disease course is outlined in Table 10.7, and a treatment algorithm is shown in Fig. 10.5.

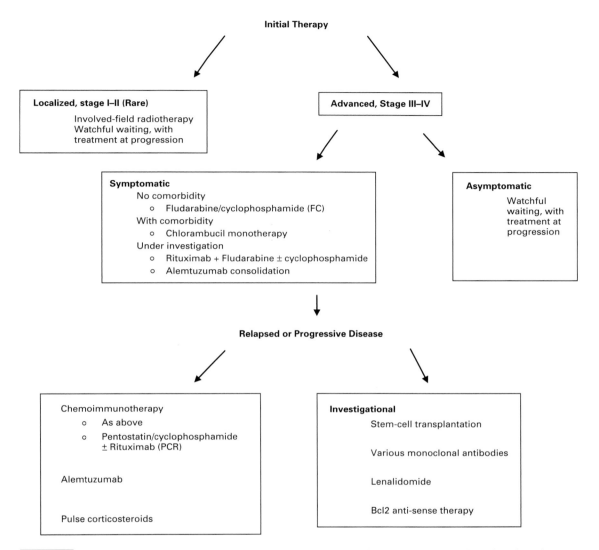

Figure 10.5. Therapeutic approaches in small lymphocytic lymphoma/CLL. As standard therapies for front-line and for relapsed or refractory disease are not yet established, treatment of these patients on a clinical trial is encouraged.

CONCLUSION

Chronic lymphocytic leukemia/small lymphocytic lymphoma is in the midst of a revolution in the understanding of the biology of the disease, and with respect to the implications this information has on the application of the novel therapeutic approaches which are being developed. We are now in a position to attempt to eradicate detectable disease in patients with CLL, but such approaches will inevitably result in additional toxicity, such as immune suppression. This necessitates the accurate assessment of which patients should be stratified into more intensive therapeutic pathways and which patients do not benefit from such an approach. Carefully designed clinical trials are currently recruiting which will attempt to answer these key questions in the management of CLL.

Table 10.7. General recommendations for the treatment of CLL.

Initial therapy in CLL	In patients without significant comorbid conditions (regardless of age) the combination of fludarabine plus cyclophosphamide (FC) should be considered standard therapy. Chlorambucil is indicated for very elderly patients and those with significant comorbid conditions.
Relapsed but not refractory CLL (fludarabine-sensitive relapse)	Consider for re-treatment with the same therapy as long as the initial remission was at least a year from the end of therapy. If the initial therapy was fludarabine alone then re-treat with FC. Patients relapsing between 6 and 12 months after completing initial therapy should be considered for alternative therapies such as FC or FCM.
Fludarabine-refractory CLL	Patients with predominantly blood and marrow disease with relatively small lymph nodes should be treated with alemtuzumab. The eradication of detectable minimal residual disease from the marrow is a reasonable endpoint. Patients with bulky lymphadenopathy should receive initial therapy to reduce the bulk of lymph nodes prior to treatment with alemtuzumab in order to eradicate detectable minimal residual disease. High-dose methylprednisolone ($1g/m^2$ per day for 5 days every 4 weeks) is effective in patients for whom high dose steroids are not contraindicated.
Autologous stem-cell transplantation	Should not be perfomed in CLL except in the context of well-designed clinical trials.
Allogeneic stem-cell transplantation	Long-term disease-free survival is achievable following allogeneic stem-cell transplantation, presumably due to active graft-versus-CLL. Patients should be considered for allogeneic transplantation if they have poor-risk CLL as defined by deleted chromosome 17 or if they have fludarabine-refractory disease.

FURTHER READING

Binet, J. L., Auquier, A., Dighiero, G. et al. A new prognostic classification of chronic lymphocytic leukaemia derived from a multivariate survival analysis. Cancer **48** (1981), 198–206.

Bosch, F., Ferrer, A., López-Guillermo, A. et al. Fludarabine, cyclophosphamide and mitoxantrone in the treatment of resistant or relapsed chronic lymphocytic leukaemia. Br. J. Haematol. **119** (2002), 976–984.

Bosch, F., Ferrer, A., Villamor, N. et al. Combination chemotherapy with fludarabine, cyclophosphamide and mitoxantrone (FCM) induces a high response rate in previously untreated CLL. Blood (ASH Annual Meeting Abstracts) **106** (2005), 718.

Catovsky, D., Richards, S. and Hillmen, P. Early results from LRF CLL4: a UK multicenter randomized trial. Blood (ASH Annual Meeting Abstracts) **106** (2005), 716.

Cheson, B. D., Bennett, J. M., Grever, M. et al. National Cancer Institute-sponsored Working Group guidelines for chronic lymphocytic leukemia: revised guidelines for diagnosis and treatment. Blood **87** (1996), 4990–4997.

Damle, R. N., Wasil, T., Fais, F. et al. IgV gene mutation status and CD38 expression as novel prognostic indicators in chronic lymphocytic leukemia. Blood **94** (1999), 1840–1847.

Doehner, H., Stilgenbauer, S., Benner, A. et al. Genomic aberrations and survival in chronic lymphocytic leukemia. N. Engl. J. Med. **343** (2000), 1910–1916.

Eichhorst, B. F., Busch, R., Hopfinger, G. et al. the German CLL Study Group. Fludarabine plus cyclophosphamide versus fludarabine alone in first-line therapy of younger patients with chronic lymphocytic leukemia. Blood **107** (2006), 885–891.

Flinn, I. W., Kumm, E., Grever, M. R. et al. Fludarabine and cyclophosphamide produces a higher complete response rate and more durable remissions than fludarabine in patients with previously untreated CLL: intergroup trial E2997. Blood (ASH Annual Meeting Abstracts) **104** (2004), 475.

Gribben, J. G., Zahrieh, D., Stephans, K. et al. Autologous and allogeneic stem-cell transplantations for poor-risk chronic lymphocytic leukemia. Blood **106** (2005), 4389–4396.

Hamblin, T. J., Davis, Z., Gardiner, A., Oscier, D. G. and Stevenson, F. K. Unmutated Ig V(H) genes are associated with a more aggressive form of chronic lymphocytic leukemia. Blood **94** (1999), 1848–1854.

Hillmen, P., Skotnicki, A., Robak, T. et al. Preliminary phase 3 efficacy and safety of alemtuzumab vs chlorambucil as front-line therapy for patients with progressive B-cell chronic lymphocytic leukemia (BCLL). J. Clin. Oncol. (ASCO Annual Meeting) **24** Suppl. (2006), 6511.

Keating, M. J., O'Brien, S., Albitar, M. et al. Early results of a chemoimmunotherapy regimen of fludarabine, cyclophosphamide, and rituximab as initial therapy for chronic lymphocytic leukemia. J. Clin. Oncol. **23** (2005), 4079–4088.

Moreton, P., Kennedy, B., Lucas, G. *et al.* Eradication of minimal residual disease in B-cell chronic lymphocytic leukemia after alemtuzumab therapy is associated with prolonged survival. *J. Clin. Oncol.* **23** (2005), 2971–2979.

Rai, K. R., Sawitsky, A., Cronkite, E. P., Chanana, A. D., Levy, R. N. and Pasternack, B. S. Clinical staging of chronic lymphocytic leukemia. *Blood* **46** (1975), 219–234.

Rai, K. R., Peterson, B. L., Appelbaum, F. R. *et al.* Fludarabine compared with chlorambucil as primary therapy for chronic lymphocytic leukemia. *N. Engl. J. Med.* **343** (2000), 1750–1757.

Rawstron, A. C., Kennedy, B., Evans, P. A. *et al.* Quantitation of minimal disease levels in chronic lymphocytic leukemia using a sensitive flow cytometric assay improves the prediction of outcome and can be used to optimize therapy. *Blood* **98** (2001), 29–35.

Wendtner, C. M., Ritgen, M., Schweighofer, C. D. *et al.* Consolidation with alemtuzumab in patients with chronic lymphocytic leukemia (CLL) in first remission: experience on safety and efficacy within a randomized multicenter phase III trial of the German CLL Study Group (GCLLSG). *Leukemia* **18** (2004), 1093–1101.

11 MANTLE CELL LYMPHOMA

Martin Dreyling and Michael E. Williams

Pathology: Andrew Wotherspoon
Molecular cytogenetics: Andreas Rosenwald and German Ott

INTRODUCTION

Mantle cell lymphoma (MCL) is a unique subtype of non-Hodgkin's lymphoma (NHL) characterized in almost all cases by the chromosomal translocation t(11;14)(q13;q32) and nuclear cyclin D1 overexpression. Most patients present with advanced-stage disease, often with extranodal dissemination, and typically pursue an aggressive clinical course, with median survival historically averaging 3–4 years. No standard curative therapy exists, even with intensive induction regimens followed by autologous stem-cell transplantation. However, a number of recent insights into the molecular and cellular biology of the disease, as well as combined immunochemotherapy and novel therapeutic approaches, hold promise for improved outcomes. Importantly, MCL provides a paradigm for therapeutic targeting in neoplasms with dysregulated cell cycle and apoptotic pathways.

MCL comprises approximately 4–8% of all NHL, with a preponderance of older males relative to other lymphoma subtypes. The male-to-female ratio is 2–3 : 1 and median age at presentation is 60–65 years. No specific etiologic factors have been identified for this disease. An increased risk of lymphoid neoplasms has been reported in first-degree relatives of MCL patients, although MCL occurrence among multiple family members appears to be quite rare.

CLINICAL PRESENTATION

MCL typically presents in advanced stage; over 90% of patients are stage III–IV at diagnosis, frequently with B symptoms. Splenomegaly is seen in half or more of patients, often in association with a leukemic phase.

In some patients disease is largely non-nodal and confined to the blood, bone marrow and spleen; these individuals may experience a more indolent clinical course than those with predominant nodal disease. Common extranodal sites of disease include the gastrointestinal tract, especially colonic polyposis; subclinical involvement of the gastric or colonic mucosa has been reported in most patients on endoscopic biopsies even in the absence of overt polyps or mucosal abnormalities. This tropism for the GI tract is as yet not fully explained, but may relate to the expression of adhesion molecules such as the mucosal homing receptor $\alpha4\beta7$. Genitourinary, pulmonary and soft-tissue (including head and neck or periorbital) sites of disease may also be observed. CNS involvement, either parenchymal or leptomeningeal, is unusual at presentation but may develop in a minority of patients. Routine CNS prophylaxis is not typically incorporated into therapeutic regimens.

PATHOLOGY

The entity now identified as MCL is relatively newly recognized among the subtypes of NHL. Designations in the older literature used descriptive terms such as "lymphocytic lymphoma of intermediate differentiation" and "mantle zone lymphoma." The first specific recognition was by Lennert, who described "diffuse germinocytoma" in 1973, renamed "centrocytic lymphoma" in the 1974 Kiel classification. As immunophenotypic characterization became more refined and, importantly, the strong correlation with the t(11;14)(q13;q32) chromosomal translocation permitted differentiation from other small-cell

Lymphoma: Pathology, Diagnosis and Treatment, ed. Robert Marcus, John W. Sweetenham and Michael E. Williams. Published by Cambridge University Press. © Cambridge University Press 2007.

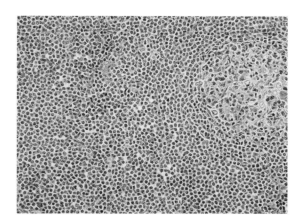

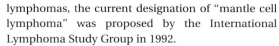

Figure 11.1. Mantle cell lymphoma (lymph node). A diffuse infiltrate of cells with scanty cytoplasm surrounding a residual germinal center. The cells have irregular nuclei and indistinct nucleoli.

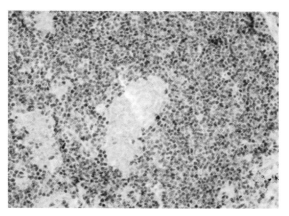

Figure 11.2. Mantle cell lymphoma (lymph node). Immunostaining for cyclin D1 gives a characteristic nuclear pattern.

lymphomas, the current designation of "mantle cell lymphoma" was proposed by the International Lymphoma Study Group in 1992.

The lymph-node architecture is usually effaced by a diffuse proliferation of lymphoid cells with monotonous appearance (Fig. 11.1). In some cases there may be a more nodular growth pattern, or the cells may be seen surrounding residual reactive germinal centers in a mantle-zone pattern. The cells are small to intermediate in size with scanty cytoplasm and with nuclei that show variable irregularity, although a subset of MCL are cytologically blastoid. The nuclear chromatin is granular and cells may have small, rather indistinct eosinophilic nucleoli. The background frequently contains hyalinized small blood vessels and may contain histiocytes. Proliferation centers are absent.

Immunophenotypically the cells have surface IgM and IgD. They are positive for CD20 and CD79a and typically co-express CD5, CD43 and FMC7. Although up to 94% of cases express CD43, as many as 20% of cases in some series are reported to be CD5-negative. MCL is negative for CD10 and bcl-6 and is usually CD23-negative. Staining for nuclear cyclin D1 is characteristically positive, reflecting the underlying t(11;14)(q13;q32) that is characteristic of this lymphoma (Fig. 11.2). Cyclin D1 positivity is also present in rare cases that appear to lack this cytogenetic abnormality; even more rarely, cyclin D2 or D3 is expressed rather than D1. Such D1-negative cases, confirmed by gene expression profiling, may present a considerable diagnostic challenge. The

cells are positive for bcl-2 protein. There is no staining for MUM1/IRF4. Proliferation marker expression is variable. Staining for follicular dendritic cells usually demonstrates an expanded and disrupted meshwork, most obvious in cases with more nodular growth but usually present even in those with a diffuse pattern. In contrast to other B-cell lymphomas, MCL is more frequently associated with lambda rather than kappa light chain expression.

MOLECULAR PATHOLOGY AND CYTOGENETICS

The molecular pathogenesis of MCL is a paradigm of dysregulated control of the cell-cycle machinery and the response to DNA damage in human cancer. Most, if not all, molecular and cytogenetic alterations described to date in MCL appear to affect these two crucial cellular pathways. The hallmark chromosomal translocation, the t(11;14)(q13;q32), can be detected in the vast majority of MCL cases and results in the overexpression of cyclin D1, which plays an important role in the regulation of the G1/S-phase transition of the cell cycle. The juxtaposition of the *Cyclin D1 (CCND1)* chromosomal locus on 11q13, designated *bcl-1* (B-cell lymphoma/leukaemia 1), to the enhancer of the immunoglobulin heavy chain joining region at 14q32 leads to upregulation of this D-type cyclin that is usually not expressed in B cells. Cyclin D1 forms a complex with the cyclin-dependent kinases 4 (CDK4) and 6 (CDK6), and over-expression of cyclin D1 in MCL leads to increased levels of cyclin D1/CDK complexes, which in turn phosphorylate the retinoblastoma protein (Rb) and thus directly facilitate cell-cycle progression. In addition, increased levels of cyclin D1/CDK complexes may sequester the CDK inhibitors p27^{kip1} and p21 that are usually bound to cyclin E/CDK2 complexes which, once activated, promote S-phase entry. These studies suggest that aberrant expression of cyclin D1 plays a crucial role in the pathogenesis of MCL. Moreover, the level of cyclin D1 expression is directly correlated with the proliferation rate of the tumor cells and therefore with the clinical aggressiveness of this lymphoma.

Besides the deregulation of cyclin D1 as a result of the translocation t(11;14), other genetic alterations have been reported that disrupt proper function of the cell cycle. Specifically, a significant proportion of MCLs harbor hemi- or homozygous deletions in the chromosomal locus 9p21 (as detected by conventional karyotyping or fluorescence *in-situ* hybridization [FISH] techniques), affecting the CDK inhibitor p16^{INK4a}. p16^{INK4a} serves as an inhibitor of CDK4 and CDK6 and thus helps to maintain the Rb protein in its dephosphorylated, antiproliferative state. Functional inactivation of this CDK inhibitor may therefore cooperate with aberrant cyclin D1 expression in MCL and enhance cell-cycle progression. It is noteworthy that MCL cases with inactivated p16^{INK4a} usually display increased proliferative activity. Rare cases of MCL with a wild-type status of the *p16^{INK4a}* locus have been described with overexpression and genomic amplification of *BMI-1*, which belongs to the Polycomb group of genes and acts as a transcriptional repressor of the *p16^{INK4a}* locus. *BMI-1* overexpression in a small subset of MCL cases may therefore represent a pathogenetic alternative to the more frequently observed deletions of its transcriptional target *p16^{INK4a}*. Finally, a few MCL cases with genomic amplification and protein overexpression of CDK4 have been reported, and this may represent yet another mechanism of disturbing the G1/S-phase cell-cycle checkpoint.

As noted above, a second major target of genetic alteration in MCL is the DNA damage response pathway. In particular, the chromosomal region 11q22–23 is frequently deleted in MCL, affecting the *ataxia-telangiectasia mutated* (*ATM*) gene. In addition to hemizygous *ATM* deletions, many MCL cases show concomitant mutations of the *ATM* gene. *ATM* encodes a kinase that belongs to the PI-3 kinase-related superfamily and plays a pivotal role in the cellular response to DNA damage. *ATM* mutations frequently affect the kinase domain of the gene or result in a truncated version of the ATM protein. Besides frequent *ATM* alterations, other molecules involved in the DNA damage response, and specifically targets of the ATM kinase itself, are also occasionally altered in MCL. Specifically, rare alterations of the kinases CHK2 and CHK1 are observed. CHK2 stabilizes and activates p53, which plays a central role in the response to DNA damage by initiating cell-cycle arrest, apoptosis or DNA repair. Decreased protein levels and occasional *CHK2* mutations, present in a subset of MCL, may compromise p53 function and are associated with a high number of chromosomal imbalances. Importantly, p53 is inactivated in approximately 30% of MCL cases with blastoid morphology and high proliferation rates, while this event is uncommon in MCL cases with classic morphology and low proliferative activity. Gene expression profiling analysis of MCL has provided a quantitative measurement of tumor cell proliferation of both pathogenetic and prognostic importance, as described below.

STAGING

The majority of patients present with advanced-stage symptomatic disease. Standard lymphoma staging approaches apply in MCL, including thorough history and physical examination, CT scans and bone-marrow aspirate and biopsy. Flow cytometry and cytogenetics with FISH for the t(11;14) should be obtained at the time of marrow biopsy. Careful attention to assessment of potential sites of extranodal disease is warranted; colonoscopy should be considered in the staging evaluation, especially if there is evidence of gastrointestinal blood loss or significant anemia. Routine upper and lower endoscopy is not required for staging in the absence of relevant signs and symptoms of involvement. Overt lymphocytosis is present in about 25% of patients, with a more subtle leukemic component in additional patients often confirmed by flow cytometry.

The role of PET scanning in initial staging and in assessment of treatment response has not been formally evaluated, although MCL is typically

Table 11.1. Prognostic markers in mantle cell lymphoma.

	Better prognosis	Poorer prognosis
Clinical presentation	Predominantly blood, marrow and splenic disease	Predominantly nodal
Nodal architecture	Nodular or mantle zone	Diffuse
Cytology	Small cleaved cell	Blastoid
Mitotic count	Low	High
Phenotypic and serologic		
Ki67	Low	High
Beta-2 microglobulin	Normal	Increased
Molecular markers		
p53	Wild type	Mutated
Chromosome 8p21	Wild type	Deleted
Chromosome 13q14	Wild type	Deleted
Chromosome 9/CDK p16^{INK4a}	Wild type	Deleted or methylated
CDK4	Wild type	Gene amplification
Proliferation signature	Low	High

PET-positive, and use of this technique to document post-therapeutic complete response is appropriate.

PROGNOSTIC FACTORS

MCL displays considerable morphologic and clinical heterogeneity. Most patients pursue an aggressive clinical course while a minority show a slow pace of disease similar to that of indolent lymphomas. The underpinnings of this variability are becoming better understood at the molecular and cellular levels via cDNA microarray and proteomic analyses, and provide new approaches to assessing individual patient prognosis (Table 11.1).

Clinical prognostic factors

The International Prognostic Index (IPI) developed for diffuse large B-cell lymphoma has relatively limited predictive value in MCL, as the majority of patients present with advanced-stage disease and frequent leukemic or extranodal sites of involvement. Patients who present with predominantly peripheral blood, bone-marrow and splenic involvement without significant lymphadenopathy may experience a more indolent clinical course, although these cases need to be carefully distinguished from splenic lymphoma with villous lymphocytes and prolymphocytic leukemia.

Morphologic subtype

Both architectural and cytologic variants of MCL have been reported to affect prognosis. Most patients show a diffuse nodal effacement, although nodular or mantle zone patterns are also observed and appear to correlate with a more indolent pace of disease. A blastoid cell type may be present at diagnosis or may develop with progression. Blastoid MCL in most series has a poorer survival of approximately 12–18 months as compared with non-blastoid MCL survival of 3–5 years. Increased mitotic activity may also be associated with more aggressive clinical behavior.

Phenotypic and molecular markers

Markers of proliferation such as Ki67 are often expressed in MCL, and the proliferation rate was identified as the most important prognostic factor in studies, supporting a two-step model with initial inhibition of apoptosis pathways and secondary cell-cycle alteration (Fig 11.3). These findings are extended by recent gene expression profiling of MCL by Rosenwald and colleagues, which has provided a quantitative measurement of tumor-cell proliferation, termed "proliferation signature," allowing for the definition of prognostic subgroups that differ in

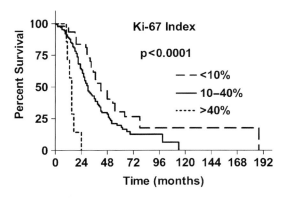

Figure 11.3. Clinical course of MCL in a large retrospective survey based upon Ki67 expression (from Tiemann *et al.* Br. J. Haematol. **131** (2005), 29).

their median survival by more than five years. Since the gene-expression-based measurement of proliferation was better at predicting the length of survival than individual molecular parameters alone or in combination (e.g. level of cyclin D1 expression, p16^{INK4a} alterations), the proliferation signature may be viewed as a quantitative integrator of oncogenic events in MCL that could be helpful in the future to test targeted therapeutic approaches and guide treatment decisions. Other markers have also been correlated with prognosis, as outlined in Table 11.1.

FIRST-LINE THERAPY

MCL remains the lymphoma subtype with the poorest long-term outcome, with a median survival of only 3–4 years and a high degree of primary and secondary refractoriness. The small number of patients with limited-stage disease potentially may achieve long-term remissions after extended- or involved-field radiation. In a recent retrospective study, five-year progression-free and overall survival of 17 patients with stage I–II MCL was 68% and 71%, respectively, after involved-field radiotherapy, either alone or in combination with conventional chemotherapy. In contrast, in stage III–IV disease the benefit of radiation therapy is not proven.

Standard chemotherapy

In advanced-stage disease, standard chemotherapy remains a non-curative approach. Due to the aggressive

clinical course in the majority of patients, a wait-and-see strategy generally should not be pursued. However, some patients who present a history consistent with very slow-paced or low-volume advanced-stage disease may be considered for cautious "watchful waiting," although even these patients typically require therapy within months rather than years, as is seen in many truly indolent lymphomas.

In the only randomized trial, no advantage of the anthracycline-containing CHOP regimen (cyclophosphamide, doxorubicin, vincristine, prednisone) in comparison to a non-anthracycline combination (COP) was detectable. Overall response after CHOP was 89%, compared to 84% in the COP arm, and median survival rates were 37 and 32 months respectively (Table 11.2). In contrast, a retrospective study suggested the superiority of anthracycline-containing regimens in patients with low and low-intermediate risk profile according to the IPI. However, because of the aggressive course of MCL, many clinicians favor CHOP-like or even more intensive regimens as initial therapy.

The efficacy of purine analogs (e.g. fludarabine, cladribine) has been investigated in various studies. Fludarabine showed only moderate efficacy in MCL when applied as a single agent, with overall response rates of approximately 30–40%. In contrast, based on an in-vitro synergism, combinations with either alkylating agents (e.g. cyclophosphamide) or anthracyclines (e.g. mitoxantrone, idarubicin) seem to achieve significantly higher remission rates (Table 11.3). Various phase II studies achieved overall response rates of more than 80% even in relapsed disease. Even more remarkably, the combination of fludarabine and cyclophosphamide achieves 70% complete and 30% partial remissions in previously untreated patients, with a median progression-free survival of 28 months, although the number of patients is rather small in most of these phase II studies and diagnosis has generally not been confirmed by central reference pathology review. Similar efficacy was achieved by a cladribine-containing combination.

Monoclonal antibody and combined immunochemotherapy

Despite high CD20 expression in MCL, rituximab monotherapy achieves only moderate response rates

Table 11.2. Anthracyclines in first-line therapy of advanced-stage MCL.

Study	Patients (n)	Regimen	ORR (CR)	PFS (mo)	OS (mo)
Meusers *et al. Hematol. Oncol.* **7** (1989), 365.	37	COP	84% (41%)	10	32
	26	CHOP	89% (58%)	7	37
Unterhalt *et al. Leukemia* **10** (1996), 836.	20	COP	80% (5%)	n.a.	n.a.
	19	PmM	80% (27%)		
Zinzani *et al. J. Clin. Oncol.* **18** (2000), 773.	18	Fludarabine/ idarubicin	61% (33%)	n.a.	n.a.
	11	Fludarabine	73% (27%)		
Lenz *et al. J. Clin. Oncol.* **23** (2005), 1984.	60	CHOP	75% (7%)	19	median not reached

ORR, overall response rate; CR, complete response; PFS, progression-free survival; mo, months; OS, overall survival; n.a., not available.

Table 11.3. Efficacy of fludarabine combinations in MCL.

Study	Regimen	Patients (n)	Disease status	ORR (CR)
Zinzani *et al. J. Clin. Oncol.* **18** (2000), 773.	Fludarabine 25 mg/m^2/d × 3 Idarubicin 12 mg/m^2/d × 1	18	First-line	61% (33%)
Flinn *et al. Blood* **96** (2000) 71.	Fludarabine 25 mg/m^2/d × 3 Cyclophosphamide 250 mg/m^2/d × 3	8	Relapsed	50% (13%)
Cohen *et al. Leuk. Lymphoma* **42** (2001), 1015.	Fludarabine 20–25 mg/m^2/d × 3 Cyclophosphamide 600 mg/m^2/d × 1	30	First-line and relapsed	63% (30%)
Seymour *et al. Cancer* **94** (2002), 585.	Fludarabine 30 mg/m^2/d × 2 Cisplatin 25 mg/m^2/d × 4 Cytarabine 500 mg/m^2/d × 2	8	Relapsed	88%
Lefrere *et al. Haematol.* **89** (2002), 1275.	Fludarabine 20 mg/m^2/d × 5 Cyclophosphamide 600 mg/m^2/d × 1	10	First-line	80% (40%)

Abbreviations as in Table 11.2.

of 20–35%. In the largest dataset available thus far, from the Swiss SAKK study group, weekly therapy at standard doses of rituximab for four weeks achieved complete and overall response rates of 2% and 27% respectively in 104 patients with newly diagnosed or relapsed MCL, resulting in a median event-free survival of 6 months only. Thus antibody monotherapy should be applied only in exceptional patients with strict contraindications for systemic chemotherapy.

In contrast, based on a proposed in-vitro synergism, a combined immunochemotherapy regimen of rituximab and CHOP achieved high overall (96%) and complete response rates (48%) in a recent phase II study. However, even patients achieving a molecular remission displayed a median progression-free survival of only 18.8 months, and there appeared to be no difference in duration of response between those who did and did not achieve molecular remission. A randomized trial confirmed that the addition

Table 11.4. Combined immunochemotherapy in MCL.

Study	Patients (n)	Regimen	Disease status	ORR (CR)	PFS	OS
Howard *et al. J. Clin. Oncol.* **20** (2002), 1288.	40	R-CHOP	First-line	96% (48%)	17 months	n.a.
Forstpointner *et al. Blood* **104** (2004), 3064.	55	R-FCM	Relapsed	62% (33%[a])	8 months	median not reached
Herold *et al. Blood* **104** (2004), 168a.	44	R-MCP	First-line	71% (32%)	20 months	median not reached
Lenz *et al. J. Clin. Oncol.* **23** (2005), 1984.	62	R-CHOP	First-line	92%[a] (32%)	19 months	median not reached

Abbreviations as in Table 11.2.

[a] Significant improvement in comparison to chemotherapy alone.

of rituximab results in a superior overall response rate of 94% versus 75% with CHOP alone ($p = 0.0054$); CR rates were also improved (34% vs. 7%, $p = 0.00024$). However, after a limited follow-up, again no major improvement of the progression-free survival was observed. Thus, R-CHOP represents a current standard approach in first-line therapy of MCL but additional consolidation concepts are warranted to translate the high response rates into long-term benefit for the patient.

In another trial by the German Lymphoma Study Group, the addition of rituximab not only resulted in significantly improved complete response rates (33% vs. 0%) and slightly higher overall response (62% vs. 49%, n.s.) in relapsed or refractory MCL, but more importantly an improved overall survival was observed after combined immunochemotherapy with R-FCM (fludarabine, cyclophosphamide, mitoxantrone) in comparison to FCM chemotherapy alone (Table 11.4). A third randomized trial compared combined rituximab immunochemotherapy to chemotherapy only with the MCP regimen (mitoxantrone, chlorambucil, prednisone), and also showed a trend towards higher complete (32% vs. 15%, $p = 0.08$) and overall response rates (71% vs. 63%) in the experimental arm; however, because of the smaller number of patients these differences were not significant and, in contrast to the previous study, no improvement of overall survival has been observed in the R-MCP arm.

Radioimmunotherapy (RIT)

Another approach is the application of radio- ([131]iodine or [90]yttrium) labeled anti-CD20 antibodies. Myeloablative regimens incorporating RIT followed by autologous stem-cell transplantation achieved high overall response rates of 100% (91% CR) and an estimated three-year overall survival of 93%. In contrast, conventional dose radioimmunotherapy delivered varying results, with 36% overall response and rapid progression, resulting in a median progression-free survival of only three months in relapsed disease. Other recent clinical trials are testing the use of RIT as consolidation following induction therapy, although results and longer-term follow-up have not yet been reported.

Dose-intensified regimens

Various studies of the efficacy of high-dose cytarabine (Ara-C) have reported promising results. More than 80% of patients obtained a complete remission following a sequential CHOP-DHAP regimen (dexamethasone, high-dose cytarabine and cisplatin). Similar encouraging results were achieved by several other study groups. Lefrere and colleagues observed a CR rate of $< 10\%$ in previously untreated patients with MCL following CHOP therapy, which was converted into an impressive 84% after four additional cycles of the high-dose cytarabine-containing DHAP regimen.

Table 11.5. Autologous stem-cell transplantation in the treatment of MCL.

Study	Patients (*n*)	Disease status	PFS	OS
Dreger *et al. Hematol. J.* **1** (2000), 87.	34	First-line	77% (2 years)	100% (2 years)
	12	Relapsed/ refractory	30% (2 years)	54% (2 years)
Andersen *et al. Eur. J. Haematol.* **71** (2003), 73.	27	First-line	15% (4 years)	51% (4 years)
Vandenberghe *et al. Br. J. Haematol.* **120** (2003), 793.	195	First-line/ relapsed/ refractory	55% (2 years)	76% (2 years)
Dreyling *et al. Blood* **105** (2005), 2677.	62	First-line	54% (3 years)	83% (3 years)

Abbreviations as in Table 11.2.

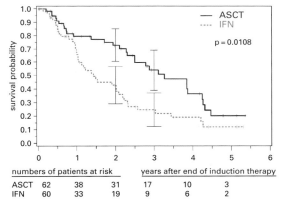

numbers of patients at risk

ASCT	62	38	31	17	10	3
IFN	60	33	19	9	6	2

Figure 11.4. Progression-free survival after high-dose radio-chemotherapy followed by autologous stem-cell transplantation (ASCT) or interferon α maintenance (IFN) in MCL (from Dreyling *et al.* 2005).

An even more dose-intensified approach by the M.D. Anderson Cancer Center used rituximab plus Hyper-CVAD (fractionated cyclophosphamide plus vincristine, doxorubicin and dexamethasone) alternating with high-dose methotrexate/cytarabine, and this again achieved impressive response rates (ORR 97%, CR 87%) and, importantly, prolonged remissions (three-year failure-free survival 64%), similar to the sequential dose-intensified approach with myeloablative consolidation. However, toxicity was significant, with 29% of patients unable to complete scheduled treatment and a therapy-associated mortality of 8%, including predominantly infectious complications and secondary myelodysplasia and/or acute myelogenous leukemia in four of 97 patients. Because of its toxicity, many MCL patients are not candidates for this regimen due to age or comorbidity, and modifications of the regimen are under study.

Sequential dose intensification and autologous transplantation

Encouraging results were obtained in various phase II studies exploring the potential of consolidation by myeloablative therapy followed by autologous stem-cell transplantation (ASCT). A randomized trial of more than 200 patients with previously untreated MCL compared the addition of myeloablative consolidation (12 Gy total-body irradiation, cyclophosphamide 2×60 mg/kg body weight) followed by ASCT after initial CHOP induction to conventional chemotherapy and interferon maintenance only (Table 11.5). This international prospective trial confirmed an impressive improvement in complete response (81% vs. 37%) and significantly longer progression-free survival rates (median PFS 39 vs. 17 months in the IFN-α study arm, $p < 0.001$, Fig. 11.4). Interestingly, the benefit of myeloablative consolidation was confirmed in several subgroup analyses, including patients with low and intermediate IPI scores, CR and PR after chemotherapy induction. However, so far no benefit of overall survival has been reported (71% vs. 51% 5-year overall survival, $p = 0.18$) and only a small number of patients included in this study received an antibody-containing regimen of combined immunochemotherapy. Despite these limitations, myeloablative radiochemotherapy followed by ASCT represents one of the standard therapeutic approaches in first-line treatment of younger MCL patients (age <65 years). However, even after such a dose-intensified consolidation, the vast majority of patients with MCL will eventually relapse.

One major obstacle of autologous stem-cell transplantation is the contamination of the harvested stem cells with circulating lymphoma cells. Thus, purging procedures have been introduced to eliminate residual lymphoma cells. Applying such a procedure with rituximab, various phase II studies have suggested an improved long-term outcome after antibody-based "in-vivo purging" and subsequent myeloablative therapy. The most favorable results have been reported by an Italian study group, with a progression-free survival of 79% after 54 months.

CONSOLIDATION AND MAINTENANCE THERAPY

Even after dose-intensified induction, a continuous relapse pattern has been observed in most series. Thus there is an urgent need for effective additional consolidation strategies to eliminate minimal residual disease after successful completion of induction.

Rituximab maintenance

Interestingly, in a recent update of a randomized trial in relapsed malignant lymphoma, a subgroup analysis revealed some benefit of rituximab maintenance even after a rituximab-containing induction in patients with relapsed MCL. The addition of eight applications of rituximab (four weekly doses after 3 and 9 months) resulted in an improvement of three-year progression-free survival from 9% to 45%. However, these data were generated in only a limited number of patients and thus have to be confirmed in larger trials before this strategy can be generally recommended. In a Swiss SAKK trial of rituximab monotherapy for newly diagnosed and relapsed or refractory MCL, no benefit of maintenance with four single doses of rituximab given every eight weeks was observed following standard weekly × 4 rituximab induction.

Radioimmunotherapy

Although first-line radioimmunotherapy induction has shown only limited efficacy, with disappointingly short durations of remissions, a recent preliminary report from the Polish study group suggested a higher efficacy in first-line treatment after an initial fludarabine-containing induction. In line with other previous observations with either unlabeled antibody or interferon maintenance, these data suggest that conventional radioimmunotherapy may be more efficient if applied as consolidation after initial tumor debulking, and may lead to longer-lasting remissions.

Interferon α maintenance

Two phase III studies investigated the value of interferon α maintenance (IFN-α) following conventional induction therapy; both of them suggested a tendency towards a prolonged progression-free survival. However, the number of patients was too low to exactly define the benefit of IFN-α.

ALLOGENEIC STEM-CELL TRANSPLANTATION

Allogeneic bone-marrow or stem-cell transplantation is still the only curative approach in patients with advanced-stage MCL. A graft-versus-lymphoma effect has been suggested to induce long-lasting complete remissions even in patients with relapsed or refractory MCL. However, transplantation-related mortality is relatively high, and graft-versus-host disease and infectious complications are especially common.

Two recent phase II studies applying a dose-reduced conditioning reported more encouraging survival rates in less intensively pretreated patients. Thus, with a minimal conditioning regimen (fludarabine and 2 Gy TBI), disease-free and overall survival in 33 patients with relapsed and refractory MCL was 60% and 65%, respectively, with non-relapse mortality of 24% at two years. Despite these promising early results, allogeneic transplantation outside of clinical trials should be applied only in relapsed disease or very selected high-risk patients not appropriately responding to dose-intensified first-line therapy.

MANAGEMENT OF RELAPSED DISEASE

The management of relapsed disease is highly dependent on the initially applied strategies, and thus

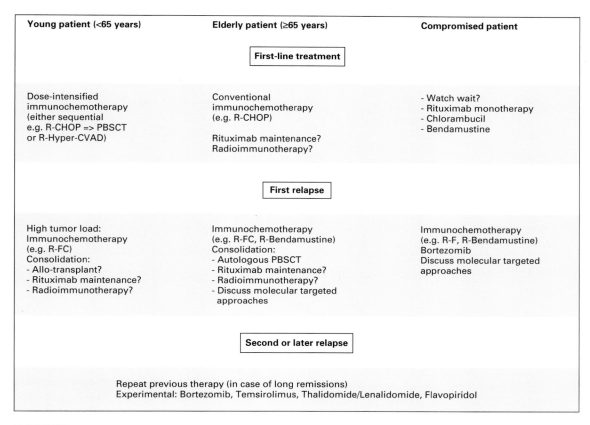

Young patient (<65 years)	Elderly patient (≥65 years)	Compromised patient
	First-line treatment	
Dose-intensified immunochemotherapy (either sequential e.g. R-CHOP => PBSCT or R-Hyper-CVAD)	Conventional immunochemotherapy (e.g. R-CHOP) Rituximab maintenance? Radioimmunotherapy?	- Watch wait? - Rituximab monotherapy - Chlorambucil - Bendamustine
	First relapse	
High tumor load: Immunochemotherapy (e.g. R-FC) Consolidation: - Allo-transplant? - Rituximab maintenance? - Radioimmunotherapy?	Immunochemotherapy (e.g. R-FC, R-Bendamustine) Consolidation: - Autologous PBSCT - Rituximab maintenance? - Radioimmunotherapy? - Discuss molecular targeted approaches	Immunochemotherapy (e.g. R-F, R-Bendamustine) Bortezomib Discuss molecular targeted approaches
	Second or later relapse	
	Repeat previous therapy (in case of long remissions) Experimental: Bortezomib, Temsirolimus, Thalidomide/Lenalidomide, Flavopiridol	

Figure 11.5. Therapeutic approaches for MCL patients (advanced stage). Since no standard therapy has been established for treatment of newly diagnosed or relapsed disease, treatment on clinical trial should be considered for all patients.

published data can hardly be compared, because of different patient risk profiles. Limited data suggest that the addition of rituximab is reasonable if a remission of at least 6–9 months has been achieved after a rituximab-containing regimen. In younger patients relapsed after dose-intensified regimens, an initial reduction of tumor load (e.g. with fludarabine-containing regimens) and subsequent allogeneic transplantation is recommended (Fig. 11.5). Alternatively, after conventional first-line therapy, dose-intensified approaches (either with sequential ASCT or the Hyper-CVAD regimen) should be discussed. In elderly patients (> 65 years), a non-cross-resistant regimen is recommended, and this has to be selected considering the patient's comorbidity. In such patients relapsed after R-CHOP first-line therapy, one might consider either fludarabine-containing regimens or other alternatives with limited side effects (e.g. bendamustine monotherapy). In patients initially treated with alkylating compounds only, a switch to more efficient induction strategies (either R-CHOP or high-dose cytarabine-containing regimens) is recommended. However, based on the expected clinical courses, with the majority of patients relapsing within 1–2 years, some additional consolidating strategies, either rituximab (or interferon) maintenance or radioimmunotherapy consolidation, is strongly encouraged. Whenever possible, in medically fit patients, dose intensification – if not applied in first line – may be rediscussed.

Bendamustine is a novel "hybrid" cytotoxic agent composed of a benzimidazole ring with an attached nitrogen mustard moiety, which acts primarily as a bifunctional alkylating agent but with activity distinct from other alkylators. Cell death is induced via

Table 11.6. Novel agents for treatment of relapsed and refractory mantle cell lymphoma.

Agent	Proposed targets	ORR (CR)	Reference
Bendamustine	Apoptosis, mitosis	75% (50%) (with rituximab)	Rummel *et al. J. Clin. Oncol.* **23** (2005), 3383.
Bortezomib	NF-κB, Bcl-2, p53, angiogenesis	33% (8%)	Fisher *et al. J. Clin. Oncol.* **24** (2006), 4867.
Thalidomide	Angiogenesis, microenvironment, and/ or cytokine pathways?	81% (30%)	Kaufmann *et al. Blood* **104** (2004), 2269.
Flavopiridol	Cyclin D1	11% (0%)	Kouroukis *et al. J. Clin. Oncol.* **21** (2003), 1740.
mTOR	PI3 kinase/Akt pathway	38%	Witzig *et al. J. Clin. Oncol.* **23** (2005), 5347.
[90]Y-ibritumomab tiuxetan	Radiotherapeutic monoclonal antibody	35% (22%)	Younes *et al. Blood* **106** (2005), 689a.

Abbreviations as in Table 11.2.

apoptosis pathways and apoptotic-independent "mitotic catastrophe." It has been utilized in Germany for over 20 years and has demonstrated single-agent activity in breast cancer and a variety of hematologic neoplasms including NHL, multiple myeloma and CLL. In a German study of bendamustine plus rituximab in 16 patients with relapsed MCL, including seven refractory to prior therapy, an overall response rate of 75% was observed, including CR in 50% (Table 11.6). The median progression-free survival was 18 months. Grade 3 leukopenia was observed in 16% of all NHL patients treated in this study, which also included indolent lymphoma. Non-hematologic toxicity was mild. Preliminary results of a recent small phase II US trial of bendamustine plus rituximab in relapsed MCL also have shown objective responses in the majority of patients treated, including CR in about a third. The most common toxicities were reversible myelosuppression and grade 1–2 non-hematologic toxicities.

Based on the promising results of various molecularly targeted regimens, which achieve similar response rates and durations of remission in comparison to chemotherapy only, one should discuss such innovative approaches preferably in a combined fashion (e.g. proteasome inhibitors, mTOR antagonists or thalidomide, as discussed below).

NOVEL THERAPEUTIC APPROACHES

MCL responds well in most cases to initial therapy. Improved overall and complete response rates have been achieved with newer immunochemotherapy approaches, compared with previous combination chemotherapy regimens. However, as discussed above, virtually all patients relapse within 1–4 years even after intensive induction therapy and/or autologous stem-cell transplantation. Second-line regimens may show high therapeutic activity, although the durability of these responses is often short-lived. There is thus a pressing need for better agents for relapsed and refractory patients, and a number of novel agents have shown clinical activity in this setting. These may be targeted to the dysregulated cell-cycle elements characteristic of this disease, or to other growth and proliferation or apoptosis pathways (Table 11.6). Many of these are already being incorporated into front-line regimens in an effort to improve complete response and progression-free survival in MCL.

Bortezomib

Bortezomib targets the ubiquitin–proteasome pathway and appears to provide therapeutic efficacy via effects on multiple cellular mechanisms in lymphoid neoplasms including NF-κB signaling, bcl-2-mediated anti-apoptosis, p53-related pathways and angiogenesis. The agent has been approved for the treatment of relapsed and refractory multiple myeloma, but has also been shown to inhibit the growth of human lymphoma cell lines, including MCL lines. Since many of the bortezomib-targeted pathways are active in MCL, it has been tested in patients with relapsed or refractory MCL. Two phase II studies, taken together, showed a 44% overall response rate, with 18% complete responses (Table 11.6). Bortezomib activity in MCL is being further tested in ongoing multicenter studies, as a single agent and in combination with rituximab, and in combination with immunochemotherapy.

Thalidomide

Thalidomide has activity in relapsed and refractory multiple myeloma and Waldenström's macroglobulinemia, with multiple potential mechanisms of action including direct antiproliferative effects, downregulation of tumor-cell/stromal-cell interactions with disruption of essential cytokine loops, immunomodulatory and anti-angiogenic effects. Given in combination with rituximab to a predominantly rituximab-naive group of 16 patients, 13 patients showed response, including five with CR (Table 11.6). The median progression-free survival was 20 months, longer than that observed for their previous chemotherapy regimen. Most patients required a dose reduction of thalidomide due to anticipated toxicities of somnolence, fatigue and constipation; two episodes of thromboembolism were observed. Ongoing studies include the use of thalidomide in combination with rituximab plus chemotherapy. There is also interest in assessing responses and toxicity of lenalidomide, the next-generation agent in this class, which appears to have more potent anti-tumor activity and a more favorable toxicity profile.

Flavopiridol

Flavopiridol is a synthetic flavone with mechanisms of action that include downregulation of cyclin D1 and cyclin D3 as well as competitive inhibition of the cyclin-dependent kinases CDK4 and CDK6. This ability to target the cell-cycle pathway renders the agent of interest for MCL, as does preclinical work in cell lines and animal models supporting its activity. Using a short-infusion protocol that appeared to decrease dose-limiting diarrhea (observed in previous flavopiridol studies in solid-tumor patients), a Canadian study found a modest 11% response rate in MCL for single-agent flavopiridol. However, after rescheduling the application based on pharmacokinetic data, impressive responses including some associated with acute tumor lysis have been reported, providing a rationale for further testing of this or other cell-cycle inhibitors in multi-agent combinations (Table 11.6).

Temsirolimus

The mammalian target of rapamycin (mTOR) is a downstream signaling molecule in the phosphatidylinositol-3 kinase (PI3K)/Akt pathway that serves a critical role in regulating mRNA translation, including that of cyclin D1. Temsirolimus (CCI-779), a derivative of rapamycin, has been tested in a phase II single-agent trial in relapsed MCL, based upon the potential ability to interrupt cyclin D1-dependent pathways. Using a flat dose of 250 mg intravenously, an overall response rate of 38% with a median time to progression of 6.5 months was observed among 34 heavily pretreated patients (median three prior therapies, range 1–11) (Table 11.6). Reversible but dose-limiting thrombocytopenia was the most frequent toxicity. A preliminary report of a follow-up study using a dose of 25 mg suggested similar activity with less toxicity, including thrombocytopenia, and there is interest in incorporating this agent into combination therapies for MCL.

Radioimmunotherapy (RIT)

RIT delivers a targeted radiotherapeutic, [90]yttrium or [131]iodine, via an anti-CD20 murine monoclonal antibody. Several applications of these agents are being investigated in MCL, as described above, including consolidation following induction immunochemotherapy and as a component of the conditioning regimen prior to stem-cell transplantation. In a preliminary report of a phase II single-agent study in relapsed and refractory MCL, responses were observed in eight of 23 patients (35%), with five patients achieving CR or CR unconfirmed (Table 11.6). The median response duration was 9.5 months, with delayed myelosuppression the most frequent toxicity.

FUTURE DIRECTIONS

Mantle cell lymphoma presents unique challenges among the non-Hodgkin's lymphomas, typically displaying an aggressive clinical course characterized by high responses to induction immunochemotherapy but with brief durations of response and overall poor survival. Current strategies for management outside clinical trials are outlined in Fig. 11.5, but treatment approaches are anticipated to evolve rapidly as a result of ongoing investigations that include stratifying patient risk by gene expression or phenotypic profiling, incorporating dose-intensified and targeted therapies front-line, and the identification of novel agents for relapsed disease which may ultimately move into front-line or consolidation therapy. Although challenging, MCL has provided important insights relevant to cancer pathogenesis and the role of cell-cycle, apoptosis and cell signaling pathways that may ultimately prove useful in other hematologic and non-hematologic neoplasms.

FURTHER READING

Dreyling, M., Lenz, G., Hoster, E. *et al.* Early consolidation by myeloablative radiochemotherapy followed by autologous stem-cell transplantation in first remission significantly prolongs progression-free survival in mantle cell lymphoma: results of a prospective randomized trial of the European MCL Network. *Blood* **105** (2005), 2677–2684.

Fang, N. Y., Greiner, T. C., Weisenburger, D. D. *et al.* Oligonucleotide microarrays demonstrate the highest frequency of ATM mutations in the mantle cell subtype of lymphoma. *Proc. Natl. Acad. Sci. USA* **100** (2003), 5372–5377.

Fernandez, V., Hartmann, E., Ott, G., Campo, E. and Rosenwald, A. Pathogenesis of mantle cell lymphoma: all oncogenic roads lead to dysregulation of cell cycle and DNA damage response pathways. *J. Clin. Oncol.* **23** (2005), 6364–6369.

Forstpointner, R., Dreyling, M., Repp, R. *et al.* The addition of rituximab to a combination of fludarabine, cyclophosphamide, mitoxantrone (FCM) significantly increases the response rate and prolongs survival as compared to FCM alone in patients with relapsed and refractory follicular and mantle cell lymphomas: results of a prospective randomized study of the German Low-Grade Lymphoma Study Group (GLSG). *Blood* **104** (2004), 3064–3071.

Forstpointner, R., Unterhalt M., Dreyling M. *et al.* Maintenance therapy with rituximab leads to a significant prolongation of response duration after salvage therapy with a combination of rituximab, fludarabine, cyclophosphamide and mitoxantrone (R-FCM) in patients with relapsed and refractory follicular and mantle cell lymphomas: results of a prospective randomized study of the German Low Grade Lymphoma Study Group (GLSG). *Blood* **108** (2006), 4003–4008.

Ghielmini, M., Schmitz Hsu, S. -F., Cogliatti, S. *et al.* Effect of single-agent rituximab given at the standard schedule or as prolonged treatment in patients with mantle cell lymphoma: a study of the Swiss Group for Clinical Cancer Research (SAKK). *J. Clin. Oncol.* **23** (2005), 705–711.

Gianni, A. M., Magni, M., Martelli, M. *et al.* Long-term remission in mantle cell lymphoma following high-dose sequential chemotherapy and in vivo rituximab-purged stem cell autografting (R-HDS regimen). *Blood* **102** (2003), 749–755.

Gopal, A. K., Rajendran, J. G., Petersdorf, S. H. *et al.* High-dose chemo-radioimmunotherapy with autologous stem cell support for relapsed mantle cell lymphoma. *Blood* **99** (2002), 3158–3162.

Hernandez, L., Bea, S., Pinyol, M. *et al.* CDK4 and MDM2 gene alterations mainly occur in highly proliferative and aggressive mantle cell lymphomas with wild-type INK4a/ARF locus. *Cancer Res.* **65** (2005), 2199–2206.

Herold, M., Pasold, R., Srock, S. *et al.* Results of a prospective randomised open label phase III study comparing rituximab plus mitoxantrone, chlorambucile, prednisolone chemotherapy (R-MCP) versus MCP alone in untreated advanced indolent non-Hodgkin's lymphoma (NHL) and mantle cell lymphoma (MCL). *Blood* **104** (2004), abstract 584.

Khouri, I. F., Lee, M. S., Saliba, R. M. *et al.* Nonablative allogeneic stem-cell transplantation for advanced/recurrent mantle-cell lymphoma. *J. Clin. Oncol.* **21** (2003), 4407–4412.

Lefrere, F., Delmer, A., Levy, V. *et al.* Sequential chemotherapy regimens followed by high-dose therapy with stem-cell transplantation in mantle cell lymphoma: an update of a prospective study. *Haematologica* **89** (2004), 1275–1276.

Lenz, G., Dreyling, M., Hoster, E. *et al.* Immuno-chemotherapy with rituximab and CHOP significantly improves response and time to treatment failure but not long-term outcome in patients with previously untreated mantle cell lymphoma: results of a prospective randomized trial of the German Low-Grade Lymphoma Study Group (GLSG). *J. Clin. Oncol.* **23** (2005), 1984–1992.

Maris, M. B., Sandmaier, B. M., Storer, B. E. *et al.* Allogeneic hematopoietic cell transplantation after fludarabine and 2 Gy total body irradiation for relapsed and refractory mantle cell lymphoma. *Blood* **104** (2004), 3535–3542.

Quintanilla-Martinez, L., Davies-Hill, T., Fend, F. *et al.* Sequestration of p27Kip1 protein by cyclin D1 in typical and blastic variants of mantle cell lymphoma (MCL): implications for pathogenesis. *Blood* **101** (2003), 3181–3187.

Romaguera, J. E., Fayad, L., Rodriguez, M. A. *et al.* High rate of durable remissions after treatment of newly diagnosed aggressive mantle-cell lymphoma with rituximab plus Hyper-CVAD alternating with rituximab plus high-dose methotrexate and cytarabine. *J. Clin. Oncol.* **23** (2005), 7013–7023.

Rosenberg, C. L., Wong, E., Petty, E. M. *et al.* PRAD1, a candidate BCL1 oncogene: mapping and expression in centrocytic lymphoma. *Proc. Natl. Acad. Sci. USA* **88** (1991), 9638–9642.

Rosenwald, A., Wright, G., Wiestner, A. *et al.* The proliferation gene expression signature is a quantitative integrator of oncogenic events that predicts survival in mantle cell lymphoma. *Cancer Cell* **3** (2003), 185–197.

Swerdlow, S. H. and Williams, M. E. From centrocytic to mantle cell lymphoma: a clinicopathologic and molecular review of 3 decades. *Human Pathol.* **33** (2002), 7–20.

Tort, F., Hernandez, S., Bea, S. *et al.* Checkpoint kinase 1 (CHK1) protein and mRNA expression is downregulated in aggressive variants of human lymphoid neoplasms. *Leukemia* **19** (2005), 112–117.

Zinzani, P. L., Magagnoli, M., Moretti, L. *et al.* Randomized trial of fludarabine versus fludarabine and idarubicin as frontline treatment in patients with indolent or mantle-cell lymphoma. *J. Clin. Oncol.* **18** (2000), 773–779.

12 DIFFUSE LARGE B-CELL LYMPHOMA

John W. Sweetenham

Pathology: Andrew Wotherspoon
Molecular cytogenetics: Andreas Rosenwald and German Ott

INTRODUCTION

Diffuse large B-cell lymphoma (DLBCL) is the most common type of non-Hodgkin's lymphoma (NHL), accounting for 35–40% of all cases of NHL. Despite high reported response rates to anthracycline-based combination chemotherapy regimens, only 50–65% of patients with this disease have achieved long-term disease-free survival with this approach. The emergence of new strategies, including monoclonal antibodies, dose-dense chemotherapy approaches and the identification of new rational therapeutic targets by gene expression profiling, has resulted in improvements in outcome for patients with this disease in recent years.

Involvement of extranodal sites, either as a primary site of disease or as sites of dissemination, is relatively common in DLBCL. With the exception of primary central nervous system lymphoma (see Chapter 14) and some other specific anatomic sites, treatment recommendations for DLBCL are generally identical for nodal and extranodal disease, with the exception of single-site non-lower limb DLBCL of the skin (see Chapter 16).

CLINICAL PRESENTATION

The clinical presentation of DLBCL, as with other types of NHL, is most commonly with painless lymphadenopathy. Approximately 25% of patients present with anatomically limited stage disease (clinical stage I or II), with the remaining 75% having more advanced disease (bulky stage II, or stage III–IV). Many patients will also experience constitutional ("B") symptoms including drenching night sweats, unexplained fevers and unexplained weight loss of more than 10% of body weight. Since extranodal disease is relatively common in DLBCL, and since almost any organ can be affected by this disease, presenting symptoms may mimic many other diseases. For example, patients with primary mediastinal large-cell lymphoma may present with chest discomfort, respiratory obstruction and symptoms and signs of superior vena cava obstruction. Patients with extranodal disease in the GI tract may present with abdominal discomfort, GI bleeding or evidence of intestinal obstruction. Patients with DLBCL may therefore be diagnosed through many different subspecialties.

PATHOLOGY

Diffuse large B-cell lymphoma replaces the nodal architecture, or that of extranodal sites of involvement, by a proliferation of large cells with a diffuse growth pattern. Several morphological variants have been described, based on the morphological appearance of the cells, the cellular background and the immunophenotype (Fig. 12.1).

The characteristically diffuse large B-cell lymphomas express CD45 with the pan-B-cell markers CD20 and CD79a. Monotypic surface and/or cytoplasmic immunoglobulin is demonstrable in a majority of cases. Combinations of staining for CD10, bcl-6 and MUM1 have been used as an immunocytochemical surrogate for the identification of germinal center phenotype (CD10+ or CD10−, bcl-6+ and MUM1−) as opposed to non-germinal center DLBCL, recapitulating the separation seen by studies using microarray techniques. The expression of bcl-2 protein is present in 30–50%. A proportion of cases express CD5 but these are negative for cyclin D1. Expression of CD30

Lymphoma: Pathology, Diagnosis and Treatment, ed. Robert Marcus, John W. Sweetenham and Michael E. Williams. Published by Cambridge University Press. © Cambridge University Press 2007.

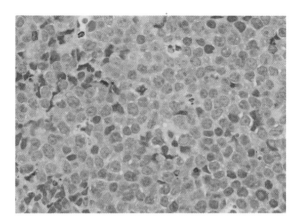

Figure 12.1. Diffuse large B-cell lymphoma. A sheet of large lymphoid cells with pale cytoplasm and large pleomorphic nuclei containing prominent nucleoli.

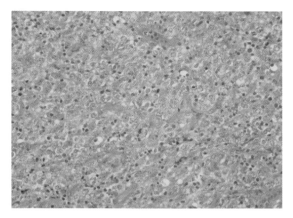

Figure 12.2. Diffuse large B-cell lymphoma. A sheet of large cells with abundant pale eosinophilic cytoplasm and nuclei that show marked lobulation.

is seen in occasional cases with non-anaplastic morphology. Staining for CD23 may also be seen in some cases (up to 16% in some series). Expression of CD138 may be seen in cases showing plasmablastic morphology but is rarely seen in other cases.

Centroblastic lymphoma

This variant is characterized by sheets of large cells with large vesicular nuclei containing prominent nucleoli that are mainly associated with the nuclear membrane. The nuclei are usually round or oval but in some cases may show prominent nuclear lobulation (polylobated centroblastic lymphoma-type) (Fig. 12.2).

Immunoblastic lymphoma

In this variant the vast majority of cells (> 90%) are immunoblasts with a moderate amount of basophilic cytoplasm and a round nucleus that contains a single, central eosinophilic nucleolus.

T-cell/histiocyte-rich B-cell lymphoma (TCHRBCL)

In this variant the neoplastic B cells form a small percentage (usually < 10%) of the cellular population while the majority of the cells are T lymphocytes and/ or histiocytes. The large cells may have a variety of appearances, including centroblastic or immuno-blastic, and in some cases they may resemble

Reed–Sternberg cells or the cells of lymphocyte-predominant Hodgkin's lymphoma. Small B cells are essentially absent. Some cases express CD30 but lack CD15, and there may be expression of epithelial membrane antigen (EMA).

These cases need to be distinguished from classical and lymphocyte-predominant Hodgkin's lymphoma. Immunophenotypic studies help distinguish them from classical HL, as the latter express CD30 and CD15 and lack the full B-cell-related antigen profile, while TCHRBCLs express CD20 and CD79a with staining for Oct-2 and Bob-1, and they are positive for CD45 with staining for EMA in a proportion of cases. The presence of nodular areas with large cells, within areas containing small B cells and follicular dendritic cell meshworks, raises the possibility of lymphocyte-predominant HL.

Anaplastic B-cell lymphoma

The cells of this variant of DLBCL have abundant cytoplasm. Their nuclei are pleomorphic and may resemble Reed–Sternberg cells or cells of anaplastic T-cell lymphoma. Multinucleate giant cells may be seen. There may be a sinusoidal pattern of infiltration within nodes.

Immunophenotypically the cells of this variant express CD30. They are distinguished from anaplastic T-cell lymphoma and Hodgkin's lymphoma by the expression of B-cell-related antigens, with absence of T-cell-associated markers or CD15. There is no staining for ALK kinase protein.

Plasmablastic lymphoma

The cells of this variant have abundant basophilic cytoplasm with eccentric nuclei that may be associated with a perinuclear clearing similar to that seen in plasma cells. The nuclear chromatin is clumped and there is usually a single prominent nucleolus.

Immunophenotypically the cells show features of plasma cell differentiation, with loss of CD45 and CD20. Staining for CD79a is retained and there is often staining for CD138.

Diffuse large B-cell lymphoma with expression of full-length ALK

The cells of this variant resemble centroblasts, immunoblasts or plasmablasts and in some cases may have a more anaplastic appearance, but in general they have more abundant cytoplasm than these more classical variants. The cells are weakly positive for CD45 and lack CD20 and CD79a. They are frequently positive for EMA but are negative for CD30. The cells contain cytoplasmic IgA. Staining for ALK kinase protein shows a granular cytoplasmic pattern. There is no expression of T-cell-related antigens.

Mediastinal (thymic) large B-cell lymphoma

There is diffuse infiltration of the mediastinum (or other extranodal sites with dissemination) by a population of cells with variable size. Most of the cells are large and in many cases the nuclei are lobulated. Characteristically the cytoplasm is abundant and pale. Sclerosis is usually present but the pattern is variable, ranging from pericellular to broad sclerotic bands separating the infiltrate into cellular nodules. Eosinophils may be associated with the neoplastic cell infiltrate and some cases may morphologically resemble Hodgkin's lymphoma of nodular sclerosis subtype (Fig. 12.3).

Immunophenotypically the cells express CD45 and the B-cell antigens CD20 and CD79a. Staining for bcl-6 is most often positive but CD10 is rarely expressed. Staining for CD5 is usually negative. There may be staining for EMA. CD30 is frequently expressed either focally or in all cells, but this is usually weaker than is seen in classical HL. Up to 70% of cases express CD23. Cytoplasmic immunoglobulin is usually absent.

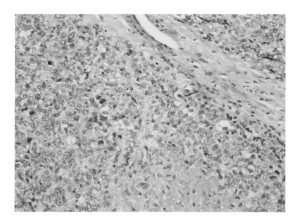

Figure 12.3. Mediastinal (thymic) large B-cell lymphoma (mediastinal mass). Sheets of large cells with pale/clear cytoplasm and large lobulated nuclei separated by fibrous bands with focal necrosis.

Intravascular large B-cell lymphoma

The cells of this lymphoma are characteristically confined within the lumen of small blood vessels, although a minor extravascular component may be observed in some cases. Cases in which the lymphoma cells are entrapped in mural thrombi are sometimes encountered. The tumor cells are large, with vesicular nuclei and prominent nucleoli. In some cases they may line the wall of the vessel, mimicking cuboidal endothelial cells. Erythrophagocytosis may be present in associated macrophages.

Immunophenotypically the cells are positive for CD45 and express the B-cell antigens CD20 and CD79a. Some cases are positive for CD10 or CD5. There is no expression of endothelial markers (e.g. CD34). Occasional cases with expression of T-cell-related antigens have been reported (Fig. 12.4).

MOLECULAR PATHOLOGY AND CYTOGENETICS

Diffuse large B-cell lymphoma is a heterogeneous disease clinically and, not surprisingly, this is also reflected at the molecular level. No unifying genetic alteration has been uncovered so far in this aggressive lymphoma; however, several chromosomal translocations, genomic copy number changes and molecular alterations occur in DLBCL with increased frequency. The hallmark translocation in follicular lymphoma, the t(14;18)(q32;q21), is present

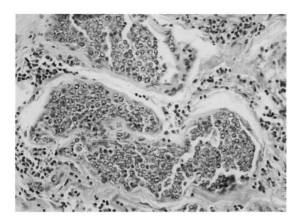

Figure 12.4. Intravascular large B-cell lymphoma. Clusters of large cells confined within vascular spaces. The cells have pleomorphic nuclei with prominent nucleoli.

in approximately 20% of DLBCL, and this genetic alteration is strongly associated with the germinal center type of DLBCL (GC-DLBCL) as defined by gene expression profiling. DLBCL carrying the t(14;18) may arise by transformation of a pre-existing follicular lymphoma, but this translocation presumably occurs also in *de novo* DLBCL. The *BCL-6* oncogene, located in the chromosomal band 3q27, is rearranged by translocation in approximately 30–40% of DLBCL cases. Translocations of *BCL-6* involve immunoglobulin heavy and light chain gene loci (in 14q32, 2p12 and 22q11) in half of the cases, whereas a number of alternative, non-immunoglobulin *BCL-6* translocation partners have also been described. *BCL-6* is typically expressed in germinal-center B cells, and *BCL-6* translocations may exert an oncogenic effect by preventing *BCL-6* downregulation, which occurs in normal B cells upon terminal differentiation. As an alternative way of Bcl-6 deregulation in DLBCL, the regulatory region of *BCL-6* can harbor mutations which may significantly deregulate Bcl-6 expression. The Burkitt translocation t(8;14)(q24;q32) involving the *C-MYC* oncogene is also encountered in a small subset of DLBCL (5–10%), and occasionally the distinction between a DLBCL carrying a *C-MYC* translocation and a *bona fide* Burkitt's lymphoma can be difficult.

An important aspect of the molecular pathogenesis of DLBCL may be the observation that 50% of these tumors show aberrant somatic mutation of various oncogenes and proto-oncogenes. Physiological somatic hypermutation occurs in normal germinal-center B cells and affects predominantly immuno-globulin genes in a process termed affinity maturation. In DLBCL, however, the hypermutation machinery appears aberrantly activated, leading to mutational events in additional genes such as *C-MYC*, *PIM1*, *PAX5* and *RhoH/TTF*, potentially resulting in their oncogenic activation.

In recent years, deeper insights into the molecular heterogeneity of DLBCL were gleaned by gene expression profiling studies using the DNA microarray technology. In particular, two major DLBCL subgroups could be discerned that differ in their underlying molecular features and in their clinical behavior. The germinal center B-cell type of DLBCL (GC-DLBCL) shows similarity in its global gene expression pattern to normal germinal-center B cells, while the other subgroup, termed activated B-cell-like DLBCL (ABC-DLBCL), displays gene expression features of mitogenically in-vitro-activated B cells. In a retrospective analysis, the clinical outcome of GC- and ABC-DLBCL patients varied considerably, with five-year survival of 60% (GC-DLBCL) and 35% (ABC-DLBCL). Beyond major differences in their global gene expression profiles, additional molecular features of the tumors point to a profound biological difference between GC- and ABC-DLBCL. In particular, as mentioned above, translocations of the *BCL-6* oncogene are strongly associated with the GC type of DLBCL, as are amplifications of a chromosomal region in 2p that harbors the *REL* and *BCL-11A* loci. Additional genetic differences between GC- and ABC-DLBCL include frequent chromosomal gains of 12q in GC-DLBCL, whereas chromosomal gains/amplifications of 3q and 18q are predominantly detected in the ABC-DLBCL subtype. In contrast to GC-DLBCL, ABC-DLBCL is characterized by constitutive activation of the oncogenic NF-κB pathway. Cell lines representative of this DLBCL subtype can be killed by blocking NF-κB, suggesting that this pathway may represent a potential new therapeutic target, e.g. for proteasome inhibitors (PS341).

Functional studies of GC- and ABC-DLBCL cell lines revealed additional molecular differences. For example, phosphodiesterase 4B (PDE4B), an inactivator of cyclic AMP (cAMP) which mediates apoptosis in B cells via AKT inactivation, is highly expressed in ABC-DLBCL. As a result, activation of the cAMP pathway in GC-DLBCL cell lines leads to apoptotic cell death, whereas there is no effect in ABC-DLBCL lines that have PDE4B expression. Likewise, the response to interleukin-4 stimulation appears to be different between the two subtypes.

The transcriptional heterogeneity of DLBCL is further highlighted by the description of additional gene expression signatures that are variably expressed between these tumors. Monti and colleagues, for example, defined "oxidative phosphorylation," "B-cell receptor proliferation" and "host response" clusters that show variable expression in DLBCL tumors. In the clinical setting, the gene expression profiling approach may also be used to predict survival of DLBCL at the time of diagnosis. By combining gene expression signatures that capture the germinal center phenotype, the proliferative activity, MHC class II expression and the host response, a powerful mathematical predictor can be constructed that identifies DLBCL patients with particularly favorable or poor prognoses. Genetic alterations such as gains of 3p may improve such survival predictors, indicating that genetic alterations may not be generally inherent in global gene expression profiles.

STAGING INVESTIGATIONS

Recommended staging investigations for newly presenting patients with DLBCL are summarized in Table 12.1.

Present treatment approaches to DLBCL are still largely based upon anatomic stage, and, particularly in the context of clinical trials, on the risk factors described by the International Prognostic Index (IPI) as described below. Emerging data on the potential value of ^{18}F-fluorodeoxyglucose positron emission tomography (FDG-PET) as a staging and response evaluation technique in this disease is likely to modify determination of disease extent in the future. It is therefore important to emphasize that new treatment strategies may emerge as new data on the value of FDG-PET appear. This subject is discussed more fully in Chapter 3.

PROGNOSTIC FACTORS

Since the introduction of the IPI, described in detail in Chapter 4, most clinical trials in DLBCL have been stratified according to this index, or have included patients with specific risk groups as defined by the

Table 12.1. Standard staging investigations in DLBCL.

Complete history and physical examination
Determination of performance status
Complete blood count and differential white-cell count
Serum biochemistry profile
Lactate dehydrogenase
Serum β_2 microglobulin
Serum protein electrophoresis and immunofixation
Chest X-ray
CT scan neck, chest, abdomen, pelvis
Bone-marrow aspirate and core biopsy for routine histopathology, flow cytometry, cytogenetics
Other imaging techniques including magnetic resonance imaging as indicated clinically
Potential future role for FDG-PET

IPI. For patients aged 60 years or less, in whom intensive treatment strategies have been widely used, the age-adjusted IPI (aaIPI) is a frequently used predictive model. Treatment strategies for clinically limited (stage I and II) disease have emerged separately from those for patients with more advanced-stage disease, and a "stage-adjusted" IPI has also been described in patients with stage I and II DLBCL (see below).

Although the IPI has proved to be a useful model for risk stratification in clinical trials in DLBCL, there is marked variability in outcome within each of the risk groups identified in the IPI, reflecting the underlying biological heterogeneity of this disease. This has limited the clinical utility of the IPI, and has led many investigators to study "biological" prognostic factors in DLBCL by the use of techniques such as gene expression profiling and tissue microarray studies. These techniques have allowed identification of distinct biological entities within DLBCLs, with possible clinical and prognostic significance, particularly related to the cell of origin of the lymphoma. There is no clear evidence at present that treatment should be modified according to cell of origin, although the findings from these techniques are likely to lead to the development of new treatments directed at rationally identified targets in the near future. At present, although some evidence suggests that distinct treatment approaches should be used in patients with early-stage compared with advanced-stage disease, there is no clear evidence that risk-adapted treatment of this disease has improved outcomes for specific risk groups. As a result, standard treatment approaches are still based primarily on anatomic stage of disease.

TREATMENT OF EARLY-STAGE DLBCL

Interpretation of clinical trials in patients with early-stage DLBCL has been complicated by the variable definition of limited disease. Many of the major clinical trials which have established treatment approaches for this disease were designed before the advent of the WHO classification and the IPI, and are heterogeneous with respect to inclusion of patients with various diffuse aggressive lymphomas. Since DLBCL is likely to be the predominant histological subtype in these trials, the results have generally been considered to be relevant to the management of DLBCL.

Early studies of the treatment of limited-stage DLBCL used involved-field radiation therapy (IF-RT), with most patients relapsing at sites distant from the irradiated area. Combination chemotherapy was therefore introduced in addition to radiation therapy in an attempt to control clinically undetected disease at distant sites. The use of combined modality therapy, with three cycles of CHOP (cyclophosphamide, doxorubicin, vincristine, prednisone) followed by involved-field radiation therapy, was compared with standard chemotherapy using eight cycles of CHOP in a study from the Southwest Oncology Group (SWOG). Localized disease was defined as non-bulky stage I or II disease. Disease bulk was defined as any mass measuring more than 10 cm in maximum diameter, or a mediastinal mass measuring more than one-third of the transthoracic diameter on a standard PA chest X-ray. The five-year progression-free survival was 77% for the combined modality arm versus 64% for chemotherapy alone ($p = 0.03$). The corresponding figures for overall survival (OS) were 82% and 72% ($p = 0.02$). This study established combined modality therapy with three cycles of CHOP chemotherapy followed by IF-RT as the standard of care for most patients with localized DLBCL. However, longer-term follow-up of this study has shown that the early survival advantage associated with combined modality therapy has not been maintained.

Other trials have investigated the need for IF-RT in this patient population. A recent study from the Groupe d'Etude des Lymphomes de l'Adulte (GELA) included 647 patients with localized aggressive NHL (81% of whom had DLBCL) who were randomized to receive either three cycles of CHOP chemotherapy followed by IF-RT, or dose-intensified chemotherapy with ACVBP (doxorubicin, cyclophosphamide, vindesine, bleomycin, prednisone) followed by sequential consolidation therapy with methotrexate, etoposide, ifosfamide and cytarabine. With a median follow up of 7.7 years, the five-year event-free survival (EFS) was 82% in the chemotherapy arm, compared with 74% in the combined modality arm ($p < 0.001$). The corresponding figures for overall survival were 90% and 81% ($p < 0.001$).

The outcomes for patients with non-bulky disease were analyzed separately, and the difference in EFS and OS in favor of the chemotherapy-only arm was maintained. The upper age limit for the GELA study was 61 years, with a median age of 46 years. By comparison, the median age in the SWOG was 59 years, with approximately 50% of the patients being over 60 years. It is therefore not clear whether an unselected patient population with limited-stage disease would tolerate or benefit from the dose-intensified chemotherapy used in the GELA study, particularly since this regimen was associated with a 25% hospitalization rate with each of the first three cycles of ACVBP chemotherapy.

Although the results of these studies suggest that chemotherapy alone may be adequate treatment for bulky disease, this was not confirmed by a study from the Eastern Cooperative Oncology Group (ECOG) in which 352 patients with clinical stage I or II disease (including bulky disease) were initially treated with eight cycles of CHOP chemotherapy. Patients in complete response after chemotherapy were randomized between 30 Gy of IF-RT or no further treatment. Patients in partial remission after chemotherapy received 40 Gy of IF-RT. For the 172 randomized patients, the six-year disease-free survival was 73% for the radiation therapy arm, compared with 56% for the observation arm ($p < 0.05$). No overall survival difference was observed. Patients with mediastinal large B-cell lymphoma (MLBCL) most commonly present with stage I or II disease, often with extranodal spread to either the pleura or pericardium. Patients with MLBCL have been included in the studies cited above. Although there is some uncertainty about the need for IF-RT in MLBCL, current evidence suggests that patients with this disease should be treated in the same manner as other patients with limited-stage DLBCL.

Table 12.2. Stage-adjusted International Prognostic Index.

Adverse factor	Stage-adjusted IPI
Stage	Bulky stage II
Age	> 60
LDH	> normal
Performance status	≥ 2
Extranodal sites	Not applicable

Primary testicular lymphoma also presents with early-stage disease in most patients. It typically affects patients in their 60s and 70s, and appears to have a worse prognosis than DLBCL at other sites. There is a relatively high incidence of CNS relapse as well as recurrence in the controlateral testis in patients who do not receive scrotal radiation therapy. These patients should therefore receive standard R-CHOP chemotherapy with scrotal irradiation. In view of the relatively high incidence of CNS relapse, intrathecal prophylaxis is often given, although there is no clear evidence that this reduces the risk of CNS recurrence.

The apparent differences in outcomes between the studies described above are, in part, related to patient selection for the various studies. Since patients with limited-stage disease represent a heterogeneous patient group, a stage-adjusted IPI has recently been proposed, to facilitate risk stratification in future studies in early-stage disease (Table 12.2). This prognostic model has been validated in other patient populations with early-stage disease. According to this model, patients with no adverse risk factors have projected five-year overall survival of approximately 95% when treated with brief-duration chemotherapy (CHOP × 3) and involved-field radiation therapy. Such combined modality therapy should therefore be considered the standard approach for this patient group, since future studies are very unlikely to demonstrate further improvements in outcome. In contrast, patients with one adverse factor have a projected five-year OS rate of around 70%, and only 50–60% of those with three or four adverse factors survive for five years. New approaches are therefore needed for these groups, although combined modality therapy as described above remains the current standard treatment.

Several studies in advanced DLBCL have now demonstrated improvements in disease-free and overall survival by the addition of the anti-CD20 monoclonal antibody rituximab to combination chemotherapy such as CHOP. No randomized studies have been reported to date in limited-stage disease. A recent phase II study from SWOG has tested the addition of rituximab to three cycles of CHOP chemotherapy plus IF-RT for diffuse aggressive B-cell NHL. The two-year progression-free survival was 94%. These results compared favorably with an historical series of patients treated with CHOP × 3 plus IF-RT using identical selection criteria. Randomized studies will be required to prospectively evaluate the benefit of the addition of rituximab to chemotherapy in this context.

Summary: early-stage DLBCL

A treatment algorithm for early-stage DLBCL is shown in Fig. 12.5.

- Combined modality therapy with brief-duration chemotherapy and IF-RT is the standard of care, irrespective of risk group according to the stage-adjusted IPI.
- The addition of rituximab to initial chemotherapy has not been formally evaluated in a randomized trial. Preliminary data suggest that it may reduce the need for IF-RT, but this requires prospective evaluation.
- Novel approaches include the addition of radio-labeled monoclonal antibodies to standard combined

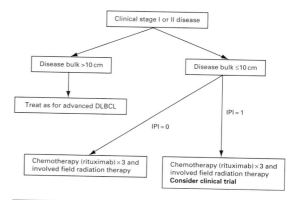

Figure 12.5. Treatment algorithm for early-stage DLBCL. The role of rituximab-containing chemotherapy in early-stage disease has not been evaluated prospectively. Use of rituximab is recommended based on results in advanced-stage disease.

modality therapy. Cooperative group trials testing this approach are under way at present.

TREATMENT OF ADVANCED-STAGE DLBCL

Approximately 75% of patients with DLBCL present with bulky stage II or stage III–IV disease, and should therefore be regarded as having advanced-stage disease. Until recently, CHOP was considered the standard first-line therapy for all patients with DLBCL, mainly on the basis of the SWOG randomized trial which compared this regimen with three more intensive regimens, showing no difference in response rates, progression-free or overall survival, but a higher toxicity rate in the regimens other than CHOP.

In recent years, a number of new approaches have been investigated, in an attempt to improve the outcome for patients with advanced-stage disease.

Dose-intensified and dose-dense therapy

Intensification of the CHOP regimen, either by reducing the treatment duration from 21 to 14 days or by the addition of etoposide to the standard regimen, has been investigated in two studies from the German non-Hodgkin's Lymphoma Study Group. Parallel studies were conducted in young and elderly patients, and in each study the comparison of CHOP-21 with CHOP-14 and CHOP with the same regimen plus etoposide (CHOEP) was performed using a 2×2 factorial design. The trial in older patients included 689 patients, 71% of whom had DLBCL, and CHOP-14 was shown to be significantly superior to CHOP-21. The five-year event-free rate for CHOP-21 was 33%, compared with 44% for CHOP-14 ($p = 0.003$). The corresponding rates for overall survival were 41% versus 53% ($p < 0.001$). The addition of etoposide had no effect in this study.

The corresponding study included 710 younger patients, aged 18 to 60 years, with stage I–IV disease and a normal LDH level. No event-free or overall survival benefit was seen in this group from reduction of the treatment interval from CHOP-21 to CHOP-14. However, an event-free survival benefit was seen for patients receiving CHOEP-14 or 21 (five-year EFS 69%) compared with those receiving CHOP-14 or 21 (five-year EFS 58%, $p = 0.004$). No overall survival benefit was observed, possibly due to the ability to "salvage" patients relapsing after first-line therapy.

The clinical relevance of these findings is unclear, and they must be evaluated in the context of rituximab-containing therapy (see below).

High-dose therapy and autologous stem-cell transplantation as a component of first-line therapy

The reported effectiveness of high-dose therapy (HDT) and autologous stem-cell transplantation (ASCT) as a salvage treatment in aggressive NHL has prompted many groups to investigate the use of ASCT as a component of first-line therapy, particularly for patients identified as having "poor risk" disease at presentation. Many trials are now published, although comparison of these studies is complicated by the variable inclusion criteria, and by the variable definition of poor-risk disease. Some of these studies are retrospective subset analyses of clinical trials which were not initially stratified according to risk groups and not statistically powered to detect differences in subgroup analysis.

Many prospective studies have subsequently been conducted, using the aaIPI to define poor-risk patients (Table 12.3). Results have been variable, although most studies have failed to show an advantage for high-dose versus conventional-dose remission consolidation.

A randomized study comparing eight cycles of CHOP chemotherapy with two cycles of a more dose-intensive first-line regimen, followed by high-dose therapy and ASCT for responding patients with advanced diffuse aggressive NHL, has recently been reported by Milpied and colleagues (Table 12.3). Eligible patients were aged 15 to 60 years with low-risk, low-intermediate-risk or high-intermediate-risk disease according to the aaIPI, and therefore represented a relatively favorable group compared with many other studies. An intent-to-treat analysis was performed, demonstrating a significantly higher EFS in the high-dose-therapy arm (55% vs. 37%, $p = 0.037$), although there was no difference in OS. Subset analysis showed a significant difference in OS in patients with high-intermediate-risk disease ($p < 0.001$).

In view of the conflicting results which have been reported in studies of first-remission transplantation

Table 12.3. Results of HDT and ASCT in first remission for DLBCL and other aggressive NHLs.

Reference	Patients (n)	Randomization	DFS (conventional chemotherapy vs. ASCT)	OS (conventional chemotherapy vs. ASCT)
Haioun *et al. J. Clin. Oncol.* **18** (2000), 3025–3030.	464	Sequential chemotherapy vs. HDT and ASCT in patients in CR after induction chemotherapy	52% vs. 59% at 3 years ($p = 0.46$)	71% vs. 69% at 3 years ($p = 0.6$)
Santini *et al. J. Clin. Oncol.* **16** (1998), 2796–2802.	124	VACOP-B vs. VACOP-B plus HDT and ASCT for responding patients	60% vs. 80% at 6 years ($p < 0.1$)	65% vs. 65% at 6 years ($p < 0.5$)
Kluin-Nelemans *et al. JNCI* **93** (2001), 22–30.	194	CHVmP/BV vs. CHVmP/BV plus HDT and ASCT for responding patients	56% vs. 61% at 5 years ($p = 0.712$)	77% vs. 68% at 5 years ($p = 0.336$)
Gianni *et al. NEJM* **336** (1997), 1290–1297.	98	MACOP-B vs. high-dose sequential therapy including HDT and ASCT	49% vs. 76% at 7 years ($p = 0.004$)	55% vs. 81% at 7 years ($p = 0.09$)
Gisselbrecht *et al. J. Clin. Oncol.* **20** (2002), 2472–2479.	370	ACVBP and sequential consolidation vs. intensive induction chemotherapy plus HDT and ASCT	76% vs. 58% at 5 years ($p = 0.004$)	60% vs. 46 at 5 years ($p = 0.007$)
Milpied *et al. NEJM* **350** (2004), 1287–1295.	207	CHOP vs. intensive induction chemotherapy plus HDT and ASCT	37% vs. 55% at 5 years ($p = 0.037$)	44% vs. 74% at 5 years ($p < 0.001$)

DFS, disease-free survival; OS, overall survival.

in aggressive NHL, a meta-analysis has recently been conducted. This study included data from 2018 patients from 13 randomized trials who were evaluable for outcome data. Although a significantly higher CR rate was reported for HDT and ASCT, no differences in EFS or OS were observed. No difference in outcome was seen according to IPI group, and analyses according to the number of patients with DLBCL, transplant conditioning regimen and response status prior to ASCT also failed to identify a group with superior outcome after HDT.

Based on these results, HDT and ASCT should not be considered a component of first-line therapy in patients with diffuse aggressive lymphoma (including DLBCL), irrespective of IPI risk group, and the addition of ASCT to standard induction therapy should still be considered experimental and used only in the context of clinical trials.

Since most of the studies reported above were conducted prior to the introduction of rituximab (see below) or dose-dense chemotherapy regimens, their

relevance to current management of diffuse aggressive NHL is unclear. The current SWOG 9704 study may help to clarify the role of remission consolidation with ASCT in patients receiving CHOP-rituximab as first-line therapy.

Addition of rituximab to chemotherapy

The benefit of adding rituximab to CHOP chemotherapy for DLBCL was initially demonstrated in a randomized trial from GELA. In this study, 399 previously untreated patients aged between 60 and 80 years with DLBCL were randomized to receive eight cycles of CHOP chemotherapy at 21-day intervals, or the same chemotherapy plus rituximab (R-CHOP) given on day 1 of each cycle. The R-CHOP arm was shown to be superior to CHOP in terms of complete response rate (76% vs. 63%, $p < 0.005$), two-year EFS (61% vs. 43%, $p < 0.002$) and two-year OS (70% vs. 57%, $p < 0.007$). Significant differences in EFS, PFS and OS were maintained in a subsequent report.

The survival advantage for R-CHOP in this trial was observed in all IPI risk groups. Subsequent analyses have suggested that the survival benefit of R-CHOP may be restricted to patients who have immunohistochemical evidence of expression of the bcl-2 protein, suggesting that rituximab may overcome the adverse prognostic significance of bcl-2 in DLBCL, possibly by modifying bcl-2-mediated chemoresistance.

The addition of rituximab to CHOP in elderly patients with DLBCL has also been investigated in an intergroup study in the USA, including patients aged over 60 years with previously untreated advanced DLBCL. Patients were randomized to receive either 6–8 cycles of CHOP, according to response, or the same chemotherapy plus rituximab. A second randomization was included for responding patients, between observation only and maintenance rituximab, given once per week for four weeks at six month intervals for a total of two years. Of 632 patients initially randomized, 415 responders were subsequently randomized to maintenance rituximab or observation only. There was a significant improvement in three-year failure-free survival (FFS) in the R-CHOP arm compared with CHOP (53% vs. 46%, $p = 0.04$) and in the maintenance rituximab arm compared with observation alone. The advantage of maintenance rituximab appeared to be limited to patients who did not receive this agent as part of their induction regimen. No overall survival differences were observed on the study, possibly because around 40% of patients randomized to receive CHOP alone received rituximab in the second randomization.

Further evidence for the benefit of addition of rituximab to chemotherapy has been reported from a retrospective population-based study from British Columbia, Canada, which has demonstrated higher event-free and overall survival rates for patients with DLBCL since the introduction of rituximab. A benefit for rituximab in younger, low-risk patients has also been shown in the MInT (MabThera International Trial). This study included patients with DLBCL with bulky stage I or stage II–IV disease, aged 18–60 years, with IPI scores of 0 or 1. Treatment comprised six cycles of CHOP, CHOEP or a comparable chemotherapy regimen with or without rituximab administered on day 1 of each chemotherapy cycle. Preliminary results have been reported for the first 326 randomized patients. The two-year time to treatment failure (TTF) was 76% for patients receiving chemotherapy plus rituximab, compared with 60% for those receiving chemotherapy alone ($p < 0.001$). The corresponding rates for overall survival were 94% versus 87% ($p < 0.001$).

These results suggest that the addition of rituximab to chemotherapy is likely to benefit all risk groups. Further studies will be required to determine whether biological markers such as bcl-2 protein expression will reliably predict those patients likely to benefit from the addition of rituximab to chemotherapy. The potential role of first-remission high-dose therapy and ASCT is uncertain for patients receiving rituximab as part of their induction regimen. The SWOG 9704 study may help to clarify its benefit in this context.

Other ongoing trials are comparing the R-CHOP combination given according to a standard 21-day or accelerated 14-day schedule.

Summary: advanced-stage DLBCL

A treatment algorithm for advanced and relapsed/refractory DLBCL is shown in Fig. 12.6.

- Rituximab-CHOP-21 should be regarded as the standard of care therapy for patients with advanced-stage DLBCL regardless of risk group.

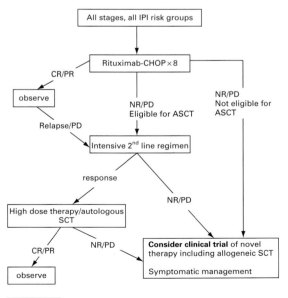

Figure 12.6. Treatment algorithm for advanced and relapsed/refractory DLBCL.

- The role of maintenance rituximab after rituximab-containing induction is unknown. It should only be used in the context of clinical trials.
- There is no current evidence to support the use of high-dose therapy and stem-cell transplantation as a component of first-line therapy, even for poor-risk patients – this approach should still be considered only in the context of prospective clinical trials.

MANAGEMENT OF RELAPSED DLBCL

Second-line therapy prior to ASCT

Although HDT and ASCT remains the standard of care for patients with relapsed DLBCL, a survival benefit for this approach has only been demonstrated convincingly in patients with disease which is responsive to second-line salvage chemotherapy. Commonly used second-line regimens, including DHAP (dexamethasone, high-dose cytosine arabinoside, cisplatin), ICE (ifosfamide, carboplatin, etoposide) and mini-BEAM (carmustine, etoposide, cytarabine, melphalan) produce overall response rates of 40–60%, and CR rates of only 25–35%. Analysis of the effectiveness of ASCT from the date of transplantation therefore overestimates the effectiveness of this approach in the entire population of relapsed patients. When analyzed by intent to treat, the event-free survival for relapsing patients with DLBCL treated with second-line salvage therapy followed by ASCT is between 20% and 35%.

The development of more effective second-line regimens has the potential advantage of increasing response rates and therefore increasing the number of patients eligible for ASCT. Two randomized studies in which rituximab-based second-line regimens are compared are in progress. The CORAL study, comparing R-DHAP with R-ICE in patients with relapsed DLBCL, is under way in Europe and the USA. The National Cancer Institute of Canada is leading a similar study comparing R-DHAP with another second-line regimen, R-GDP (rituximab, gemcitabine, dexamethasone, cisplatin).

Optimal second-line therapy therefore remains uncertain. Patients who do not achieve at least a partial remission on this therapy have a poor outcome when treated with HDT and ASCT in most series. These patients should be considered for trials of novel treatment approaches. A recent retrospective analysis from the UK has demonstrated that patients who do not respond to one conventional-dose salvage regimen are not rescued by subsequent conventional-dose salvage therapy.

High-dose therapy and ASCT

The use of HDT and ASCT has been regarded as the standard of care for patients with relapsed DLBCL for over a decade. This is based on the results of the PARMA randomized trial, a study that included 215 patients with relapsed aggressive NHL (mostly DLBCL), initially treated with two cycles of salvage chemotherapy with DHAP. Responding patients were randomized to receive further DHAP chemotherapy, or to proceed to high-dose therapy using BEAC (carmustine, etoposide, cytarabine, cyclophosphamide) and autologous bone-marrow transplantation. Significantly superior five-year event-free (46% vs. 12%, $p < 0.0001$) and overall survival (53% vs. 32%, $p = 0.038$) rates were observed for the transplant arm compared with the conventional chemotherapy arm. No formal follow-up analysis of the PARMA study has been published. Although this study established ASCT as the standard approach for patients with relapsed chemosensitive DLBCL, the results should be interpreted cautiously. Of the 215 patients entered onto the study, only 109 were randomized, the commonest reason for exclusion being that a patient did not achieve an adequate response to second-line therapy with DHAP (only 56% of patients responded to this chemotherapy). All subsequent survival analyses were restricted to randomized patients only, and no intent-to-treat analysis was performed.

In addition to these limitations, the relevance of the study in the present context is unclear. Improved supportive care, including the use of peripheral blood progenitor cells, has reduced the morbidity associated with high-dose therapy and extended its use to older patient groups, typically up to 70 or 75 years old. Most centers will now accept patients for transplantation if they achieved a PR to prior therapy, unlike the PARMA study, in which a previous CR was required for eligibility. The population of patients now receiving ASCT is therefore less defined than that in the original PARMA study, raising questions concerning the current relevance of this trial. The addition of rituximab to combination chemotherapy regimens, and the advent of accelerated 14-day regimens for first-line treatment, have improved disease-free and overall survival in DLBCL. It is not clear whether patients whose disease relapses after one of these regimens will have the same salvage rates as those treated without monoclonal antibodies as part of their initial treatment. A recent retrospective comparison of outcomes following ASCT for patients receiving first-line CHOP or R-CHOP has recently been reported from the University of Nebraska. No difference in event-free or overall survival following ASCT was observed according to initial therapy, although the total study population was only 103 patients.

In contrast, a recent report of dose-adjusted EPOCH-R as primary therapy in DLBCL has shown a two-year progression-free survival rate of 83%, with a very similar overall survival, indicating the high activity of this regimen and the apparent inability to salvage relapsed patients with a standard transplant approach.

Although high-dose therapy and ASCT remains the standard of care for patients with relapsed DLBCL which is still sensitive to second-line chemotherapy, the true benefit of this approach in the context of modern first-line therapies is unclear and requires re-evaluation.

Allogeneic stem-cell transplantation in DLBCL

Current data on the role of allogeneic SCT in aggressive lymphoma, using either myeloablative or non-myeloablative conditioning regimens, are limited. Comparative studies of allogeneic and autologous SCT in aggressive NHL have not shown a survival advantage for allogeneic SCT, despite the lower relapse rate in allogeneic recipients. The lower relapse rate has been offset by the increased therapy-related mortality associated with allogeneic transplantation. In the absence of clear evidence of a clinically relevant graft-versus-lymphoma effect in aggressive NHL, the use of allogeneic SCT should be restricted to research protocols.

Allogeneic transplantation for patients who relapse after autologous transplantation is increasing in use, although there are few data to confirm its benefit. A recent retrospective study from the International Bone Marrow Transplant Registry analyzed results for 114 patients with various subtypes of NHL who received allogeneic SCT after relapse following autologous SCT. All patients underwent myeloablative conditioning. The therapy-related mortality was 22% at three years, and the five-year OS and PFS were 24% and 5% respectively. No analysis was performed according to NHL subtype, but the study suggests that the curative potential for this approach is low and that its use should be restricted to patients in prospective trials.

Prognostic factors for relapsed DLBCL

Multiple early single-institution and registry studies of ASCT in aggressive NHL demonstrated the importance of sensitivity of disease to second-line therapy as a predictive factor for outcome after transplantation. Short (less than one year) remission duration and disease bulk at the time of ASCT were also identified as adverse factors in many studies.

The age-adjusted International Prognostic Index (aaIPI) has been shown to have predictive value in a follow-up report of the PARMA study. It proved highly predictive of response to DHAP. Patients with an aaIPI score of 0 had an overall response rate of 77%, compared to only 42% for those with three adverse factors. The aaIPI was predictive of overall survival for the entire patient cohort. When randomized patients were analyzed separately, the aaIPI was predictive for those receiving DHAP, but not in those undergoing ASCT. In a subset analysis, there was no difference in overall or progression-free survival according to randomized arm for patients with an aaIPI score of 0, although a significant difference remained for those with scores of 1–3. Similar results have been reported from other centers.

These subset analyses should be interpreted cautiously, but question whether ASCT offers a survival advantage to low-risk patients. In both studies, results are poor in the high-risk patients, underlining the need for novel strategies. One recent study has also addressed the potential value of cell of origin, as defined by tissue microarrays, as a prognostic factor for patients undergoing salvage therapy with HDT and ASCT. In this study, no difference in overall survival was observed when patients with germinal center or non-germinal center phenotypes were compared.

The potential value of functional imaging using FDG-PET, following salvage therapy but prior to

HDT and ASCT, has also been assessed. In patients with Hodgkin's lymphoma, PET-scan positivity prior to ASCT has been shown to be highly predictive of outcome. In the case of DLBCL, limited data have been published from small studies, and the predictive value of PET in this context therefore remains unclear.

Other treatment approaches for relapsed disease

Radiolabeled monoclonal antibodies

Both ^{131}I-tositumomab (Bexxar) and ^{90}Y-ibritumomab tiuxetan (Zevalin) are active agents in indolent and transformed CD20-positive B-cell lymphomas. Few data are available for these agents in DLBCL. A phase II study of ^{90}Y-ibritumomab tiuxetan in 104 patients with relapsed or refractory DLBCL, not eligible for HDT and ASCT, has shown an overall response rate of 44%. The response rate was higher in patients who had not had prior therapy with rituximab, compared with those who had been previously treated with rituximab and chemotherapy as their primary treatment. Median PFS was around six months for patients who were rituximab-naive, compared with only about two months for those previously treated with rituximab.

These agents have also been studied in high-dose regimens used with ASCT. Most studies to date have included patients with mixed histologic subtypes of NHL. Early results indicate that both ^{131}I-tositumomab and ^{90}Y-ibritumomab tiuxetan can be combined with standard high-dose chemotherapy regimens without additional toxicity or prolongation of engraftment times. In view of the emerging data on the use of rituximab as maintenance therapy in DLBCL, new studies are currently being planned to assess the use of radioimmunotherapy to consolidate remission after induction therapy with R-CHOP and other rituximab–chemotherapy combinations in DLBCL.

Summary: relapsed DLBCL

See Fig. 12.6 for a treatment algorithm for relapsed/refractory DLBCL.
- High-dose therapy and autologous stem-cell transplantation is the standard of care for patients with chemosensitive relapse.
- The true impact of stem-cell transplantation in patients relapsing after rituximab-containing therapy is unclear.

Table 12.4. Potential therapeutic targets in DLBCL.

CD22
Histone deacetylase (HDAC)
HLA-DR
Proteasome
Bcl-6
Bcl-2
mTOR/Akt
CD40
TRAIL
PKC-β

- Allogeneic stem-cell transplantation has no proven benefit in relapsed DLBCL and should be used only in the context of prospective clinical trials.
- Patients with refractory disease do not benefit from stem-cell transplantation. Other experimental strategies should be considered.
- New treatment approaches are required for patients who relapse after stem-cell transplantation, or who are ineligible for transplantation.

NEW THERAPEUTIC TARGETS IN DLBCL

The use of molecular techniques including gene expression profiling has identified many potential rational therapeutic targets which are now under investigation in DLBCL. Some of these are listed in Table 12.4.

Histone deacetylase (HDAC) inhibitors may have several potential mechanisms of action in DLBCL. Acetylation of histones in the nucleosome is a major determinant of the regulation of many genes. Deacetylation of histones results in condensed chromatin structure and repression of gene transcription. Inhibitors of HDAC such as suberoylanilide hydroxamic acid (SAHA) have been shown to induce differentiation and/or apoptosis in various tumor cell lines, and this agent has demonstrated clinical activity in heavily pretreated patients with NHL. HDAC inhibitors may exert some of their activity in DLBCL through *BCL-6*. This gene is thought to be important in the pathogenesis of DLBCL, and has been shown to be anti-apoptotic in tumor cells through inhibition of transcription of the *p21WAF1* gene. In the presence of HDAC inhibitors, *p21WAF1* transcription results in growth inhibition, apoptosis and differentiation. Various HDAC inhibitors are now in early-phase clinical trials in DLBCL and results are awaited. The anti-VEGF monoclonal antibody, bevacizumab, has been shown to be active in phase II studies in relapsed DLBCL, presumably acting through inhibition of angiogenesis. A clinical non-progression rate of 25% was observed for the 51 patients in this study, with a median time to progression of five months (range 4–18 months). This agent is now being assessed in combination with R-CHOP in phase II studies by ECOG and SWOG.

Mammalian target of rapamycin (mTOR) is a serine/threonine protein kinase involved in the regulation of cell growth in response to multiple nutrients. It is phosphorylated via the PI3/Akt pathway and plays a role in the regulation of apoptosis. It also appears to be involved in the regulation of angiogenesis through effects on production of VEGF. Clinical studies of various agents which target mTOR are now under way, including CCI-779.

The expression of protein kinase C β (PKC-β) by immunohistochemistry has been shown to be an adverse prognostic factor in DLBCL, and in-vitro studies of inhibitors of PKC-β, including bryostatin, have validated this molecule as a target in DLBCL. Preliminary phase I data confirm the clinical activity of agents directed against this target, and phase II studies are in progress.

FURTHER READING

Coiffier, B., Lepage, E., Briere, J. *et al.* CHOP chemotherapy plus rituximab compared with CHOP alone in elderly patients with diffuse large B-cell lymphoma. *N. Engl. J. Med.* **346** (2002), 235–242.

Fisher, R. I., Gaynor, E. R., Dahlberg, S. *et al.* Comparison of a standard regimen (CHOP) with three intensive chemotherapy regimens for advanced non-Hodgkin's lymphoma. *N. Engl. J. Med.* **328** (1993), 1002–1006.

Greb, A., Schiefer, D. H., Bohlius, J. *et al.* High-dose chemotherapy with autologous stem cell support is not superior to conventional-dose chemotherapy in the first-line treatment of aggressive non-Hodgkin's lymphoma: results of a comprehensive meta-analysis. *Blood* **104** (2004), 263a [abstract].

Habermann, T. M., Weller, E. A., Morrison, V. A. *et al.* Phase III trial of rituximab-CHOP (R-CHOP) vs. CHOP with a second

randomization to maintenance rituximab (MR) or observation in patients 60 years of age and older with diffuse large B-cell lymphoma (DLBCL). *Blood* **102** (2003), 6a [abstract].

Hans, C. P., Weisenberger, D. D., Greiner, T. C. *et al.* Conformation of the molecular classification of diffuse large B-cell lymphoma by immunohistochemistry using a tissue microarray. *Blood* **103** (2004), 275–282.

Horning, S. J., Weller, E., Kim, K. *et al.* Chemotherapy with or without radiotherapy in limited-stage diffuse aggressive non-Hodgkin's lymphoma: Eastern Cooperative Oncology Group Study 1484. *J. Clin. Oncol.* **22** (2004), 3032–3038.

Miller, T. P., Dahlberg, S., Cassady, J. R. *et al.* Chemotherapy alone compared to chemotherapy plus radiotherapy for localized intermediate- and high-grade non-Hodgkin's lymphoma. *N. Engl. J. Med.* **339** (1998), 21–26.

Miller, T. P., Unger, J. M., Spier, C. *et al.* Effect of adding rituximab to three cycles of CHOP plus involved field radiotherapy for limited-stage aggressive diffuse B-cell lymphoma (SWOG-0014). *Blood* **104** (2004), 48a [abstract].

Pfreundschuh, M., Trumper, L., Gill, D. *et al.* First analysis of the completed MabThera International (MInT) trial in young patients with low-risk diffuse large B-cell lymphoma (DLBCL): addition of rituximab to a CHOP-like regimen significantly improves outcome of all patients with the identification of a very favorable subgroup with IPI = 0 and no bulky disease. *Blood* **104** (2004), 48a [abstract].

Pfreundschuh, M., Trumper, L., Kloess, M. *et al.* Two-weekly or 3-weekly CHOP chemotherapy with or without etoposide for the treatment of young patients with good-prognosis (normal LDH) aggressive lymphomas: results of the NHL-B1 trial of the DSHNHL. *Blood* **104** (2004), 626–633.

Pfreundschuh, M., Trumper, L., Kloess, M. *et al.* Two-weekly or 3-weekly CHOP chemotherapy with or without etoposide for the treatment of elderly patients with aggressive lymphomas: results of the NHL-B2 trial of the DSHNHL. *Blood* **104** (2004), 634–641.

Philip, T., Guglielmi, C., Hagenbeek, A. *et al.* Autologous bone marrow transplantation as compared with salvage chemotherapy in relapses of chemotherapy-sensitive non-Hodgkin's lymphoma. *N. Engl. J. Med.* **333** (1995), 1540–1545.

Reyes, F., Lepage, E., Ganem, G. *et al.* ACVBP versus VHOP plus radiotherapy for localized aggressive lymphoma. *N. Engl. J. Med.* **352** (2005), 1197–1205.

Rosenwald, A., Wright, G., Chan, W. C. *et al.* The use of molecular profiling to predict survival after chemotherapy for diffuse large B-cell lymphoma. *N. Engl. J. Med.* **346** (2002), 1937–1947.

Sehn, L. H., Donaldson, J., Chhanabhai, M. *et al.* Introduction of combined CHOP plus rituximab therapy dramatically improved outcome of diffuse large B-cell lymphoma in British Columbia. *J. Clin. Oncol.* **23** (2005), 5027–5033.

Alan S. Wayne and Wyndham H. Wilson

Pathology: Andrew Wotherspoon
Molecular cytogenetics: Andreas Rosenwald and German Ott

INTRODUCTION AND PRESENTATION

Burkitt's (BL) and lymphoblastic lymphomas (LBL) are highly aggressive diseases with distinct natural histories and clinical presentations. BL mostly occurs in the first two decades of life and accounts for 1–2% of all lymphomas. Three clinical variants are recognized: endemic BL, which is primarily found in equatorial Africa and Papua New Guinea, sporadic BL, which presents worldwide but is the most common type in Western countries, and immunodeficiency-associated BL, which is associated with HIV infection. There are important clinical differences in these variants (Table 13.1), with endemic BL involving the jaw, orbit and paraspinal regions in half of the cases as well as the mesentery and gonads, while sporadic BL mostly involves the distal ileum, cecum and/or mesentery, and rarely the jaw. When bulky or disseminated disease is present, extranodal involvement of the ovaries, kidney, breasts and/or central nervous system (CNS) may be seen. Clinical presentation in a Berlin–Frankfurt–Munster Group (BFM) series of 152 pediatric patients included advanced-stage (III/IV) disease in 38%, bone-marrow involvement in 33% and CNS disease in 4%. Overall, 27% of the patients in this series presented as acute leukemia and are usually referred to as the L3 subtype of acute lymphoblastic leukemia (ALL) within the French–American–British (FAB) classification. BL infrequently presents in adults, but does occur with increased frequency in patients with HIV infection.

LBL is most commonly a malignancy of T-cell precursor cells, and as such it is identical to T-cell acute lymphoblastic leukemia (T-ALL). The World Health Organization (WHO) classifies these as a single entity, with the exception that blasts make up < 25% of nucleated bone-marrow cells in LBL. T-ALL makes up approximately 15% of pediatric and 25% of adult ALL. Most individuals without frank leukemia present with advanced-stage disease (III/IV), and bulky adenopathy, anterior mediastinal mass, pleural effusion and/or massive organomegaly are common. Patients should be closely evaluated for emergent complications such as airway obstruction, superior vena cava syndrome and pericardial tamponade. Marrow involvement may result in cytopenias and/or hyperleukocytosis, and CNS involvement is frequent (5–15%) at diagnosis. Rare individuals with B-lineage LBL (i.e. B-precursor ALL/LBL and < 25% marrow blasts) present with more confined disease (e.g. bone, skin). LBL/T-ALL has historically faired poorer than B-precursor ALL; however, intensified treatment has minimized this difference. Currently, the outcome for children with LBL is excellent, although older individuals have lower relapse-free survival rates.

PATHOLOGY

Burkitt's lymphoma

Burkitt's lymphoma is characterized by a diffuse proliferation of rather monotonous intermediate-sized cells with little pleomorphism. Within the sheet of neoplastic cells are dispersed macrophages containing apoptotic nuclear debris that give the so-called "starry sky" appearance to this lymphoma at low magnification (Fig. 13.1). The cells have deeply basophilic cytoplasm containing small vacuoles (best seen on imprint/cytology sections but which can sometimes be seen at the edge of tissue sections) that contain fat. The nuclei are not usually larger than those of the associated macrophages and are

Lymphoma: Pathology, Diagnosis and Treatment, ed. Robert Marcus, John W. Sweetenham and Michael E. Williams. Published by Cambridge University Press. © Cambridge University Press 2007.

Table 13.1. Comparison of endemic, sporadic, and HIV-associated Burkitt's lymphoma.

	Endemic	Sporadic	HIV-associated
Epidemiology	Equatorial Africa and Papua New Guinea. Geographic association with malaria.	United States and Europe	United States and Europe
Incidence	5–10 per 100 000	2–3 per million	6 per 1000 AIDS cases
Age and gender	Malignancy of childhood Peak incidence 4–7 years Male : female ratio 2 : 1	Malignancy of childhood and young adults Median age 30 years Male : female ratio 2–3 : 1	Malignancy of adults Associated with higher CD4 counts $> 100/mm^3$
Clinical presentation	Jaw and facial bones in *c*.50%. Also involves mesentery and gonads. Increased risk of CNS dissemination.	Abdomen most common presentation, often involving the ileo-cecal region. Other extranodal sites include bone marrow, ovaries, kidneys, breasts. Increased risk of CNS dissemination.	Nodal presentation most common, with occasional bone marrow. Increased risk of CNS dissemination.

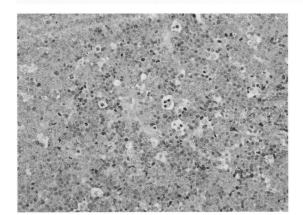

Figure 13.1. Burkitt's lymphoma. A diffuse proliferation of cells and scattered macrophages with apoptotic debris giving a "starry sky" appearance.

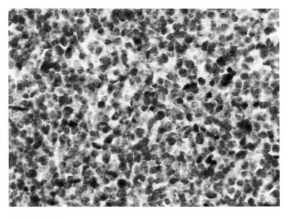

Figure 13.2. Burkitt's lymphoma. The proliferation marker Ki-67 stains > 98% of tumour cell nuclei.

characteristically round with a smooth contour and little variation in size or shape. The nuclear chromatin is granular and there are 2–5 rather indistinct small nucleoli. Mitoses are frequent.

Immunophenotypically the cells are positive for CD45 and express the B-cell markers CD20 and CD79a. They are positive for markers of germinal-center origin CD10 and bcl-6, but always lack bcl-2 protein expression, and they are negative for CD5 and CD23. The proliferation marker Ki67 stains > 98% of tumor cell nuclei (Fig. 13.2). The cells are negative for terminal deoxynucleotidyl transferase (TdT).

Precursor B-lymphoblastic lymphoma/leukemia

This is predominantly a disease of bone marrow, where there is effacement of the intertrabecular space by a sheet-like diffuse proliferation of cells. In lymph nodes the infiltrate usually effaces the nodal architecture with a diffuse pattern but there are usually occasional residual reactive germinal centers within the diffuse blastic infiltrate. Scattered histio-cytes may be seen within the infiltrate.

Morphologically the lymphoma cells are medium-sized blast cells with scanty cytoplasm. The nuclei are

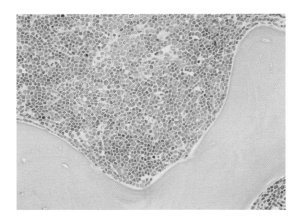

Figure 13.3. Precursor B-lymphoblastic lymphoma. Expression of TdT and other markers of immaturity such as CD34, CD117 and CD99. Proliferation is high, but does not reach 95%.

either monotonous or may show a degree of pleo-morphism. They are usually round with indentations but may be convoluted. The chromatin is classically finely granular ("salt and pepper" chromatin). Nucleoli are not usually prominent but may be seen in some cases. Mitoses are easily seen. Distinction of reactive hematogones from subtle marrow infiltration by lymphoblastic lymphoma is essential, and may be problematic, as hematogones may be numerous in children and following chemotherapy.

Immunophenotypically the cells frequently do not express CD45 and are most frequently negative for CD20. The majority of cases are positive for CD79a and CD10, with expression of bcl-2 protein. The precursor nature of the lymphoid cells is indicated by expression of TdT and other markers of immaturity such as CD34, CD117 and CD99. Proliferation is high, but does not reach 95% (Fig. 13.3).

Precursor T-lymphoblastic lymphoma/leukemia

Infiltration is usually as a sheet, with linear infiltration of cells into surrounding soft tissue at the periphery.

Morphologically T-lymphoblastic lymphoma is indistinguishable from the B-cell counterpart. The cells are medium-sized blasts with scanty cytoplasm and nuclei that may be round, indented or more obviously convoluted. Chromatin is finely granular ("salt and pepper"). Nucleoli are usually indistinct or small. Mitoses are frequent and there may be

scattered histiocytes in the infiltrate. In mediastinal lesions remnants of normal thymus may be seen. Distinction from normal thymus and lymphocyte-rich thymomas is essential and may be difficult morphologically, particularly when the biopsies are small. This is helped by the demonstration of intimately admixed epithelial proliferations in thymomas using antigens to high-molecular-weight cytokeratin, while the T cells of lymphoblastic lymphoma extend well away from any residual epithelial structures and into fatty connective tissue.

Immunophenotypically the cells are usually negative for CD45. There is variable expression of T-cell antigens CD2, CD3, CD5 and CD7. Cells may express CD4 or CD8 but frequently express both and may express neither. The cells are usually positive for bcl-2 protein. Expression of CD79a (usually associated with B-cell phenotype) is frequent, and expression of CD10 may also be seen. The immature nature of the cells is confirmed by expression of TdT, CD34, CD117 and CD99. There is variable expression of CD1a. Occasionally myeloid-associated antigens (CD13, CD33) may be expressed. Proliferation is high but does not exceed 95%.

MOLECULAR PATHOLOGY AND CYTOGENETICS

The progress in molecular profiling of Burkitt's and Burkitt-like lymphoma, together with precursor lymphoblastic lymphoma/leukemia, not only promotes our understanding of the mechanisms involved in the pathogenesis of these lymphomas and related leukemias, but also provides an important tool for the definition of prognostic subgroups and therapy stratification.

Burkitt's lymphoma

Although BL comprises only 1–2% of all lymphomas in western Europe and the USA, it represents 30–50% of childhood lymphomas in the same parts of the world and 25–35% of all HIV-associated lymphomas. In endemic areas, it is the most common childhood malignancy.

Epstein–Barr virus (EBV) infection is reported in nearly 100% of endemic BL patients, 20–30% of sporadic BL patients and approximately 40% of HIV-BL, characteristically as a latency I phenotype with restricted EBV nuclear antigen 1 (EBNA1) expression.

The chromosomal translocations involving 8q24/ *MYC* represent a cytogenetic hallmark of all three clinical forms of BL and result in the deregulation of the *MYC* gene by juxtaposition to immunoglobulin regulatory sequences and loss or disruption of its 5′ regulatory sequences. In approximately 85% of BL cases, the translocation partner of *MYC* is the immunoglobulin heavy chain (IgH) locus on chromosome 14, whereas in the remaining 15% the κ and λ light chain loci on chromosomes 2 and 22, respectively, are involved. Interestingly, the position of the breakpoints in both the 8q24/*MYC* and 14q32/IgH loci varies between geographical regions. In most sporadic BL the *MYC* breakpoints are located within intron 1 or the region immediately 5′ of *MYC*, whereas in endemic cases they are dispersed over a large genomic area 5′ of *MYC*. The 14q32/IgH breakpoints are characteristically located in the switch region of the IgH locus in sporadic tumors, whereas endemic BLs harbor breakpoints in the rearranged VDJ region of the IgH locus that contains somatic hypermutations. This observation suggests different pathogenetic mechanisms for the generation of chromosomal breakpoints in endemic and sporadic BL patients (namely translocation events during the process of IgH hypermutation or during IgH class switch recombination, respectively) and points to a derivation from different stages of B-cell development.

The *MYC* gene represents a key regulator of various cell-cycle checkpoints and, most importantly, provides strong proliferation signals. On the other hand, apoptosis is promoted as well through induction of the *ARF–MDM–p53* pathway and the activation of the BH3-only protein Bim, which acts as a powerful inhibitor of bcl-2. Transforming events that are able to circumvent pro-apoptotic properties of *MYC* upregulation in BL cells include the inactivation of p53 by mutation, which can be detected in approximately 30% of primary tumors, as well as *MDM2* overexpression and *p14/ARF* deletion. Recent data have shown that mutations in codons 57 and 58 of the translocated *MYC* result in inefficient induction of Bim, thus providing additional survival stimuli.

In cytogenetic analysis, BLs are characterized by a relatively simple karyotype; when present, complex karyotypic alterations are associated with a poor clinical prognosis. Abnormalities of chromosome 1, including 1q duplication or balanced translocation, and of chromosomes 13q, 17 and 22 have been reported in substantial subsets of BL. Concomitant *MYC* and *BCL-2* chromosomal translocations can occasionally be detected, and are usually associated with very aggressive disease.

Two recent gene expression profiling studies revealed a distinct global molecular signature of Burkitt's lymphoma that allows for a clinically relevant discrimination from diffuse large B-cell lymphoma (DLBCL) on molecular grounds. As expected, BL is characterized by high expression levels of c-myc target genes, but also by a subgroup of germinal-center-associated B-cell genes that differs significantly from the physiologic expression profile of normal germinal-center B cells. In addition, low expression of MHC class I molecules and NF-κB target genes are a hallmark feature of BL. Importantly, a subset of aggressive B-cell lymphomas was identified that according to current classification criteria was diagnosed as DLBCL, whereas a gene expression-based classification approach clearly placed these cases in the BL category. Although the number of these cases was low and clinical data were obtained retrospectively, these patients appeared to benefit from intensified chemotherapy regimens. Genomic profiling using array-based comparative genomic hybridization (array CGH) revealed that BL is characterized by a low chromosomal complexity score, whereas DLBCL patients, including cases harboring a *C-MYC* rearrangement, had a high chromosomal complexity score.

Precursor B-lymphoblastic lymphoma/leukemia

The translocation t(12;21)(p13;q22), resulting in a *TEL–AML1* fusion transcript, is detected in up to 25% of childhood ALL. Both *TEL* and *AML1* (also known as *RUNX1*) genes are involved in other leukemia-associated translocations as well, for example by generating fusion transcripts with *RDGFRβ*, *MN1*, *ABL*, *EVI1*, *JAK2* and *CBFβ*. In contrast to childhood ALL, the *TEL–AML1* translocation represents a relatively rare genetic aberration in adult ALL patients (3% of adult B-ALL). In both age groups, however, the translocation confers a highly favorable prognosis, with event-free survival (EFS) rates close to 90%. Microarray-based gene expression profiling has revealed a distinctly homogeneous expression pattern in ALL cases with *TEL-AML1* translocations, suggesting that tumors harboring this aberration represent a unique leukemia subtype. Interestingly, the tumor cells have been shown to overexpress the erythropoietin receptor which potentially affects proliferation and survival signaling of the tumor cells. Hyperdiploidy (more than 50 chromosomes per leukemic cell) is also a common genetic alteration detected in about 30% of pediatric and 9% of adult B-ALL cases. This condition also defines a patient subgroup with an excellent clinical outcome. In addition, pediatric cases with trisomies 4, 10 and 17 may have a specifically favorable prognosis. In about 20% of patients with hyperdiploid chromosome clones, activating mutations in the receptor tyrosine kinase gene *FLT3* have been demonstrated, suggesting a possible therapeutic benefit from the administration of small tyrosine kinase inhibitor molecules in this group.

The translocation t(9;22) encoding the BCR–ABL fusion protein can be detected in about 30% of adult and 5% of pediatric B-ALL tumors and confers an adverse prognosis in both age groups. The different incidence of the t(9;22) in pediatric and adult B-ALL may, at least in part, account for the overall difference in clinical outcome between the two age groups, and bone-marrow transplantation during first remission is often recommended in B-ALL patients with a *BCR-ABL* fusion transcript. In contrast to hyperdiploidy, hypodiploidy (fewer than 45 chromosomes) is an infrequent finding in B-ALL patients (< 2%) which has been associated with poor outcome. The tumors in about 6% of B-ALL patients may harbor the t(1;19)(q23;p13) chromosome translocation that generates the *E2A-PBX1* fusion transcript. This chimeric protein interferes with hematopoietic differentiation by disrupting the HOX-gene-dependent regulatory network.

Aberrations involving the chromosomal band 11q23 are detected in lymphoblastic and acute myeloid leukemias. The *mixed-lineage leukemia* (MLL) gene in 11q23 is involved in translocations with more than 40 different translocation partners, generating fusion proteins harboring the NH_2 terminus of the *MLL* gene and COOH terminus of the partner genes. Translocations involving *MLL* probably play a role in leukemogenesis via deregulation of the HOX pathway. The most common *MLL* translocation, the t(4;11)(q21;q23), results in an AF4–MLL fusion protein. It is present in almost 50% of infant ALL cases, and less frequently in other age groups, and is associated with a poor prognosis. Approximately 20% of

the cases with *MLL* translocations show a high expression of the FLT3 receptor tyrosine kinase, due to a mutation in the activation loop region. This finding suggests that MLL fusion proteins may cooperate with activated tyrosine kinases in promoting leukemogenesis. In keeping with this concept, FLT3 inhibitors are anti-tumor effective in vitro and in mouse models.

Precursor T-lymphoblastic lymphoma/leukemia

Chromosomal rearrangements in precursor T-lymphoblastic lymphoma/leukemia frequently result in proto-oncogene deregulation by juxtaposing them to T-cell receptor (TCR) regulatory elements. Important genes involved in such rearrangements are *TAL1*, *MYC*, *LYL1*, *LMO1*, *LMO2*, *HOX11*, and *HOX11L2*. *TAL1* overexpression is induced by the translocation t(1;14)(1p32;q11) or by deletion of upstream regulatory elements of the gene, and occurs in about 25% of pediatric T-ALL. The deregulated expression of TAL1 probably activates a set of genes that are normally quiescent in T-cell progenitors or, alternatively, may inactivate E2A homo- and heterodimers. The translocations t(11;14)(p15;q11) and t(11;14)(p13;q11) are thought to affect similar pathways via the ectopic expression of the *LMO1* and *LMO2* genes. LMO1 and LMO2 proteins are highly expressed in the central nervous system but nearly inactive in T cells and their progenitors.

The deregulated expression of *HOX11* in T cells, as a consequence of either the t(10;14)(q24;q11) or the t(7;10)(q35;q24), promotes transformation via disruption of normal cellular regulatory networks. These aberrations occur in approximately 30% of adult T-ALL patients and in only 3% of childhood ALL cases. In both age groups, abundant ectopic HOX11 protein expression is associated with a favorable clinical outcome. The *HOX11L2* gene located in the chromosomal band 5q35 is deregulated in a subset of T-ALL patients by either the t(5;14)(q35;q11) or the t(5;14)(q35;q32). The latter translocation results in HOX11L2 overexpression by juxtaposing it to the *BCL-11b* gene that is differentially expressed during T-cell development. Using molecular techniques, *HOX11L2* translocations are detected in about 20% of T-ALL patients, but are an infrequent finding in adults.

Recently, microarray-based gene expression studies have revealed that T-ALL cases overexpressing

Table 13.2. Staging systems.

Stage	St. Jude	Ann Arbor
I	Single site (excluding abdomen or mediastinum)	Single node region or extranodal site (I_E)
II	Single extranodal site with regional nodes ≥ 2 node regions, same side of diaphragm 2 extranodal sites, same side of diaphragm Primary GI, completely resected (II_R)	≥ 2 nodal sites, same side of diaphragm $\pm$ Localized contiguous extranodal site (II_E)
III	2 extranodal sites, both sides of diaphragm ≥ 2 nodal sites, both sides of diaphragm Primary thoracic Primary GI, extensive Paraspinal, epidural	≥ 2 nodal regions, both sides of diaphragm $\pm$ Localized contiguous extranodal site (III_E) Spleen (III_S) or Both (III_{ES})
IV	CNS and/or bone marrow ($< 25\%$ blasts)	Bone marrow or liver Diffuse extranodal disease not encompassed in a single radiation field E: Single extranodal site contiguous with a known nodal site A: No symptoms B: Fever, weight loss, night sweats

HOX11 and *HOX11L2*, as well as T-ALL with *MLL* fusion genes, share the same expression pattern, characterized by a global *HOXA* gene deregulation signature. The translocation t(11;19)(q23;p13), resulting in an *MLL–ENL* fusion transcript, occurs in acute myeloid leukemia patients, but also in patients with B-ALL and T-ALL. In T-ALL patients, the translocation is associated with a favorable prognosis and long-term survival. T-ALL with a *CALM–AF10* fusion, generated by the t(10;11)(p13;q14), characteristically displays immature phenotypic features, either lacking TCR expression or expressing TCRγ/δ.

While the *NOTCH1* gene is rarely targeted by chromosomal translocations, activating mutations in this gene have been detected in approximately 50% of T-ALL tumors of all different molecular subtypes. The *NOTCH1* gene encodes a transmembrane receptor involved in the regulation of normal T-cell development, and chromosomal aberrations involving *NOTCH1* have been shown to induce T-ALL in mouse models.

STAGING

Staging is a critical component of treatment for lymphomas. In particular, the recognition that early-stage BL and LBL require less treatment than advanced-stage disease has led to risk-adaptive strategies that are dependent on the accuracy of the staging classification systems. The Ann Arbor staging system, which is the most commonly used system for lymphomas, was initially developed for radiation treatment of Hodgkin's lymphoma. As such, it is relatively useful for identifying nodal and extranodal regions involved by disease, but much less so for disease bulk or specific disease sites. The occurrence of BL and LBL in pediatrics led to the St. Jude staging system, which was developed to more accurately reflect tumor bulk and high-risk disease sites (Table 13.2). The St. Jude staging classification recognizes early-stage (I and II) disease as low risk but, unlike the Ann Arbor system, requires resection of abdominal disease, which is an adverse site in BL. Stage III disease is identified by disease on both sides of the diaphragm, similar to the Ann Arbor classification, but also includes primary intrathoracic or unresected abdominal disease. Stage IV in both classifications involves the bone marrow and/or CNS. Overall, the St. Jude staging system is most commonly used for risk-adaptive treatment of BL and LBL.

Standard staging entails the use of whole-body computerized tomography (CT) scans, with particular attention to the bowel in the case of BL, where involvement may not be readily apparent. FDG-PET (positron emission tomography) scans are not standard but may yield additional staging information. Evaluation of the central nervous system with magnetic resonance imaging (MRI) and cerebral spinal fluid analysis for cytology are essential to rule out active involvement by Burkitt's lymphoma or lymphoblastic lymphoma. Patients should also undergo bone-marrow biopsy, and flow cytometry of the blood may be useful to rule out a leukemic phase. Serologies for HIV and hepatitis B are also indicated, given the increased incidence of BL in the former and the risk of hepatitis B reactivation in patients with a carrier state.

TREATMENT PRINCIPLES FOR BURKITT'S LYMPHOMA

BL is a systemic disease and requires chemotherapy for all disease stages. Importantly, locoregional radiation does not improve survival and should be avoided. While older studies showed that surgical resection of abdominal disease improves outcome, indicating the importance of tumor volume, more effective and risk-adapted treatments have made surgical resection unnecessary except for specific complications like obstruction, perforation, fistula or bleeding.

Early treatment strategies for BL were modeled on ALL regimens employing dose-intensified and prolonged treatment with induction, consolidation and maintenance phases. These approaches stood in contrast to the significantly less dose-intensified regimens used in adults with "intermediate-grade" lymphoma, such as CHOP and CHOP-based regimens, which only produced a 50–60% EFS. While dose intensity and dose density are important treatment components for BL, later studies indicated that shorter treatment durations were equally successful and less toxic. Furthermore, the recognition that tumor volume is an important prognostic feature led to the use of risk-adaptive approaches and a further reduction in treatment for early-stage patients.

Several biological characteristics of BL have helped guide treatment strategies, including its high proliferative fraction. It has been recognized for years that BL is sensitive to multiple chemotherapy classes, and in endemic BL "cures" were occasionally achieved with single-agent cyclophosphamide. Despite initial sensitivity, however, patients frequently relapsed, particularly those with higher volume disease. This apparent dichotomy can potentially be explained by the high tumor proliferative rate. The role of tumor cell kinetics was raised some 30 years ago by Skipper and colleagues, who observed that the fraction of cells undergoing DNA replication, termed the "growth fraction," greatly influenced drug sensitivity – a finding that likely reflects the greater sensitivity during S phase to many drug classes. Although a high growth fraction would predict greater drug sensitivity, it could also lead to greater tumor proliferation between cycles. Depending on the relative impact of these two effects, cure could increase due to higher fractional cell kill or decrease if tumor proliferation between cycles leads to a "kinetic" failure. One strategy to overcome "kinetic" failure is to increase dose density through frequent chemotherapy administration, a strategy employed by most BL regimens. Another strategy is to increase the fractional cell kill or efficacy of chemotherapy, thereby reducing the number of tumor cells which can survive and proliferate between cycles. Hence, BL regimens are relatively high-dose and employ multiple chemotherapy agents administered in alternating cycles. They typically include anthracyclines, epipodophyllotoxins, vinca alkaloids and alkylators, as well as methotrexate and cytarabine, which are cell-cycle-specific agents and take advantage of the high rate of tumor proliferation. These agents, however, are administered in a variety of combinations and schedule, indicating the empiric nature of the actual combinations (Table 13.3). Indeed, the optimal dose and schedule of cyclophosphamide, methotrexate and cytarabine remain unknown, and vary among the major regimens (Table 13.4).

The risks of tumor lysis syndrome and propensity for CNS dissemination in BL also have important treatment implications. To reduce tumor lysis, which can produce life-threatening electrolyte imbalances and renal failure, many regimens employ a pre-phase in which relatively low-dose cyclophosphamide and prednisone are administered. This strategy has been incorporated into the regimens of the Société

Table 13.3. Comparison of dose and dose intensity among Burkitt's lymphoma regimens.

	CODOX-M/IVAC	LMB 89	BFM 90	Dose range
Doxorubicin				
Dose	40	60	50	40–60
Dose intensity	13	20	25	13–25
Cyclophosphamide				
Dose	1600	1500	1000	1000–1600
Dose intensity	533	500	500	500–533
Vincristine				
Dose	3	2	1.5	1.5–2
Dose intensity	1.0	0.63	0.75	0.63–1.0
Etoposide				
Dose	300	800	200	200–800
Dose intensity	100	266	100	100–266
Methotrexate				
Dose	6720	8000	5000	5000–8000
Dose intensity	2240	2666	2500	2240–2666
Cytarabine				
Dose	8000	9000	600	600–9000
Dose intensity	2666	3000	200	200–3000
Ifosfamide				
Dose	7500	—	4000	4000–7500
Dose intensity	2500	—	2000	2000–2500
Other drugs	—	Prednisone	Dexamethasone	—

Dose is expressed as mg/m^2. Dose intensity is expressed as planned dose intensity and calculated as mg/m^2 per week.

Française d'Oncologie Pédiatrique (SFOP), German Multicenter Study Group for Adult ALL (GMALL) and BFM, but not CODOX-M or Hyper-CVAD (Table 13.4). The high risk of CNS involvement is handled by the use of relatively high-dose intravenous methotrexate and cytarabine, both of which have CNS penetration, and intrathecal administration. An important advance has been to reduce intrathecal treatment and eliminate whole-brain radiation for prophylaxis, which has significantly reduced CNS toxicity.

TREATMENT OF BURKITT'S LYMPHOMA

Beginning in 1981, the SFOP developed a series of protocols to refine the treatment of BL and L3 ALL (LMB).

These studies demonstrated that short dose-intensified treatment was effective in patients without CNS involvement, and that dose intensification of methotrexate, cytarabine and etoposide with cranial irradiation improved the EFS of patients with CNS involvement to 75%. Based on these findings, a risk-adapted protocol (LMB 89) was developed in which treatment was based on tumor burden and early response to chemotherapy (Table 13.4). Using the St. Jude staging, group A included stage I or II with abdominal resection; group B included unresected stage I, non-abdominal stage II, any stage III or IV disease and/or L3 ALL (CNS negative and < 70% marrow blasts); and group C patients had CNS involvement and/or > 70% marrow blasts. Based on these risks, group A only received induction, group B received pre-phase, induction, consolidation and limited maintenance, and group C also

Table 13.4. Selected regimens for Burkitt's lymphoma.

Regimen	Patients (n)	Histology (n)	Median age (yrs) (range)	Stage (%)	CR (%)	EFS (%)	OS (%)
LMB 89	561	Burkitt's and L3 ALL (420)	8 (0.17–18)	III–IV 79%	97%	92% at 5 yrs	92% at 5 yrs
Modified LMB	72	Burkitt's and L3 ALL	33 (18–76)	III–IV 67%	72%	65% at 2 yrs	70% at 2 yrs
GMALL B-NHL 86	35	L3 ALL	36 (18–65)	—	74%	71% at 4 yrs for DFS	51% at 4 yrs
Modified GMALL (CALGB)	92	Burkitt's and L3 ALL	47 (17–78)	III–IV 89%	74%	45–52% at 3 yrs	50–54% at 3 yrs
BFM 90	413	Burkitt's and L3 ALL (322)	9 (1.2–17.9)	III–IV 60%	N/A	89% at 6 yrs	14 deaths
CODOX-M/IVAC	21 pediatric 20 adult	Burkitt's	12 (3–17) 25 (18–59)	III–IV 78%	95%	85% (ped.) and 100% (adults) at 2 yrs	2 deaths
CODOX-M/IVAC	52	Burkitt's	35 (15–60)	III–IV 61%	77%	65% at 2 yrs	73% at 2 yrs
Hyper-CVAD	26	L3 ALL	58 (17–79)	—	81%	61% at 3 yrs for DFS	49% at 3 yrs
Intensive sequential and ASCT	27	Burkitt's	36 (15–64)	III–IV 44%	81%	73% at 5 yrs	81% at 5 yrs

CR, complete response; EFS, event-free survival; OS, overall survival; DFS, disease-free survival.

received extended maintenance and cranial irradiation if the CNS was involved. If a CR was not achieved in groups B and C after the third or fourth induction–consolidation course, patients underwent autologous transplant. This strategy was highly successful in pediatric patients, with five-year event-free and overall survivals of 92% (Table 13.4). The success of LMB 89 in pediatrics led to its testing in adults with minor modifications (Table 13.4). The outcome in 72 adult patients, mostly with advanced disease, was favorable, with EFS and OS of 65% and 70%, respectively, at two years. Toxicity remains a problem for advanced-stage patients due to the treatment intensity. Therapy-related deaths from infection were higher in adults than in children, with incidences of 5% and 1.6%, respectively, among patients in groups B and C. Myelosuppression was the primary treatment complication, with over 40% of adults experiencing febrile neutropenia. Tumor lysis syndrome requiring dialysis was prevented by the pre-phase treatment and associated supportive care.

The GMALL reported excellent results with an intensive 18-week regimen in adult patients with L3 ALL. In an effort to reduce CNS toxicity, the Cancer and Leukemia Group B (CALGB) studied a modified version in which intrathecal methotrexate was reduced and cranial radiation was only administered to high-risk patients (Table 13.4). These patients were compared to another cohort, who received the standard CNS prophylaxis. Overall, with 92 patients enrolled in the two cohorts, there were no differences in outcome, with EFS and OS of 45–52% and 50–54%, respectively, at three years. This study suggested that short-duration treatment with less intensive CNS prophylaxis was equally effective as more aggressive prophylaxis, and with significantly less neuroxicity.

Another highly effective regimen for BL was developed by the BFM (Table 13.4). Like other regimens for BL, the BFM approach was based on short, intensive cycles and over the course of several protocols led to a reduction in the number of cycles based on risk stratification. The BFM 90 protocol continued to further refine the risk stratification and to improve the outcome of patients who had an incomplete initial response with further treatment intensification. Among 322 pediatric patients with BL or L3 ALL treated with the BFM 90 regimen, the overall EFS was 89% at six years. Importantly, this represented a significant advance for advanced-stage patients compared to the previous BFM 86 protocol.

Two clinical trials conducted at the National Cancer Institute (NCI protocols 77-04 and 89-C-41) diverged from the leukemia model of treatment and investigated the role of more limited treatment (Table 13.4). In the 77-04 protocol, three cycles of intravenous cyclophosphamide, vincristine, doxorubicin, methotrexate and leucovorin rescue with cytarabine intrathecal prophylaxis (CODOX-M) showed that intensive combination chemotherapy produced an EFS of 66% in patients with low-risk disease. However, patients with high-risk disease (i.e. St. Jude stage IV) fared poorly, with a 19% EFS. Based on the observation that some patients were salvaged with combination ifosfamide, etoposide and cytarabine (IVAC), a successor protocol 89-C-41 was developed in which CODOX-M was alternated with IVAC and administered for four cycles in high-risk patients. This approach yielded an overall EFS of 85%, compared to 55% for all patients treated on CODOX-M alone, with no difference between low- and high-risk disease. When the CODOX-M/IVAC regimen was tested in an adult cooperative group trial, however, they only achieved an EFS of 65% at two years.

The Hyper-CVAD regimen was based on a modification of a regimen developed by Murphy *et al.* for pediatric L3 ALL (Table 13.4). In this regimen, hyper-fractionated cyclophosphamide, vincristine, doxorubicin and dexamethasone were alternated with methotrexate and cytarabine for a total of eight cycles. The results in 26 adults with L3 ALL were quite favorable, with EFS of 73% at five years. Based on these results in L3 ALL, this regimen is also used for BL.

In an effort to improve the outcome of BL, investigators have explored the role of autologous stem-cell transplantation (ASCT) consolidation. One study investigated the role of two courses of intensive chemotherapy, without high-dose methotrexate or cytarabine, followed by BEAM (BCNU, etoposide, cytarabine and melphalan) and ASCT (Table 13.4). In a multicenter study of 27 adult patients with BL

without CNS or extensive bone marrow involvement, the EFS was 73% at five years. While these results are encouraging, they are not significantly different from other regimens, and question the added benefit of ASCT over current approaches.

While current treatments are quite effective in BL, improvements are needed in patients in advanced-stage disease. Furthermore, toxicity of the regimens for advanced-stage disease is high, particularly in older adults, and treatment-related mortality is excessive. Because all BL regimens are very aggressive, there are no specific recommendations regarding which ones to use in adults. However, the treating physician must be cognizant of their toxicity, particularly in patients over 50 years of age. Hence, new strategies are needed to improve the therapeutic index of treatment and to increase efficacy. The success of rituximab in DLBCL has prompted its testing in BL. Rituximab has been incorporated in the Hyper-CVAD regimen with a one-year disease-free survival of 86% in 20 patients, most of whom had advanced-stage disease. Rituximab has also been incorporated into an ongoing CALGB protocol for BL. Preliminary results with the NCI Dose-Adjusted EPOCH-R regimen, a pharmacodynamic-based infusional regimen with etoposide, prednisone, vincristine, cyclophosphamide, doxorubicin and rituximab, suggest that optimizing the schedule may significantly improve the therapeutic index of chemotherapy and reduce toxicity. Preliminary results in 12 HIV-negative untreated BL patients treated with DA-EPOCH-R has shown a 100% complete remission and survival rate at 31 months median follow-up. Such results suggest that DA-EPOCH-R may be an excellent and well-tolerated alternative to dose-intensified regimens for HIV-positive patients and older adults with BL where toxicity is a major concern. Multiple new targeted agents are also currently under development and may have utility in BL. However, these agents are in early clinical development and have yet to demonstrate activity in BL.

MANAGEMENT OF RELAPSED BURKITT'S LYMPHOMA

The salvage treatment of relapsed or refractory BL is usually unsuccessful. Early-stage patients who relapse after having received limited treatment, however, may still be curable, whereas advanced-stage patients who have received intensive treatment or are primary induction failures are rarely curable. In general, patients with chemosensitive disease received ASCT consolidation. A review from the European Group for Blood and Marrow Transplantation (EBMT) by Sweetenham and colleagues reported an OS of 37% at three years for patients with chemosensitive relapse but only 7% for those with resistant disease following ASCT. An analysis of allogeneic transplantation in BL did not find any relationship between survival and graft-versus-host disease, suggesting no graft-versus-tumor effect, and the overall survival was lower than that of matched patients treated with autologous transplant.

HIV-ASSOCIATED BURKITT'S LYMPHOMA

BL comprises 13–18% of HIV-associated lymphomas, a significant decrease since the development of highly active antiretroviral therapy (HAART). Clinically, BL in HIV-infected patients is similar to sporadic BL, and typically occurs before the development of severe immunodeficiency. Unlike other HIV-associated lymphomas, there has been no improvement in the outcome of BL since the development of HAART. A retrospective analysis of HIV-associated BL diagnosed between 1982 and 2003 from the University of Southern California showed no change in median survivals of 6.4 and 5.7 months, respectively, in the pre- and post-HAART eras. This contrasts with the outcome of DLBCL during these periods, which revealed an improvement in median survival from 8.3 to 43.2 months. This improvement is likely due to a more favorable DLBCL pathobiology occuring at higher CD4 cell counts in the HAART era. This does not seem to be the case with BL, which occurs at a high median CD4 cell count and does not have such a variable pathobiology.

The relatively poor outcome of HIV-associated BL is likely due to the use of CHOP-based regimens, which are known to have a poor outcome in this disease. In contrast, dose-intensified regimens such as Hyper-CVAD have shown encouraging results in HIV-associated BL, with 92% complete remission, but are quite toxic. BL highlights the necessity to balance treatment efficacy and toxicity in patients with HIV infection. Dose-intensified BL regimens

are considered too toxic to warrant their general use in HIV-positive patients, and have led to the use of CHOP-based treatment. The excellent results achieved with the DA-EPOCH-R regimen in HIV-associated lymphoma overall, and in BL in HIV-negative patients, suggest it may be an excellent regimen in HIV-positive patients due to its relatively low toxicity.

TREATMENT RECOMMENDATIONS IN BURKITT'S LYMPHOMA

Multiple regimens, as discussed above, have shown equivalent efficacy in BL and may be used. Current treatment plans should include risk-adaptive strategies and reduced CNS prophylaxis in order to minimize toxicity. Adults may be effectively treated with pediatric regimens, although the CODOX-M/IVAC, CALGB and Hyper-CVAD regimens have been specifically investigated in adults and shown to be effective and relatively well tolerated. Treatment with DA-EPOCH-R is promising but results are too preliminary for its clinical use except in patients of advanced age who cannot tolerate aggressive regimens and in HIV-positive patients. The benefit of rituximab in BL is unknown, and is currently the subject of clinical investigation.

TREATMENT PRINCIPLES FOR LYMPHOBLASTIC LYMPHOMA

Therapy consists predominantly of combination chemotherapy. The most commonly employed regimens include phases of induction, consolidation, CNS sterilization and maintenance. Induction with four or more drugs is often given as a 28-day course, although there are alternative approaches. A variety of consolidation blocks, also known as intensification blocks, have been shown to improve long-term outcome for high-risk pediatric subgroups, including those with slow or incomplete responses to induction. All patients with LBL require CNS sterilization, to decrease the risk of meningeal relapse, and a prolonged maintenance phase. Shortening maintenance to less than two years appears to compromise outcome for both adults and children.

Most patients with LBL present with advanced-stage (III/IV) disease. Although less intensive treatment is commonly employed for patients with low-stage (I/II) LBL, randomized clinical trials confirm the need to treat with aggressive, prolonged ALL-type therapy. For example, an early Pediatric Oncology Group (POG) trial demonstrated an advantage of the addition of a 24-week maintenance phase for pediatric patients with low-stage disease. Reducing therapy for low-stage LBL increases the risk of relapse, although salvage rates are better for such patients in comparison to those who relapse after more intensive regimens. No apparent difference in outcome has been seen within low-stage (i.e. I vs. II) or advanced-stage (i.e. III vs. IV) LBL in pediatric series. Bone-marrow involvement was associated with poor outcome in the LMT 89 trial in adults. However, subgroup numbers are small in all series, preventing firm conclusions. Rare individuals with B-precursor phenotype LBL are treated according to B-precursor ALL-specific regimens, which are not considered in detail in this chapter.

TREATMENT OF LYMPHOBLASTIC LYMPHOMA

Sequential pediatric cooperative group trials in the setting of LBL/T-ALL have led to the development of highly effective specific regimens (Table 13.5). Initial studies in the 1970s demonstrated the advantage of ALL-type therapy over CHOP-like regimens. In a trial conducted by the Children's Cancer Group (CCG) in North America, the Memorial Sloan-Kettering Cancer Center (MSKCC) LSA_2L_2 regimen was shown to be superior to COMP (cyclophosphamide, vincristine, methotrexate and prednisone) with 64% vs. 35% event-free survival (EFS). An early study conducted by the BFM group also demonstrated efficacy of ALL-type therapy for children with LBL (70% EFS). Serial BFM trials have led to steady improvements, with EFS exceeding 90% on the most current pediatric protocols. The BFM regimen "backbone" has been incorporated into recent North American studies through the CCG and Children's Oncology Group (COG).

Clinical trials have also demonstrated the advantage of ALL-type therapy for adults with LBL (Table 13.6). The pediatric BFM regimen has been applied successfully to adult patients in serial trials of the GMALL. Investigators at the M.D. Anderson Cancer Center (MDACC) have achieved good results with the Hyper-CVAD regimen. However, although remission induction rates on these trials exceed 90%, relapse-free survival rates (44–62%) are lower than in pediatric series. In the case of the GMALL studies, this is likely due at least in part to the use of less intensive and shorter-duration chemotherapy in comparison to the most effective pediatric BFM regimen.

A number of specific chemotherapy agents, doses and schedules are particularly effective against LBL/T-ALL. Increasing the intensity of induction above and beyond the standard four-drug regimen (corticosteroids, vincristine, anthracyclines, asparaginase) by the addition of other agents (e.g. cyclophosphamide) appears to improve complete remission rates in children and adults. High doses of methotrexate (MTX) are required to achieve adequate intracellular concentrations of MTX-polyglutamates in T lymphoblasts. Early French studies (LMT 81) added high-dose MTX to the LSA_2L_2 regimen with improved outcome (80% EFS). The value of intensive L-asparaginase in LBL/T-ALL has been demonstrated in POG and Dana Farber Cancer Institute (DFCI) cooperative group studies. High-dose cytarabine (Ara-C) has also been shown to have specific activity against T-NHL/ALL. Results of series with the best reported outcomes are summarized in Tables 13.5 and 13.6. Currently, treatment can be expected to result in EFS rates of approximately 80–90% for children and 50–60% for adults.

In order to maximize therapeutic benefits, and in the absence of prohibitive toxicity, attempts should be made to deliver specified doses of all prescribed chemotherapy agents. Furthermore, doses of MTX and 6-mercaptopurine (6-MP) during maintenance should be dose-escalated to achieve a targeted degree of myelosuppression. In the event of significant chemotherapy-related toxicity, specific agents should be dose-reduced or discontinued as clinically indicated. Those individuals with thiopurine S-methyltransferase deficiency ($\sim$10% incidence) require dose reduction of 6-MP in order to avoid toxicity.

Recent studies have been designed to eliminate local radiation to bulky sites of disease. A randomized trial conducted by the POG failed to show benefit for involved-field radiation for pediatric patients with low-stage disease. Mediastinal irradiation was eliminated from the treatment of advanced-stage disease on the pediatric BFM 90 study without an apparent increase in the local recurrence rate (7%). Notably, the mediastinum was the primary site of relapse

Table 13.5. Selected regimens for lymphoblastic lymphoma in children.

Regimen	Treatment	Patients (n)	Relapse-free survival by stage				
			All	I/II	III/IV	III	IV
BFM 86	7-drug induction, consolidation, re-induction, maintenance; 24 months	54			83% (5 yr)		
BFM 90	7-drug induction, consolidation, re-induction, maintenance; 24 months	109	90% (5 yr)		90% (5 yr)	90% (5 yr)	95% (5 yr)
BFM 95	7-drug induction, consolidation, re-induction, maintenance; 24 months	156			82% (5 yr)		
CCG 123 – New York I and BFM arms	4–6 drug induction, consolidation, re-induction, maintenance; 24 months	371	67% (6 yr)				
DFCI 87/91/95	4–5-drug induction, consolidation, maintenance; 24 months	15			87% (5 yr)		
EORTC 58881	4-drug induction, consolidation, re-induction, maintenance; 24 months	60			76% (6 yr)		
LMT 81	5-drug induction, consolidation, maintenance; 24 months	82	75% (5 yr)	73% (5 yr)		79% (5 yr)	72% (5 yr)
LSA$_2$L$_2$	4-drug induction, consolidation, maintenance; 24–36 months	68	75% (5 yr)	88% (5 yr)		85% (5 yr)	74% (5 yr)
POG 8704 – Intensive L-asparaginase arm	6-drug induction, consolidation, maintenance; 24 months	84			78% (4 yr)		

(17%) in adults treated on recent GMALL trials, despite the fact that most had received 2400 cGy of local irradiation, suggesting that chemotherapy is the critical determinant of bulky-site disease control. In contrast, adjuvant radiation did appear to decrease the risk of mediastinal recurrence for adults treated with the MDACC Hyper-CVAD regimen. Although males with testicular ALL/LBL have historically been treated with radiation, recent results with regimens containing intermediate- or high-dose MTX suggest that radiation may not be needed. Thus, in the absence of a protocol-specified role, radiation should be reserved for emergency management of life- or organ-threatening complications. Even in that setting, however, corticosteroids are commonly adequate to induce rapid disease reduction.

Table 13.6. Selected regimens for lymphoblastic lymphoma in adults.

Regimen	Treatment	Patients (n)	Relapse-free survival (All stages)
GMALL 89/93	7-drug induction, consolidation, re-induction, maintenance; 6–12 months	45	62% (7 yr)
Hyper-CVAD	4-drug induction, consolidation, repeated × 4, maintenance; 24–36 months	26	62% (3 yr)
LMT 89	5-drug induction, consolidation, maintenance; 12–24 months	27	44% (5 yr)

There have been few studies designed to evaluate the relative efficacy of high-dose therapy with ASCT for LBL. Most published series represent single-institution or registry studies, which often include mixed lymphoma subtypes and/or patients with high-risk features. The European Group for Blood and Marrow Transplantation and the United Kingdom Lymphoma Group conducted a randomized trial of ASCT versus conventional chemotherapy as post-remission treatment for adults with LBL. Although there was a trend towards improved relapse-free survival on the ASCT arm, no overall survival benefit was demonstrated. Thus there is no current evidence to suggest that ASCT is more effective than standard LBL-specific chemotherapy regimens.

Studies of allogeneic SCT are also limited in the setting of LBL. Most prospective trials compare allogeneic to autologous stem-cell rescue. In general, relapse rates are lower after allogeneic SCT; however, much of this advantage is offset by increased treatment-related mortality. Consequently, allogeneic SCT is usually reserved for those with specific high-risk features. In light of the excellent outcome for children and adolescents with LBL, allogeneic SCT is rarely used for pediatric patients except for those with poor response to or relapse after standard treatment.

CNS TREATMENT OF LYMPHOBLASTIC LYMPHOMA

LBL has a high rate of CNS involvement compared to other subtypes of lymphoma and leukemia. Approximately 5–15% of patients have meningeal disease at presentation. CNS-directed prophylaxis is required for all patients with LBL, due to the high risk of CNS relapse even in those without overt meningeal involvement. Historically, craniospinal irradiation has been relied upon for CNS prophylaxis for patients with advanced-stage LBL/T-ALL. In order to reduce the neurocognitive dysfunction encountered in survivors of childhood ALL, regimens that limit radiation exposure have been designed over the past two decades. Initial trials led to reductions in the cranial radiation dose and replacement of spinal irradiation with intensive intrathecal chemotherapy. Recently, cranial radiation has been eliminated in all but the highest-risk patients. Thus, CNS prophylaxis for patients with ALL now consists primarily of intrathecal chemotherapy in combination with systemic agents that have good CNS penetration, most notably high-dose MTX and dexamethasone. It must be emphasized that most of these data are derived from patients with B-precursor ALL. However, initial results from EORTC 58881, BFM 95 and COG A5971 suggest that this approach may be applied effectively to LBL/T-ALL. Nonetheless, follow-up remains relatively short for radiation-free regimens, and cranial irradiation is still considered the standard treatment for individuals with active meningeal leukemia. It is notable that in the BFM 95 study the elimination of cranial radiation prophylaxis was associated with an increase in bone-marrow relapse, the cause of which is not completely understood. Finally, in light of both the poorer overall outcome and the lower risk of neurologic toxicity in older individuals, cranial irradiation is still commonly employed for adults with ALL and LBL.

A number of practical aspects of intrathecal administration are worthy of comment. In order to minimize the risk of meningeal contamination due to traumatic lumbar puncture, spinal taps should be performed by experienced practitioners. Furthermore, it is recommended that intrathecal chemotherapy be administered at the time of the initial diagnostic lumbar puncture, especially when there are circulating blasts in the peripheral blood. To improve chemotherapy distribution, the volume of CSF removed should equal the volume administered, and patients should remain prone for approximately 30 minutes after administration. The use of an Omaya reservoir may improve delivery to the ventricles, although this approach is not routinely employed. Finally, intrathecal chemotherapy should be dosed according to age, because of age-related CSF volume changes.

MANAGEMENT OF RELAPSED LYMPHOBLASTIC LYMPHOMA

In general, the outcome after relapse is poor for both children and adults with LBL. Those patients with low-stage disease who received abbreviated therapy have higher salvage rates. Allogeneic SCT is recommended for patients with HLA-matched related donors. In addition, matched unrelated donor transplantation should be considered for young individuals. Agents targeted to T-cell malignancies hold promise. Recently, nelarabine (compound 506U78), a water-soluble prodrug of ara-G, was approved by the FDA for treatment of relapsed LBL/T-ALL.

TREATMENT RECOMMENDATIONS FOR LYMPHOBLASTIC LYMPHOMA

Therapy should be instituted as soon as possible after diagnosis, and should be directed by practitioners experienced with the specific regimen and the management of expected complications. It is highly recommended that patients be treated on clinical trials whenever possible. The best reported outcome for LBL is with aggressive ALL-type regimens, and the recent BFM regimen appears superior. In general, treatment is similar for adult and pediatric patients, although, as detailed above, therapy is often stratified based on risk of relapse and organ toxicity.

SUPPORTIVE CARE OF BURKITT'S AND LYMPHOBLASTIC LYMPHOMA

Aggressive supportive care and surveillance for complications during and after treatment is critical to successful outcome.

Antiemetics

Routine prophylaxis and treatment of nausea and vomiting are required during induction, consolidation and CNS-directed therapy phases.

Tumor lysis syndrome

As LBL and BL frequently present with a large tumor burden, and cell turnover is extremely rapid, tumor lysis syndrome is commonly encountered during initiation of therapy. Some regimens include a "prephase" of treatment to allow gradual induction, for example with a few day courses of corticosteroids alone. Tumor lysis prophylaxis should be started as soon as possible after diagnosis and at least 12 hours prior to the initiation of induction chemotherapy. Prophylaxis and monitoring should continue until disease burden is reduced and it is apparent that no complications of lysis have developed (usually 3–7 days). The following is recommended:

- Allopurinol. Oral dose 100 mg/m^2 three times a day. Urate oxidase (rasburicase) is a new alternative for the management of extreme hyperuricemia.
- Hydration. IV fluids at a rate of ≥ 2 times maintenance (≥ 120 ml/m^2 per hour) adjusted to maintain urine specific gravity ≤ 1.010 and normal urine output. Due to the risk of hyperkalemia, potassium should be avoided.
- Alkalinization. To decrease the risk of uric acid nephropathy, urine may be alkalinized with sodium bicarbonate titrated to maintain the urine pH between 6.5 and 7.5. However, extreme alkalinization should be avoided since this may be associated with hypoxanthine crystallization. In addition, to decrease the risk of calcium/phosphate precipitation, alkalinization should be minimized or avoided entirely if possible in the setting of hyperphosphatemia.
- Serum potassium, phosphorous, calcium, creatinine, BUN, and uric acid should be assayed every 4–6 hours for the first 24–48 hours, then less frequently once stable.

Transfusions

Blood transfusion therapy is usually required to counter severe cytopenias associated with the induction and consolidation phases of therapy. Specialized blood products should be employed in an attempt to decrease the risk of transfusion-associated complications.

- Platelets. To prevent bleeding, platelet counts should routinely be maintained above 10×10^9/L. Higher levels may be needed to manage active bleeding, prior to invasive procedures, and to reduce the risk of leukostasis-induced CNS hemorrhage in the setting of hyperleukocytosis. Single-donor platelets are recommended whenever possible to decrease donor exposure and the risk of HLA-alloimmunization.
- Red blood cells. Concomitant anemia often partially offsets the hyperviscosity associated with severe hyperleukocytosis. Thus, red-blood-cell transfusion should be avoided if possible when the WBC is $> 100 \times 10^9$/L. If red-cell transfusion is needed, the hemoglobin should be increased slowly using small aliquots of packed red cells until the peripheral blast count is reduced.
- Irradiation. All cellular blood products should be irradiated in order to prevent transfusion-associated graft-versus-host disease.
- Leukodepletion. Platelets and red cells should be leukocyte-reduced to decrease the risk of febrile reactions and platelet-refractoriness due to HLA-alloimmunization.

Infectious prophylaxis

Aggressive surveillance, prophylaxis and treatment for bacterial, fungal, viral and opportunistic infections is required throughout therapy.

- *Pneumocystis carinii pneumonia* (PCP). All patients should receive prophylaxis against PCP until approximately six months after completion of chemotherapy.
- Neutropenic fever. Patients with fever in the setting of an absolute neutrophil count (ANC) $< 0.5 \times 10^9$/L require emergent evaluation and management for possible infection. Immediate, empiric, broad-spectrum, intravenous antibiotics are indicated. Antifungal therapy should be initiated for persistent neutropenic fever beyond 5–7 days. Antibiotics should be continued until the ANC rises to $> 0.5 \times 10^9$/L, fever resolves, cultures are negative and any infection is fully treated.
- Myeloid growth factors. Myeloid growth factor support (e.g. G-CSF) is commonly employed as part of treatment of BL in both children and adults. However, the benefits of such have not been proved in the setting of LBL therapy.

Chemotherapy prophylaxis

Agent-specific prophylaxis should be utilized as clinically indicated (e.g. gastritis prophylaxis during corticosteroids).

Nutritional support

Nutritional status should be monitored and supplementation provided as needed. Routine folic acid use should be avoided around the time of MTX administration as this may counteract the therapeutic efficacy of folate antagonism. In contrast, leucovorin rescue is required after intermediate- and high-dose MTX.

Response and toxicity evaluations

Serial monitoring for response and therapy-associated toxicity should be conducted during and after treatment. Lifelong follow-up for possible late effects is indicated for long-term survivors, including the following.

- Cardiomyopathy. To decrease the risk of cardiotoxicity, cumulative anthracycline doses are usually limited to < 400 mg/m^2. Left-ventricular function should be monitored.
- Neurologic toxicity. Children are at high risk of neurotoxicity from CNS-directed therapy, and neurodevelopmental assessment is required.
- Endocrinologic dysfunction. Patients should be monitored for endocrinopathies including growth retardation, infertility and hormone deficiencies.
- Osteonecrosis. Corticosteroids are associated with a high incidence of osteonecrosis.
- Secondary malignancy. Long-term survivors are at risk of secondary malignancies even beyond the first decade after treatment.

FURTHER READING

Amylon, M. D., Shuster, J., Pullen, J. *et al.* Intensive high-dose asparaginase consolidation improves survival for pediatric patients with T cell acute lymphoblastic leukemia and advanced stage lymphoblastic lymphoma: a Pediatric Oncology Group study. *Leukemia* **13** (1999), 335–342.

Burkhardt, B., Woessmann, W., Zimmermann, M. *et al.* Impact of cranial radiotherapy on central nervous system prophylaxis in children and adolescents with central nervous system-negative stage III or IV lymphoblastic lymphoma. *J. Clin. Oncol.* **24** (2006), 491–499.

Dave, S. S., Fu, K., Wright, G. W. *et al.* Molecular diagnosis of Burkitt's lymphoma. *N. Engl. J. Med.* **354** (2006), 2431–2442.

Divine, M., Casassus P., Koscielny S. *et al.* Burkitt lymphoma in adults: a prospective study of 72 patients treated with an adapted pediatric LMB protocol. *Ann. Oncol.* **16** (2005), 1928–1935.

Gaynon, P. S., Trigg, M. E., Heerema, N. A. *et al.* Children's Cancer Group trials in childhood acute lymphoblastic leukemia: 1983–1995. *Leukemia* **14** (2000), 2223–2233.

Goldberg, J. M., Silverman, L. B., Levy, D. E. *et al.* Childhood T-cell acute lymphoblastic leukemia: the Dana-Farber Cancer Institute acute lymphoblastic leukemia consortium experience. *J. Clin. Oncol.* **21** (2003), 3616–3622.

Hoelzer, D., Ludwig, W. D., Thiel, E. *et al.* Improved outcome in adult B-cell acute lymphoblastic leukemia. *Blood* **87** (1996), 495–508.

Hoelzer, D. & Gokbuget, N. Treatment of lymphoblastic lymphoma in adults. *Best Pract. Res. Clin. Haematol.* **15** (2002), 713–728.

Hummel, M., Bentink, S., Berger, H. *et al.* A biologic definition of Burkitt's lymphoma from transcriptional and genomic profiling. *N. Engl. J. Med.* **354** (2006), 2419–2430.

Jabbour, E., Koscielny, S., Sebban, C. *et al.* High survival rate with the LMT-89 regimen in lymphoblastic lymphoma (LL), but not in T-cell acute lymphoblastic leukemia (T-ALL). *Leukemia* **20** (2006), 814–819.

Jaffe, E. S., Harris, N. L., Stein, H. and Vardiman, J. W. *World Health Organization Classification of Tumours. Pathology and Genetics of Tumours of Hematopoietic and Lymphoid tissues* (Lyon: IARC Press, 2001).

Magrath, I., Adde, M., Shad, A. *et al.* Adults and children with small non-cleaved-cell lymphoma have a similar excellent outcome when treated with the same chemotherapy regimen. *J. Clin. Oncol.* **14** (1996), 925–934.

Mead, G. M., Sydes, M. R., Walewski, J. *et al.* An international evaluation of CODOX-M and CODOX-M alternating with IVAC in adult Burkitt's lymphoma: results of United Kingdom Lymphoma Group LY06 study. *Ann. Oncol.* **13** (2002), 1264–1274.

Millot, F., Suciu, S., Philippe, N. *et al.* Value of high-dose cytarabine during interval therapy of a Berlin-Frankfurt-Munster-based protocol in increased-risk children with acute lymphoblastic leukemia and lymphoblastic lymphoma:

results of the European Organization for Research and Treatment of Cancer 58881 randomized phase III trial. *J. Clin. Oncol.* **19** (2001), 1935–1942.

Mora, J., Filippa, D. A., Qin, J. and Wollner, N. Lymphoblastic lymphoma of childhood and the LSA2-L2 protocol: the 30-year experience at Memorial-Sloan-Kettering Cancer Center. *Cancer* **98** (2003), 1283–1291.

Murphy, S. B., Bowman, W. P., Abromowitch, M. *et al.* Results of treatment of advanced-stage Burkitt's lymphoma and B cell (SIg+) acute lymphoblastic leukemia with high-dose fractionated cyclophosphamide and coordinated high-dose methotrexate and cytarabine. *J. Clin. Oncol.* **4** (1986), 1732–1739.

Neri, A., Barriga, F., Knowles, D. M. *et al.* Different regions of the immunoglobulin heavy chain locus are involved in chromosomal translocations in distinct pathogenetic forms of Burkitt lymphoma. *Proc. Natl. Acad. Sci. USA* **85** (1988), 2748–2752.

Patte, C., Kalifa, C., Flamant, F. *et al.* Results of the LMT81 protocol, a modified LSA2L2 protocol with high dose methotrexate, on 84 children with non-B-cell (lymphoblastic) lymphoma. *Med. Pediatr. Oncol.* **20** (1992), 105–113.

Patte, C., Auperin, A., Michon, J. *et al.* The Société Française d'Oncologie Pédiatrique LMB89 protocol: highly effective multiagent chemotherapy tailored to the tumor burden and initial response in 561 unselected children with B-cell lymphomas and L3 leukemia. *Blood* **97** (2001), 3370–3379.

Pelicci, P. G., Knowles, D. M., Magrath, I. *et al.* Chromosomal breakpoints and structural alterations of c-MYC locus differ in endemic and sporadic forms of Burkitt lymphoma. *Proc. Natl. Acad. Sci. USA* **83** (1986), 2984–2988.

Pilozzi, E., Pulford, K., Jones, M. *et al.* Co-expression of CD79a (JCB117) and CD3 by lymphoblast lymphoma. *J. Pathol.* **186** (1998), 140–143.

Reiter, A., Schrappe, M., Ludwig, W. D. *et al.* Intensive ALL-type therapy without local radiotherapy provides a 90% event-free survival for children with T-cell lymphoblastic lymphoma: a BFM group report. *Blood* **95** (2000), 416–421.

Reiter, A., Schrappe, M., Tiemann, M. *et al.* Improved treatment results in childhood B-cell neoplasms with tailored intensification of therapy: A report of the Berlin-Frankfurt-Munster Group Trial NHL-BFM 90. *Blood* **94** (1999), 3294–3306.

Rizzieri, D. A., Johnson, J. L., Niedzwiecki, D. *et al.* Intensive chemotherapy with and without cranial radiation for Burkitt leukemia and lymphoma: final results of Cancer and Leukemia Group B Study 9251. *Cancer* **100** (2004), 1438–1448.

Schrappe, M., Reiter, A., Ludwig, W. *et al.* Improved outcome in childhood acute lymphoblastic leukemia despite reduced use of anthracyclines and cranial radiotherapy: results of trial ALL-BFM 90. *Blood* **95** (2000), 3310–3322.

Shiramizu, B., Barriga, F., Neequaye, J. *et al.* Patterns of chromosomal breakpoint locations in Burkitt's lymphoma:

relevance to geography and Epstein–Barr virus association. *Blood* **77** (1991), 1516–1526.

Steinherz, P. G., Gaynon, P. S., Breneman, J. C. *et al.* Treatment of patients with acute lymphoblastic leukemia with bulky extramedullary disease and T-cell phenotype or other poor prognostic features: randomized controlled trial from the Children's Cancer Group. *Cancer* **82** (1998), 600–612.

Thomas, D. A., Cortes, J., O'Brien, S. *et al.* Hyper-CVAD program in Burkitt's-type adult acute lymphoblastic leukemia. *J. Clin. Oncol.* **17** (1999), 2461–2470.

van Imhoff, G. W., van der Holt, B., MacKenzie, M. A. *et al.* Short intensive sequential therapy followed by autologous stem-cell transplantation in adult Burkitt, Burkitt-like and lymphoblastic lymphoma. *Leukemia* **19** (2005), 945–952.

Andrés J. M. Ferreri and Lisa M. DeAngelis

Pathology: Andrew Wotherspoon
Molecular cytogenetics: Andreas Rosenwald and German Ott

INTRODUCTION

A variety of lymphomas can involve the central nervous system (CNS), at different phases of their evolution, in both immunocompetent and immunocompromised individuals. They represent a heterogeneous group of malignancies, with variable clinical and behavioral characteristics, requiring different therapeutic approaches. In this chapter, the therapeutic management of these malignancies will be analyzed separately in three main entities: primary CNS lymphomas (PCNSL), secondary CNS lymphomas (SCNSL) and other, less common, forms of CNS lymphomas.

PATHOLOGY

The vast majority of CNS lymphomas are diffuse large B-cell lymphomas (DLBCL) that share the morphological and immunophenotypic characteristics similar to those of DLBCLs encountered elsewhere. They may show a perivascular growth pattern. The perivascular infiltrate is associated with increased reticulin fibres and the periphery of areas of involvement frequently shows astrocyte gliosis. Many immunocompromised patients show features similar to Burkitt's lymphoma, while others show a more immunoblastic morphology.

Rare cases of small lymphocytic, lymphoplasmacytic and T-cell lymphoma similar to those seen in tissue outside the CNS have been described. Secondary involvement by lymphoma originating elsewhere is also encountered.

Immunophenotypically CNS lymphomas recapitulate the staining pattern of similar lymphomas encountered outside the CNS. The DLBCLs are positive for CD20 and CD79a with expression of bcl-2 protein. A proportion express CD10 and bcl-6, but they are usually negative for CD5 and CD23. Large B-cell lymphomas in immunocompromised patients frequently contain Epstein–Barr virus (EBV).

MOLECULAR PATHOLOGY AND CYTOGENETICS

The analysis of IgV$_H$ gene sequences in PCNSL has shown that these tumors harbor highly mutated immunoglobulin genes with frequent ongoing mutations, and they are therefore derived from germinal-center B cells in most of the cases. In addition, analyses of V-region genes have revealed a preferential use of the *VH4-34* gene. DLBCLs arising in the CNS are targeted by aberrant somatic hypermutation of non-immunoglobulin genes.

PCNSLs are, like their testicular DLBCL counterparts, a paradigm of lymphoid tumors arising at extranodal immune-privileged sites with particular immune reactions and a differing microenvironment. Interestingly, PCNSLs show loss of heterozygosity (LOH) at high frequency at the chromosome segment 6p21.3, where the HLA region is located. Deletions in these chromosomal regions predispose to the inactivation of genes essential for immune recognition, and may therefore contribute to the development of escape mechanisms from immune surveillance. In keeping with these findings, loss of HLA expression is frequently encountered in primary cerebral and testicular DLBCL. Interestingly, a recent study of

Lymphoma: Pathology, Diagnosis and Treatment, ed. Robert Marcus, John W. Sweetenham and Michael E. Williams. Published by Cambridge University Press. © Cambridge University Press 2007.

lymphomas not arising at immune-privileged sites has revealed that HLA locus deletions are not a feature of these (mostly systemic) lymphomas.

Comparative genomic hybridization (CGH) studies have revealed recurrent genomic imbalances in PCNSL, with gains frequently involving 1q, 7q, 12q and 18q, and deletions clustering in 6q. Indeed, chromosome 6q seems to suffer frequent deletions in these tumors, with 6q22–23 representing the minimally deleted region.

A recent microarray-based gene expression study of PCNSL has demonstrated a unique expression profile in these tumors that distinguishes them from nodal/systemic counterparts. In particular, PCNSL showed high expression of regulators of the unfolded protein response signaling pathway (ATF-6, XBP1), oncogenes (*Pim-1, MYC*) and apoptosis regulators (caspase-8 and FADD-like apoptosis regulator).

PRIMARY CNS LYMPHOMAS

Conventional therapeutic strategies

PCNSLs are aggressive malignancies arising within and confined to the CNS. They comprise 3% of intracranial neoplasms, and in the past two decades their incidence has risen in both immunocompromised and immunocompetent individuals, especially in those over 50 years of age. The main patient characteristics at presentation are summarized in Table 14.1. Current therapeutic knowledge in PCNSL results from a small number of non-randomized phase II trials, meta-analyses and large retrospective, multicenter series. The shortage of randomized trials limits comparison between new approaches and has produced limited therapeutic progress. Moreover, the use of divergent study designs and entry criteria in prospective trials, as well as the presence of some methodological pitfalls, make comparisons unreliable. Although results from prospective trials suggest progress in the treatment of PCNSL, improvements are not reflected in studies of population-based cohorts, and survival has not improved consistently in the past three decades.

The optimal treatment of PCNSL requires a multidisciplinary approach. If neuroimaging suggests the possibility of PCNSL (Fig. 14.1), then a stereotactic biopsy is the most appropriate surgical approach. Aggressive surgical resection should be avoided

Table 14.1. Patient characteristics in a retrospective multicenter series of 378 immunocompetent patients with PCNSL.

Age	
median	61 years
range	14–85
age > 70 years	14%
Male:female ratio	1.4:1
Performance status (ECOG score)	
0–1	35%
2–3	50%
4	15%
Prior cancer	4%
Histology	
indolent	5%
diffuse large B-cell lymphoma	60%
highly aggressive	15%
unclassified	20%
Presenting symptoms	
non-specific motor and/or sensory focal deficit	50%
cognitive and personality changes	40%
headache	25%
intracranial hypertension (nausea, vomiting, papilledema)	30%
seizures	15%
ocular symptoms	15%
T phenotype	2%
Elevated LDH serum level	35%
Intraocular disease	13%
Positive CSF cytology examination	16%
High CSF protein concentration	61%
Multiple lesions	34%
Involvement of deep structures of the brain (basal ganglia and/or brainstem and/or cerebellum)	36%

because it does not improve survival and may result in neurological deterioration and chemotherapy delay. Next, complete staging work-up and prognostic-factor assessment should be performed (Table 14.2). The International Prognostic Index does not discriminate between risk groups in PCNSL, but the combination of five independent predictors of response and survival (age, performance status, serum lactate dehydrogenase level, cerebrospinal-fluid protein concentration,

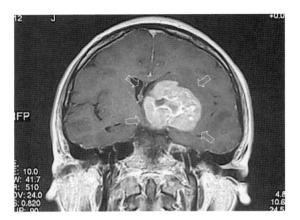

Figure 14.1 Gadolinium-enhanced MRI of lesion involving the basal ganglia and periventricular area (arrows). These are common radiological features of primary CNS diffuse large B-cell lymphoma in immunocompetent patients.

Table 14.2. Staging work-up and pre-treatment evaluations in PCNSL.

Staging

Physical examination

Routine blood studies

Whole-brain MRI

Contrast total-body CT scan

Ophthalmologic evaluation (including slit-lamp
  examination)

Cerebrospinal-fluid cytology

Cerebrospinal-fluid biochemical examination

Bone-marrow biopsy

Testicular ultrasonography (older men)

FDG-PET (investigational role)

Suspicion of vitreal infiltration may require confirmation
  by vitrectomy

Prognostic factors

Age

Performance status (PS)

Lactate dehydrogenase (LDH) serum level

Cerebrospinal-fluid protein concentration

Involvement of deep regions of the brain

Pre-treatment assessment

Neurological examination

Biochemical serum profile

Baseline neuropsychiatric tests

Renal and hepatic functionality tests (creatinine
  clearance)

Cardiac function tests[a]

HIV, hepatitis B & C virus evaluation

[a] Echocardiography with left ventricular ejection fraction evaluation is advisable in elderly patients eligible for HD-MTX-based chemotherapy, considering that the administration of this drug requires adequate hydration (near 3 L/day, the days before and after MTX).

involvement of deep structures of the brain) distinguishes three different risk groups based on the presence of 0–1, 2–3 or 4–5 unfavorable features. Use of this prognostic index, named the IELSG score, will allow the separation of patients into risk groups, which could result in the application of risk-adjusted therapeutic strategies.

Even if diverse therapeutic strategies for PCNSL are now available, some of these strategies are associated with an increased risk of severe treatment-related neurotoxicity, especially among elderly patients. A dilemma in PCNSL treatment is therefore the choice between strategies designed to intensify therapy, to improve the cure rate, and strategies of treatment de-escalation, to avoid severe neurotoxicity.

Corticosteroids

Corticosteroids, which are routinely started in any patient with a new intracranial mass, have a potent and rapid oncolytic effect, causing radiographic regression in up to 40% of patients. This condition, named "ghost" or "vanishing" tumor, is strongly suggestive of PCNSL. However, it is important to underline that only half of "vanishing tumors" are PCNSLs, while sarcoidosis, multiple sclerosis, acute disseminated encephalomyelitis and some other malignancies can exhibit a dramatic response to steroids. Because of the risk of unreliable biopsies during steroids, this therapy should be withheld in any patient with a presumptive diagnosis of PCNSL until tissue has been obtained.

Radiotherapy alone

PCNSL is a radiosensitive tumor, and whole-brain radiotherapy (WBRT) has been the standard treatment for many years. However, WBRT alone is rarely curative in PCNSL patients since response is usually short-lived, with median survivals ranging from 10 to 18 months. WBRT is necessary because of the diffuse infiltrative nature of PCNSL, and attempts to treat with focal brain radiotherapy have resulted in high rates of recurrences within and outside the radiated port. Although microscopic CSF dissemination is common, more extensive craniospinal irradiation does not confer additional survival benefit and is associated with significant morbidity; this strategy plays only a palliative role in leptomeningeal lymphoma.

The optimal dose of WBRT is controversial, but the results of several studies suggest a dose of 40–50 Gy, while WBRT doses greater than 50 Gy are associated with an increased risk of neurotoxicity. A prospective Radiation Therapy Oncology Group (RTOG) study of 40 Gy WBRT followed by a 20 Gy focal boost demonstrated a radiographic response in 62% and a complete response in 19%. The addition of a boost did not improve local tumor control or survival. A more recent RTOG study failed to show a clear benefit in terms of disease control or reduced neurotoxicity when hyperfractionated WBRT was used.

Consolidation after chemotherapy may represent the best role for radiotherapy; WBRT 40–50 Gy as exclusive treatment appears advisable in PCNSL patients who cannot be treated with primary chemotherapy (see Fig. 14.3).

Combined chemoradiotherapy

Even though not confirmed in a randomized trial, there is a consensus that combined chemoradiotherapy is superior to radiotherapy alone. Data from a large multicenter retrospective series suggest that high-dose methotrexate (HD-MTX)-based chemotherapy followed by WBRT is preferred to radiotherapy alone. With this strategy, the five-year survival remains approximately 20–25%, and it is not known whether more intensive combined treatment will improve outcome.

Similar to systemic non-Hodgkin's lymphoma (NHL), PCNSL is a chemosensitive tumor; however, the standard agents used to treat NHL are not effective in PCNSL because of their inability to penetrate the blood–brain barrier (BBB). Several studies have examined the role of CHOP or MACOP-B regimens and have found survival to be similar to that achieved with WBRT alone. While many patients have an immediate radiographic response, most experience progression after two to three cycles. This may be explained by PET studies that demonstrate normalization of the disrupted BBB three to four weeks after initial chemotherapy, suggesting that the bulky tumor

not protected by the BBB responds, but microscopic tumor is not adequately treated and progresses.

HD-MTX is the most active agent in the treatment of PCNSL. MTX doses $\geq 1\,g/m^2$ result in tumoricidal levels in the brain parenchyma and doses $\geq 3\,g/m^2$ yield tumoricidal levels in the CSF. Therefore, most treatment regimens incorporate HD-MTX ($1–8\,g/m^2$) alone or in combination with other cytostatics followed by WBRT, resulting in response rates of over 90% and median survivals ranging between 30 and 60 months. HD-MTX, when used alone, is a safe treatment even in patients older than 70. Creatinine clearance and glomerular filtration rates have been proposed to tailor MTX dose. The issues that remain unresolved are whether to give HD-MTX alone or in combination, and what is the optimal administration schedule and dose of MTX.

Late neurotoxicity is a major complication in patients treated with HD-MTX in combination with WBRT. The cumulative incidence varies from 5% to 10% at one year, and 25% to 35% at five years. White-matter abnormalities on MRI correlate with the degree of neuropsychologic impairment. Long-term impairment in the areas of attention, executive, memory and psychomotor speed are the most commonly reported. One-third of these patients died of complications related to the neurotoxicity. The mechanisms by which treatment produces CNS damage are unknown, but demyelination, tissue necrosis and microcavitary changes have been described; contributing factors are advanced age, neurological comorbidity, genetic predisposition and treatment characteristics. Treatment-related neurotoxicity in PCNSL patients has not been defined clearly because prospective assessment of neurotoxicity has been performed rarely, assessed series are small and exposed to selection biases, and there is no agreement about neurotoxicity definition, tests and scores useful to measure neurocognitive functioning as well as approaches to radiographic monitoring of treatment effect in PCNSL. The potential neurotoxicity of combined modality treatment is difficult to determine, particularly when each modality can produce CNS damage individually. To use MTX-based chemotherapy alone, and delay WBRT until relapse, has been proposed as the main strategy to minimize the incidence of this severe complication. Some small experiences suggest that this approach is feasible even in older patients, with an overall survival similar to a chemoradiotherapy combination. However, patients treated with chemotherapy alone may be more likely to relapse, and a larger experience is needed to confirm these findings.

Experimental therapeutic strategies

High-dose chemotherapy supported by autologous stem-cell transplantation (ASCT)

High-dose chemotherapy supported by ASCT can be used to dose-intensify chemotherapy as well as to replace WBRT in an effort to avoid treatment-related neurotoxicity. Preliminary results indicate that this strategy is feasible in PCNSL patients (Table 14.3). Activity data are, however, controversial because of the different induction and conditioning combinations used. The use of HD-MTX-based induction followed by thiotepa-based conditioning seems to be more active than the same induction followed by BEAM conditioning regimen. The lack of cross-resistance with MTX has been an advantage when this strategy has been used as salvage therapy, but previously irradiated patients had a higher risk of neurotoxicity. The role of this strategy in PCNSL remains to be defined, considering that worldwide experience is limited, and further studies are needed to identify the optimal induction and conditioning regimens.

Blood–brain barrier disruption

Reversible BBB disruption (BBBD) by intra-arterial infusion of hypertonic mannitol followed by intra-arterial chemotherapy is a strategy that leads to increased drug concentrations in the lymphoma-infiltrated brain and thus may improve survival. In institutions with adequate expertise, BBBD plus HD-MTX has been associated with acceptable morbidity, high tumor response and survival rates, and only a 14% loss of cognitive function at one year. In relapsed patients, carboplatin-based chemotherapy plus BBBD produced a 31% response rate, with a median duration of seven months. BBBD may prove most useful in the delivery of agents unlikely to traverse an intact BBB, such as unconjugated or radiolabeled monoclonal antibodies. However, this strategy is a procedurally intensive treatment, requiring monthly vascular interventions under general anesthesia over one year. Its role needs further clarification in PCNSL.

Investigational drugs

The small number of available active drugs limits further improvements in chemotherapy efficacy. It is important that patients with relapsed or refractory PCNSL be entered onto phase I/II trials assessing new drugs and combinations. Some drugs have emerged recently from prospective and retrospective studies and are now being incorporated into ongoing phase II trials assessing new HD-MTX-based combinations.

Temozolomide is an oral alkylating agent that spontaneously undergoes chemical conversion to MTIC (5-(3-methyl-1-triazeno)imidazole-4-carboxamide), resulting in 0–6 methylguanine-DNA methyltransferase depletion. This drug displayed excellent tolerability and a 26% response rate, mostly complete remissions, in a multicenter phase II trial on PCNSL relapsed or refractory to HD-MTX. Considering that it permeates the BBB, is well tolerated even in elderly patients, and exhibits additive cytotoxic activity with radiotherapy, temozolomide may be used as induction, maintenance or radiosensitivity treatment against PCNSL. The latter application is supported by the experience in high-grade gliomas, but the risk of severe neurotoxicity in PCNSL patients should be adequately monitored. Preliminary data suggest that a rituximab–temozolomide combination is well tolerated and active. High doses of rituximab, a chimeric monoclonal antibody directed against the B-cell-specific antigen CD20, can be safely infused to attain higher CSF concentrations. Anecdotal experience with intravenous rituximab has shown disappointing results, but promising effects have been reported in a few cases of leptomeningeal lymphoma treated with intraventricular rituximab.

Topotecan, a camptothecin derivative that inhibits the enzyme topoisomerase I, produced an objective response in one-third of patients with refractory or relapsed PCNSL, with a one-year progression-free survival (PFS) of 13%. Some retrospective evidence suggested a positive effect with the addition of high-dose cytarabine to HD-MTX. The latter observation constitutes the primary endpoint of one of the only two ongoing randomized trials in PCNSL.

Particular clinical conditions

Leptomeningeal lymphoma

PCNSL tends to infiltrate the subependymal tissues, disseminating through the CSF to the meninges; leptomeningeal lymphoma in the absence of a parenchymal

Table 14.3. Prospective phase II trials on high-dose chemotherapy supported by ASCT in PCNSL.

Authors	Year	Therapy line	Patients (n)	Induction regimen	Conditioning regimen	CR (%)	Median follow-up (months)	Survival data	Lethal toxicity
Soussain, C. et al.	2001	2nd	22	araC-VP16	thiotepa, CTX, busulfan	73%	41	3-yr EFS 53%	23%
Abrey, L. et al.	2003	1st	28	MTX-araC	BEAM	18%	27	mEFS 9 mo.	0%
Stewart, D. et al.	2004	1st	11	MTX	thiotepa, CTX, busulfan	82%	22	3-yr OS 61%	18%
Illerhaus, G. et al.	2005	1st	24	MTX	thiotepa, araC, BCNU + RT	79%	20	2-yr OS 75%	0%
Colombat, P. et al.	2003	1st	25	MVBP	araC, ITX, BEAM + RT	64%	25	3-yr OS 55%	6%
Montemurro, M. et al.	2005	1st	23	MTX	thiotepa, busulfan ± RT	81%	15	mEFS 17 mo.	13%

CR, complete response; EFS, event-free survival; mEFS, median event-free survival; OS, overall survival; MTX, methotrexate; araC, cytarabine; CTX, cyclophosphamide; ITX, ifosfamide; BEAM, carmustine, etoposide, cytarabine, melphalan; RT, radiotherapy; MVBP, methotrexate $3 \, g/m^2/day$, d1,5, VP16 $100 \, mg/m^2$ on d2, BCNU $100 \, mg/m^2$ on d3, methylprednisolone $60 \, mg/m^2/day$, d1-5, and intrathecal prophylaxis.

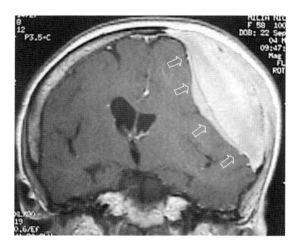

Figure 14.2 MRI showing dural lymphoma of the left parietotemporal region (arrows) infiltrating the skull and the surface of the brain. The lesion was entirely resected because the main clinical suspicion was meningioma. Histological diagnosis was diffuse large B-cell lymphoma.

mass represents less than 5% of all PCNSL (Fig. 14.2). Malignant lymphocytes can be detected in the CSF of 15–20% of PCNSL patients. An autopsy study demonstrating meningeal involvement in 100% of the cases suggests that leptomeningeal dissemination is underestimated with current methods. Prognosis of leptomeningeal lymphoma is variable due to the difficulty of delivering effective treatment to the subarachnoid space. Drug delivery using an Ommaya reservoir permits good drug distribution in the subarachnoid space. However, indications for intrathecal chemotherapy are debatable, given that its efficacy has not been studied prospectively and an international study showed that patients with PCNSL do not benefit from intrathecal drugs. Moreover, the theoretical advantage of intraventricular drug administration may not outweigh the additional risk of reservoir infectious complications and the increased risk of neurotoxicity and chemical meningitis associated with this strategy. Finally, therapeutic MTX concentrations can be achieved in CSF using intravenous doses $\geq 3\,g/m^2$, and preliminary data suggest that systemic HD-MTX is able to clear the CSF of neoplastic cells.

Intraocular lymphoma

In 5–20% of patients, PCNSL involves the eyes. Intraocular lymphoma (IOL) can occur in isolation (primary ocular lymphoma) or as a component of more extensive PCNSL. Since the eye is an extension of the CNS, its involvement is not considered systemic dissemination, even if bilateral. The neoplastic cells can infiltrate the vitreous humor, the retina, the choroid and, less frequently, the optic nerve. Patients typically present with floaters and blurred vision and are often misdiagnosed as having a benign ophthalmologic condition. Patients treated for isolated IOL have an 80% risk of developing cerebral involvement up to 10 years or more after initial diagnosis.

There is no standard treatment for isolated IOL. Systemic administration of MTX and cytarabine can yield therapeutic levels of drug in the intraocular fluids, and clinical responses have been documented; however, relapse is common. The efficacy of cytostatics is dependent on intraocular pharmacokinetics that are not well understood. Preliminary data suggest that micromolar concentrations of MTX are achieved in the aqueous and vitreous humors when the drug is given at $8\,g/m^2$. Nevertheless, a high rate of persistent ocular disease has been reported in patients treated with this strategy, perhaps because the MTX concentration in the vitreous humor, the main site of IOL, is usually lower than that obtained in the anterior chamber of the eyes. Importantly, the enrollment of patients with IOL in trials assessing the activity of chemotherapy as exclusive treatment should be critically discussed.

Better disease control combining ocular irradiation with HD-MTX-based chemotherapy has been reported. Irradiation of the posterior two-thirds of the globes with 35–45 Gy has been recommended, and more recent experience suggests using radiotherapy of the entire orbit up to 20 Gy, followed by an additional 10 Gy after shielding the anterior chamber of the eyes. Even in the presence of unilateral disease, both eyes should be irradiated because microscopic bilateral involvement occurs in 80% of patients. The actual incidence of ocular complications (cataract, dry eyes, punctate keratopathy, retinopathy, optic atrophy) is not reported because of the short follow-up of published series; however, cataract occurs in virtually all patients within several years of ocular irradiation.

The prognosis of IOL is similar to that of PCNSL without ocular involvement. The poor results obtained with conventional strategies have induced investigators to identify new therapeutic approaches. Intriguing results with intravitreal injections of MTX and high-dose chemotherapy supported by ASCT in patients with relapsed or refractory IOL have been reported.

Spinal cord lymphoma

Primary lymphomas of the spinal cord are the rarest manifestation of PCNSL. These lymphomas often arise in the upper thoracic or lower cervical regions of the spinal cord. Presenting symptoms depend on the spinal cord level involved. Myelography shows a widened spinal cord. MRI reveals hyperintensity on T2-weighted images and homogeneous enhancement after gadolinium administration on T1-weighted images. Increased CSF protein concentration is common. Lymphomas arising in the spinal nerves and ganglia ("neurolymphomatosis"), cauda equina and the sciatic nerve are extremely rare and should be distinguished from neural infiltration by a systemic lymphoma. Therapeutic results are strongly affected by pre-treatment neurological status. Prognosis of patients with spinal cord lymphoma is poor mainly due to delayed diagnosis. As with other PCNSL, corticosteroids and radiotherapy are associated with lymphoma regression and clinical improvement. Only sparse data on chemotherapy efficacy are available; however, spinal cord lymphomas should be treated similarly to other PCNSL. Because neurolymphomatosis is a condition outside the CNS, there may be a rationale for incorporating rituximab (in CD20-positive lymphomas) and CHOP chemotherapy in combination with agents that penetrate the blood–nerve barrier in the treatment of this entity.

Relapsed disease

Median survival for patients with recurrent or refractory disease without treatment is two months, but salvage treatment may substantially prolong survival. Unfortunately, the optimal salvage regimen has not been defined and a variety of possible strategies have been reported. The choice of the optimal salvage strategy should take into consideration the patient's age, performance status, site of relapse and prior therapy. Radiotherapy may be used at recurrence in previously non-irradiated patients; salvage WBRT has been associated with an overall response rate of 74% and a median survival after relapse of 11 months in patients who experienced failure after initial HD-MTX. Salvage chemotherapy is often used in an effort to improve disease control while reducing neurotoxicity. Re-induction with HD-MTX resulted in a response in approximately 50% of patients with a median PFS of 10 months. Preliminary experiences showed encouraging but unconfirmed results with combinations of procarbazine, lomustine, vincristine, etoposide, ifosfamide and cytarabine. Patients with relapsed or refractory PCNSL constitute the optimal context to identify potentially new active drugs (see *Investigational drugs*, above).

Treatment strategies for PCNSL in immunocompetent patients are summarized in Fig. 14.3.

CNS involvement in HIV-related lymphomas

PCNSL in immunocompromised patients has different characteristics and behavior compared to the immunocompetent population (Table 14.4). In HIV patients, EBV infection and *C-MYC* translocation result in the proliferation of malignant lymphocytes; a CD4 count < 50 cells/μL and high peripheral HIV viral load are the main risk factors for PCNSL development. Since the introduction of highly active antiretroviral therapy (HAART), the incidence of AIDS PCNSL has declined.

AIDS PCNSL is typically ring-enhancing on MRI (Table 14.4). Cerebral toxoplasmosis, abscesses and progressive multifocal leukoencephalopathy are the main differential diagnoses. SPECT, positron emission tomography and proton MR spectroscopy may distinguish tumor from infectious processes, but are not always definitive. Thus, a brain biopsy is often required for diagnosis, particularly if the patient has rapid neurologic deterioration, negative CSF cytology, negative *Toxoplasma* serology, radiographic features atypical for toxoplasmosis, and progressing symptoms within the first two weeks of anti-toxoplasmosis therapy. Surgical biopsy could be avoided in AIDS patients with brain lesions that have both increased thallium uptake on SPECT scanning and a positive CSF for EBV DNA. The combination of these procedures is associated with 100% sensitivity and specificity. SPECT is insufficient as a sole diagnostic modality and may give a false negative result in lesions < 0.6 cm, located near the skull or ependyma, or after steroid therapy.

Because they are profoundly immunocompromised, these patients have a much worse prognosis than non-AIDS patients. They tolerate cytotoxic chemotherapies poorly and develop more infectious complications. Before HAART, the mean survival was 1–2 months without treatment. WBRT improved survival to 3–4 months, but it may exacerbate or accelerate the risk of HIV-related dementia.

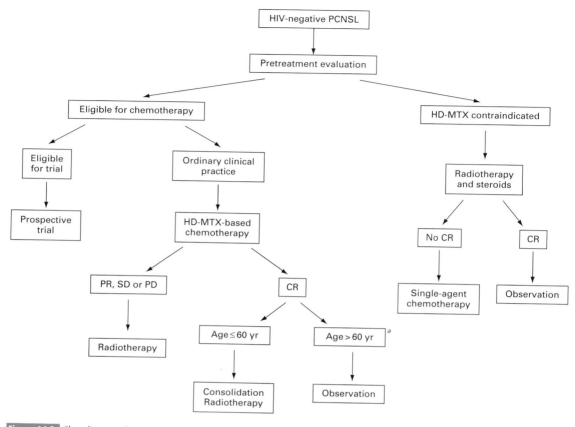

Figure 14.3. Flow diagram of recommended therapy for PCNSL according to eligibility for chemotherapy, trial availability and age. [a]The disputes on the impact on survival and neurotoxicity of consolidation radiotherapy in elderly patients in complete remission after primary chemotherapy play a central role in the design of a risk-tailored treatment against PCNSL. The best cutoff of age to distinguish subgroups of patients with different risk of neurotoxicity after consolidation radiotherapy remains to be defined. HD-MTX, high-dose methotrexate; CR, complete response; PR, partial response; SD, stable disease; PD, progressive disease.

Since the advent of HAART, the ability to deliver adequate chemotherapy to AIDS patients has improved. However, only 10% of AIDS patients with PCNSL are eligible for chemotherapy because of comorbidity or poor neurological condition. While data remain scarce, median survivals approaching or exceeding one year in patients receiving HAART, with or without other therapy, have been published, which is in contrast to earlier data that indicated a one-year survival of 10%. Therefore, patients with HIV-related PCNSL should be started on HAART (or have their HAART regimen optimized) and receive appropriate prophylaxis for opportunistic infections. This approach is adequate in patients who are retroviral-naïve, but most patients require additional specific anti-tumor therapy. HD-MTX, alone or in combination, with or without intrathecal drug delivery, has been associated with a response rate of 33–57% and a median survival of 3–4 months. The combination of oral zidovudine and HD-MTX resulted in a 46% complete response rate and a median survival of 12 months. In contrast, the use of CHOP followed by WBRT has been associated with a 12% response rate and a median survival of less than three months. In a small group of highly selected patients with HIV-related PCNSL, WBRT associated with hydroxyurea followed by PCV chemotherapy has been associated with a 100% response rate and a median survival of 13 months.

Table 14.4. Clinical, radiological and histological features of PCNSL in HIV-infected patients.

Incidence	Decreasing since HAART
Pathogenesis	EBV infection, *C-MYC* translocation
Male:female ratio	7.4:1
Median age (years)	30
Interval from symptoms to diagnosis	<2 months
Clinical presentation	Mental status changes in >50%
Number of lesions	Multiple in >50%
CSF cytological examination	Positive: 25%
Histotype	DLBCL: 75% Small noncleaved: 25%
T-cell phenotype	Very rare
EBV genomic DNA	Positive
MRI appearance	Multifocal and heterogeneous lesions Small perilesional edema and mass effect Ring enhancement common[a]
Sites of disease	Peripheral or cortically based Rarely involve the corpus callosum

[a] Ring enhancement results from central necrosis and subacute hemorrhage.

Virtually all AIDS PCNSLs are associated with EBV infection, so strategies that directly target this virus may be effective. Some investigational approaches include combinations of zidovudine, ganciclovir and interleukin 2, monoclonal antibodies or cytotoxic T lymphocytes, episomal replication inhibition by hydroxyurea or antisense oligonucleotides, and drug activation by tumor cells using thymidine kinase to phosphorylate ganciclovir or a similar molecule. Clinical experience with these interesting experimental models is still limited and successes are exceptional. In the future, it is possible that EBV-related lymphomagenesis could be blocked in high-risk patients by depleting the viral reservoir (i.e. B lymphocytes) with rituximab.

Table 14.5. Relevant clinical aspects of SCNSL.

Incidence of CNS recurrence according to histotype	
Indolent lymphomas	<3%
Aggressive lymphomas (DLBCL and PTCL)	5%
Highly aggressive lymphomas (Burkitt's and lymphoblastic)	24%
Interval between NHL diagnosis and CNS recurrence	
Median	3–6 months
Range	0–44 months
Later than one year of follow-up	4%
Site of recurrence (% of relapses)	
CNS + systemic recurrence	20%
CNS recurrence followed by systemic progression	30%
Isolated CNS recurrence	5%
Survival data	
One-year survival after CNS recurrence	25%
Median survival after relapse	4–5 months

SECONDARY CNS LYMPHOMAS

Prophylaxis against CNS relapse

CNS dissemination is an almost uniformly fatal complication of hematological malignancies. The risk of CNS relapse ranges between 5% and 30% in all NHL subtypes. The most relevant clinical aspects of this heterogeneous condition are summarized in Table 14.5. Given the high morbidity and mortality associated with CNS dissemination of NHL, a prophylactic strategy, analogous to that employed successfully for acute lymphoblastic leukemia (ALL), is indicated. However, the incidence of CNS recurrence in NHL is not sufficiently high to warrant the use of CNS prophylaxis in all patients. The analysis of risk factors for CNS relapse in NHL is biased by differences in the definition criteria and the retrospective nature of reported studies. Nevertheless, advanced disease, increased LDH serum levels, certain extranodal sites of disease and highly aggressive lymphomas (HA-NHL; Burkitt's and lymphoblastic lymphomas) have been associated with an increased risk for CNS recurrence in NHL. Patients displaying involvement of multiple extranodal organs and increased LDH serum levels have a one-year risk for CNS recurrence of 20%. The risk is increased for patients with a high IPI score, but CNS recurrence occurs in all IPI risk groups.

In HA-NHL, the five-year CNS recurrence rate was substantially higher among patients who did not receive CNS prophylaxis (32–78%) than in those who did (19%). The variable proportion of T-cell lymphoblastic lymphoma (LBL) patients within the study cohorts may explain in part this wide variation. Similar to T-cell ALL, patients with T-cell LBL may have a higher risk for CNS relapse. The inclusion of CNS-directed prophylaxis led to a substantial reduction in CNS relapse rates in LBL patients: 0–36% with intrathecal chemotherapy alone, 3–21% with intrathecal chemotherapy and WBRT, <5% with intrathecal chemotherapy, WBRT and systemic HD-MTX and high-dose cytarabine. The latter combination is the conventional CNS prophylaxis in HA-NHL.

For aggressive lymphomas, CNS prophylaxis is currently used in 10–15% of cases; however, there is still no uniformity of practice, which reflects the fact that the published data are open to differing interpretations. Patients with a high IPI score, particularly those with a high serum LDH level, involvement of more than one extranodal site, testicular lymphoma or paranasal sinus involvement, should be assessed for CNS involvement at diagnosis. Intrathecal chemotherapy and the addition of systemic HD-MTX or high-dose cytarabine to conventional chemotherapy reduce the CNS relapse rate and appear to be as effective as and less toxic than WBRT. A trial of 708 NHL patients aged 61–69 years with at least one adverse IPI feature compared an intensive chemotherapy, incorporating both intrathecal MTX and consolidation with systemic HD-MTX, ifosfamide and cytarabine, with a standard CHOP regimen. The frequency of CNS recurrence was significantly lower in the experimental arm (2.7% vs. 8.3%, $p < 0.002$). Meninges have been involved in 60% of CNS relapses, the brain parenchyma in 23% and both in 17%. These results are in line with an earlier analysis suggesting a positive impact of prophylaxis with intrathecal and intravenous MTX.

The addition of conventional-dose rituximab to CHOP in the treatment of patients with DLBCL did not influence the probability of CNS relapse in a randomized trial, with CNS relapse rates of 5.4% and 4.5% respectively ($p = 0.68$) for rituximab-CHOP and CHOP groups.

Treatment of SCNSL

In a large proportion of patients, CNS relapse is accompanied or rapidly followed by systemic relapse, and the patient's outcome is determined equally by the control of systemic and CNS disease, even in patients with isolated CNS recurrence. Therefore, treatment should be directed at the entire craniospinal axis, and also provide control of systemic disease. Systemic high-dose chemotherapy is the most effective strategy that meets these requirements. As with PCNSL, the choice of drugs is based on the ability to cross the BBB and have anti-lymphoma activity. Most first-line combinations against SCNSL contain HD-MTX or high-dose cytarabine, but the most effective administration schedules for these drugs in SCNSL remain to be defined. Most lymphoma patients with an increased risk of CNS relapse receive these drugs as first-line treatment, so salvage options may be limited because few other drugs cross the BBB. Some anecdotal experience with cisplatin-based regimens has been reported, and autologous or allogeneic transplantation may prove beneficial for selected patients.

Patients with leptomeningeal involvement without focal neurological deficits are usually treated with intrathecal chemotherapy (MTX, cytarabine and hydrocortisone), twice a week, through an Ommaya reservoir. Although this strategy invariably results in a decrease in the number of tumor cells in the CSF, symptomatic improvement occurs in fewer than 20% of cases. A slow-release formulation of cytarabine, injected once every two weeks, produces a higher response rate and a better quality of life relative to that produced by free cytarabine injected twice a week. Patients with focal neurological deficits, or with intraparenchymal lesions in the brain, cranial nerves or spinal cord, are commonly treated with radiation therapy, which results in transient symptomatic improvement in over 65% of cases; however, CNS or systemic progression is the rule. The optimal approach to managing overt CNS disease at diagnosis in children with large-cell lymphoma is controversial because of the low frequency and high heterogeneity of this group of malignancies. The BFM regimen, derived from a Burkitt's lymphoma strategy, and the APO regimen associated with intrathecal MTX deserve to be mentioned. In children with Burkitt's lymphoma, HD-MTX and cytarabine and intrathecal chemotherapy are currently used for both CNS prophylaxis and treatment.

Some of the most successful treatment regimens against HA-NHL have excluded WBRT. In children there is a trend toward reducing the use of radiotherapy for CNS disease and prophylaxis to reduce late sequelae such as second cancer, endocrinopathy and neuropsychological defects. In recent clinical trials, the prophylactic WBRT dose has been reduced to 12 Gy and the therapeutic dose to 18 Gy, while the safety of WBRT omission is being assessed in current trials on LBL in children. In recent trials, the elimination of WBRT has not been associated with an excessive rate of CNS relapse.

Autologous stem-cell transplantation

Some reports conclude that 20–40% of adults with NHL and CNS disease can achieve durable remissions after high-dose chemotherapy and autologous transplantation, primarily patients with HA-NHL in first remission at the time of transplantation. On the other hand, attempts to transplant adults with active CNS disease at the moment of autologous transplantation have had disappointing results, with a PFS of 9% at 71 months (HA-NHL). Moreover, it is difficult to estimate the exact contribution of autologous transplantation to survival in patients with HA-NHL and CNS involvement at diagnosis, which may be curable with conventional-dose treatment. In some series, overall results with high-dose chemotherapy and autologous transplantation are disappointing, which could be partially explained by a high incidence of fatal CNS complications in previously irradiated patients.

Conditioning regimens are not specifically designed for patients with CNS disease. Ideally, drugs should be chosen on the basis of anti-lymphoma activity and capacity to cross the BBB. Total-body irradiation (TBI) is highly immunosuppressive, has good antitumor activity and is not affected by the BBB. However, this strategy is associated with an increased risk of severe neurotoxicity, especially when combined with intrathecal chemotherapy or systemic HD-MTX or cytarabine. Combinations of busulfan and cyclophosphamide are good alternatives to TBI. At appropriate doses, busulfan is able to cross the BBB, while data regarding CNS penetration of cyclophosphamide are conflicting. These drugs, with or without thiotepa, can be curative in children with HA-NHL and CNS

involvement, but risk of severe neurotoxicity is high in previously irradiated patients. Some lymphoma patients with CNS involvement have been treated with nitrosourea-based conditioning regimens, obtaining a five-year PFS similar to those obtained with TBI-containing regimens (20% vs. 42%, $p = 0.3$). Novel conditioning combinations need to be investigated, given the disappointing results with this strategy.

Allogeneic stem-cell transplantation

There is some evidence to suggest that allogeneic transplantation is superior to autologous transplantation for the prevention or treatment of CNS recurrence in HA-NHL and ALL, both in children and in adults. Moreover, consolidation with allogeneic transplantation is associated with significantly improved outcome in children with early CNS recurrence of ALL. It is conceivable that graft-versus-lymphoma effects may extend to the CNS and contribute to eradication of CNS disease. However, survival benefit with this strategy is obscured by increased treatment-related mortality. Moreover, the real impact of allogeneic transplantation in CNS recurrence is difficult to define because of the interpretation bias related to the effect of immunosuppressive therapy used for prevention or treatment of graft-versus-host disease. Anecdotal experience with allogeneic transplantation in a few patients with different hematological malignancies and active CNS disease confirms the dismal prognosis of this condition, and better results can be obtained in patients whose CNS disease is in remission at transplant.

RARE FORMS OF CNS LYMPHOMA

Rare histopathological variants of CNS lymphomas exist. The most relevant clinical and therapeutic features of these CNS lymphoproliferative disorders are summarized in Table 14.6. Diagnostic, staging and therapeutic approaches to these malignancies are variable, and clinical evidence supporting therapeutic decisions is anecdotal.

Indolent lymphomas

Low-grade marginal zone B-cell lymphoma of MALT type primarily involving the CNS usually arises in the dura (Fig. 14.4). These lymphomas have excellent long-term prognosis with local

Table 14.6. Rare forms of CNS lymphoproliferative disorders.

Category	% of PCNSL	Age/gender	Stage (usually)	Clinical features	Therapeutic management
T-cell lymphomas	1–4%	M > F, 60 yr	I_EA	Systemic symptoms 11%	Similar to B-cell PCNSL, similar outcome
Anaplastic large-cell lymphomas	<1%	M > F, 29 yr	I_EA	T-cell; common meningeal disease; normal LDH levels; ↑ CSF protein	Similar to PCNSL + CSF prophylaxis; better outcome in young ALK1+ patients
Intravascular lymphomas	<1%	M > F, 70 yr	IVA	Poor performance status, B symptoms, anemia, and ↑ LDH levels; multiorgan failure; exclusive CNS involvement is rare	Anthracycline-based chemotherapy ± rituximab ± drugs with high CNS bioavailability; 3-yr OS of 25%
Low-grade marginal zone B-cell lymphoma of MALT type	5%	M < F, young	I_EA	Usually arises in dura; favorable clinical outcomes; meningioma is differential diagnosis	Excellent prognosis with local therapy; consolidation RT may be unnecessary after complete resection
Immunocytoma	4–13%	M < F, young	I_EA	Indolent course	HD-MTX has poor activity (anecdotal); good control with WBRT
Plasmacytoma	<1%	M > F, elderly	I_EA/IVA	Trend to remain within CNS; favorable outcome if solitary	Radiotherapy 50 Gy alone if solitary; chemotherapy in large lesions[a]
Hodgkin's lymphoma	1.4%	M = F, 50–85 yr	I_EA/IVA	Isolated brain or meningeal lesion; nodular sclerosis in 50% of cases	WBRT has provided acceptable DFS; intrathecal therapy in CSF+ patients

[a] Disseminated plasmacytoma with CNS disease should be treated like multiple myeloma with the addition of drugs with high CNS bioavailability.

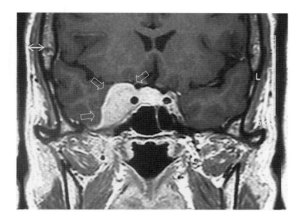

Figure 14.4 MRI showing lymphoma (arrows) of the parasellar region. The well-limited lesion was entirely resected; histological diagnosis was low-grade marginal zone B-cell lymphoma.

therapy alone, and consolidation radiotherapy may be unnecessary after complete resection (Table 14.6). Immunocytoma has been listed as accounting for up to 13% of all PCNSL (Table 14.6). However, many CNS immunocytoma cases reported before the WHO classification likely represent examples of MALT lymphomas. This indolent malignancy can be treated with radiotherapy with acceptable disease control; experience with HD-MTX-based chemotherapy is anecdotal and suggests modest activity.

Aggressive lymphomas

PCNSL of T-cell phenotype is more common in Japan (8% of PCNSL) than in Western countries. The diagnosis of T-cell PCNSL can be difficult, and its incidence is possibly overestimated because of the frequent infiltration of reactive perivascular T cells, which could interfere with the interpretation of immunophenotyping, particularly after steroid administration. The analysis of an international retrospective series of 45 cases concluded that T-cell PCNSL should be treated in an identical fashion to standard PCNSL, with the expectation of similar results, at least in Western countries. The overall therapeutic approach to primary CNS anaplastic large-cell lymphoma, usually displaying T-cell immunophenotype, is similar to the current therapy of PCNSL; meningeal prophylaxis appears advisable. Young

patients and ALK1-positive lymphomas seem to have a better outcome.

Intravascular lymphoma is an aggressive and disseminated malignancy (Table 14.6), characterized by rapidly progressing manifestations of multiorgan failure due to multiple infarcts, with CNS involvement in 34% of cases. Intravascular lymphoma involving the CNS has a worse prognosis, requiring intensive multidrug combinations containing agents with high CNS bioavailability.

CNS involvement by plasmacytoma is rare (Table 14.6), being the sole site of disease in half of cases. Intracranial plasmacytoma is unlikely to develop systemic disease in patients with initial negative staging. Involved-field irradiation with 50 Gy has been reported as an acceptable strategy in patients with solitary intracranial plasmacytoma; patients with large lesions have obtained clinical benefit from chemotherapy.

Primary CNS Hodgkin's lymphoma may present as an isolated brain lesion, as meningeal dissemination with subdural infiltration, or as a calvarial lesion with meningeal or cerebral infiltration. One-half of reported cases had nodular sclerosis. The detection of Reed–Sternberg cells or eosinophilia in the CSF is uncommon. WBRT (35–45 Gy) followed by a tumor-bed boost (5–15 Gy) has provided acceptable disease-free survival. The role of systemic chemotherapy remains to be defined, while the use of intrathecal chemotherapy in patients with CSF-positive disease has been suggested.

FURTHER READING

Abrey, L. E., Batchelor, T. T., Ferreri, A. J. *et al.* Report of an international workshop to standardize baseline evaluation and response criteria for primary CNS lymphoma. *J. Clin. Oncol.* **23** (2005), 5034–5043.

DeAngelis, L. M. and Hormigo, A. Treatment of primary central nervous system lymphoma. *Semin. Oncol.* **31** (2004), 684–692.

DeAngelis, L. M., Seiferheld, W., Schold, S. C. *et al.* Combination chemotherapy and radiotherapy for primary central nervous system lymphoma: Radiation Therapy Oncology Group Study 93–10. *J. Clin. Oncol.* **20** (2002), 4643–4648.

Ferreri, A. J., Abrey, L. E., Blay, J. Y. *et al.* Summary statement on primary central nervous system lymphomas from the Eighth International Conference on Malignant Lymphoma, Lugano, Switzerland, June 12 to 15, 2002. *J. Clin. Oncol.* **21** (2003), 2407–2414.

Ferreri, A. J., Reni, M., Pasini, F. *et al.* A multicenter study of treatment of primary CNS lymphoma. *Neurology* **58** (2002), 1513–1520.

Hoffmann, C., Tabrizian, S., Wolf, E. *et al.* Survival of AIDS patients with primary central nervous system lymphoma is dramatically improved by HAART-induced immune recovery. *AIDS* **15** (2001), 2119–2127.

Hollender, A., Kvaloy, S., Nome, O. *et al.* Central nervous system involvement following diagnosis of non-Hodgkin's lymphoma: a risk model. *Ann. Oncol.* **13** (2002), 1099–1107.

Kasamon, Y. L. and Ambinder, R. F. AIDS-related primary central nervous system lymphoma. *Hematol. Oncol. Clin. North Am.* **19** (2005), 665–687.

van Besien, K., Forman, A. and Champlin, R. Central nervous system relapse of lymphoid malignancies in adults: the role of high-dose chemotherapy. *Ann. Oncol.* **8** (1997), 515–524.

van Besien, K., Ha, C. S., Murphy, S. *et al.* Risk factors, treatment, and outcome of central nervous system recurrence in adults with intermediate-grade and immunoblastic lymphoma. *Blood* **91** (1998), 1178–1184.

15 T-CELL LYMPHOMA

Mujahid A. Rizvi, Andrew M. Evens, Beverly P. Nelson and Steven T. Rosen

Pathology: Andrew Wotherspoon
Molecular cytogenetics: Andreas Rosenwald and German Ott

INTRODUCTION

T-cell non-Hodgkin's lymphomas (NHL) are uncommon malignancies, representing approximately 12% of all lymphomas. Various geographic frequencies of T-cell NHL have been documented, ranging from 18.3% of NHL diagnosed in Hong Kong to 1.5% in Vancouver, Canada. This may in part reflect increased exposure to pathogenic factors such as human T-cell leukemia virus 1 (HTLV-1) and Epstein–Barr virus (EBV) in Asian nations. T-cell NHL commonly presents with extranodal disease and often contains varying amounts of necrosis/apoptosis on biopsy specimens, making differentiation between a reactive process and lymphoma challenging. Immunophenotypic, cytogenetic and molecular analyses have enhanced diagnostic capabilities as well as improved classification and prognostication for T-cell NHL.

The current World Health Organization/European Organisation for Research and Treatment of Cancer (WHO/EORTC) classification recognizes nine distinct clinicopathologic peripheral T-cell NHLs. The broad spectrum of pathologic subtypes with varied clinical behavior poses a challenge to the systematic study of these diseases. Furthermore, these distinct T-cell NHL subtypes have unique characteristics and often warrant individualized diagnostic and therapeutic treatment strategies. The primary cutaneous T-cell lymphomas are reviewed in Chapter 16. Here we review the etiology, pathology, diagnosis and treatment strategies for patients with peripheral T-cell lymphomas (Table 15.1).

ETIOLOGY

Genetic alterations involved in lymphoma oncogenesis include chromosome rearrangements, disruption of tumor suppressor genes and an increase in the number of copies of genes (gene amplification). Moreover, infection of cells by viruses and bacteria such as HTLV-I, human herpesvirus 8 (HHV-8), hepatitis C and *Helicobacter pylori* may also contribute to lymphomagenesis.

Chromosome rearrangements contribute to altered gene function through varied mechanisms such as proto-oncogene activation and deregulation of gene expression. The primary mechanism of proto-oncogene activation in lymphoma is reciprocal and balanced chromosomal translocations. These translocations are mostly recurrent and non-random in NHL. The majority of chromosome translocations in NHL involve the juxtaposition of a proto-oncogene from one chromosome next to regulatory sequences of a partner chromosome. This contributes to control of the proto-oncogene by a promoter associated with an immunoglobulin (Ig) or T-cell receptor (TCR) gene. The two subtypes of TCRs that T-cell lymphocytes express are gamma–delta ($\gamma\delta$) or alpha–beta ($\alpha\beta$). Approximately 95% of normal T lymphocytes express the $\alpha\beta$ heterodimer, while a minority of T lymphocytes express the $\gamma\delta$ heterodimer. Alpha–beta T cells develop predominantly in the thymus, while $\gamma\delta$ T cells may develop in extra-thymic locations such as the skin, intestinal epithelium and spleen. The four TCR genes are arranged in germline configuration in non-continuous segments of variable (V), diversity (D), joining (J) and constant (C) regions. The precise mechanism by which translocation of TCR and Ig genes occur is not known, but it appears in part to involve dysfunctional gene remodeling including V–D–J recombination, isotype switching and somatic hypermutation. T-cell

Lymphoma: Pathology, Diagnosis and Treatment, ed. Robert Marcus, John W. Sweetenham and Michael E. Williams. Published by Cambridge University Press. © Cambridge University Press 2007.

Table 15.1. Peripheral T-cell non-Hodgkin's lymphomas according to WHO/EORTC classification.

Leukemic/disseminated

Adult T-cell leukemia/lymphoma

Nodal

Peripheral T-cell lymphoma, unspecified

Angioimmunoblastic T-cell lymphoma

Anaplastic large-cell lymphoma, T/null-cell, primary systemic type

Other extranodal

Subcutaneous panniculitis-like T-cell lymphoma

Cutaneous gamma–delta T-cell lymphoma

Hepatosplenic gamma-delta T-cell lymphoma

Extranodal NK/T-cell lymphoma, nasal type

Enteropathy-type T-cell lymphoma

From Rizvi *et al.* 2006. © American Society of Hematology.

neoplasms may have rearrangements involving the site of TCR α and δ genes on chromosome 14, or more rarely, chromosome 7 (7q34–36 and 7p15), the site of TCR β and γ genes. Many of the genes located at the breakpoints of recurring chromosome translocations have been identified. The majority of translocated genes encode transcription factors. Transcription factors are involved in the initiation of gene transcription and cell differentiation. The most common result of chromosome translocations in lymphomas that involve TCR and/or Ig genes is deregulation of gene expression with irregular or overexpression in cells that normally do not express this gene. Few lymphomas have been recognized to contain translocations that produce a fusion protein, such as the t(2;5)(p23;q35) translocation in anaplastic large-cell lymphoma (ALCL) that results in expression of the nucleophosmin–anaplastic lymphoma kinase (NPM–ALK) protein.

Inactivation of tumor suppressor genes may also play a role in lymphomagenesis. The most common mechanism of tumor suppressor inactivation occurs through the Knudson two-hit model, where a reduction of homozygosity leads to tumor formation, for example following germline deletion of one allele and somatic mutation of the other. Tumor suppressor genes identified with NHL include *p53*, *p15* and *p16*. Moreover, specific chromosomal deletions that have

been detected in NHL (including some T-cell lymphomas), such as 3p, 6q, 13q and 17p, may represent sites of yet-to-be-identified tumor suppressor loci. Other mediators that may be involved in lymphomagenesis include the cyclin-dependent kinase (CDK) inhibitors, such as p21$^{(Waf1)}$. A function of the p21$^{(Waf1)}$ protein includes the arrest of cells in G_1-phase checkpoint by associating with cyclin-CDK complexes, but the exact factors critical for apoptosis have not been clearly defined. The gene for the p21$^{(Waf1)}$ protein has been identified as a downstream target of p53 in regulating cell-cycle progression through G_1. Induction of p21$^{(Waf1)}$ has also been demonstrated to occur through a p53-independent pathway.

Gene amplification leads to an increase in the number of copies of a gene in the genome of a cell, which may contribute to lymphomagenesis. Gene amplification has been identified mostly in B-cell lymphomas (e.g. *REL* gene), although amplification of TCR genes in varied T-cell lymphomas has been described. Random genomic instability, as seen in many epithelial cancers, is not a characteristic of the more stable lymphoma genome. Defects in DNA mismatch repair that manifest as genomic microsatellite instability are also less recognized in lymphoma, as compared to various hereditary solid tumor syndromes and rare sporadic cancers.

PROGNOSIS

The optimal therapeutic strategy for T-cell NHL remains unclear. Few randomized or multi-institution clinical trials comparing chemotherapeutic or other treatment modalities for T-cell NHL have been reported. This is in part due not only to the overall lower incidence and prevalence compared to other malignancies, but also to the heterogeneity of disease and the infrequent documentation of a clonal immunophenotypic marker for T cells, which often makes a timely and definite diagnosis difficult.

Several studies have documented that a T-cell phenotype is an independent poor prognostic factor among all NHL diagnoses on multivariate analysis. When analyzing T-cell NHL populations, five-year overall survival (OS) rates have ranged from 26% to 41%. Moreover, recent studies have demonstrated significantly worse survival when T-cell NHLs (all histologies) have been directly compared to aggressive B-cell NHLs, with five-year OS rates of 39–41%

versus 52–63%, respectively. There is limited data on whether this holds true in limited-stage peripheral T-cell NHL. Canadian researchers recently found that limited-stage peripheral T-cell NHL had outcomes comparable to limited-stage diffuse large B-cell lymphomas (DLBCL) and were less likely to have late relapses. Analysis of PTCL-u patients showed that the number of factors – age > 60, Eastern Cooperative Oncology Group (ECOG) performance status 2–4, LDH above normal, bone-marrow involvement – independently predicted for survival (no adverse factors = five-year and ten-year OS of 62.3% and 54.9%, respectively; one factor = 52.9% and 38.8%; two factors = 32.9% and 18.0%; three or four factors = 18.3% and 12.6%).

When large populations of T-cell NHL have been analyzed, some have documented variable survival rates among different T-cell histologies (anaplastic large cell lymphoma [ALK-positive] > peripheral T-cell lymphoma, unspecified > extranodal NK/T-cell lymphoma-nasal type > angioimmunoblastic lymphoma > subcutaneous panniculitis-like T-cell lymphoma > hepatosplenic T-cell lymphoma > enteropathy-type intestinal T-cell lymphoma), while others have not. The majority of T-cell NHL studies have established that the International Prognostic Index (IPI) significantly predicts outcome in patients. However, it is important to recognize that few reports have included sufficient numbers of less common T-cell NHL diagnoses such as subcutaneous panniculitis-like T-cell lymphoma, hepatosplenic T-cell lymphoma and enteropathy-type intestinal T-cell lymphoma to allow sufficient prognostic and survival comparisons. One report showed that within the entire subset of T-cell lymphoma EBV positivity was associated with significantly inferior survival rates compared to EBV-negative T-cell lymphoma.

SPECIFIC DISEASE TYPES

Table 15.2 summarizes the characteristics of each specific T-cell NHL.

Adult T-cell leukemia/lymphoma (ATLL)

The retrovirus HTLV-1 is critical to the development of ATLL. In endemic areas in Japan, approximately 6–37% of the population is infected with HTLV-1. The United States and Europe are considered low-risk

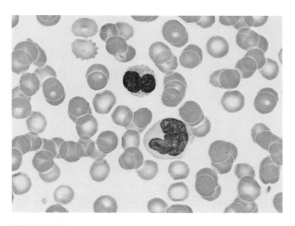

Figure 15.1. Adult T-cell leukemia/lymphoma (peripheral blood). Two lymphoma cells, one displaying a lobated nucleus with clumped chromatin, the other larger with more dispersed chromatin and cerebreform shaped nucleus. (From Rizvi et al. 2006. © American Society of Hematology.)

areas, with less than 1% of the population seropositive. Only 2–4% of patients who are carriers of the HTLV-1 virus develop ATLL. HTLV-1 is transmitted through sexual intercourse, blood products containing white blood cells, shared needles, breast milk and from mother to child during childbirth. Transfusion of HTLV-1-contaminated blood products results in seroconversion in approximately 30–50% of patients at a median of 51 days.

The median age at presentation is 55 years. Patients present with lymphadenopathy (72%), skin lesions (53%), hepatomegaly (47%), splenomegaly (25%) and hypercalcemia (28%).

Pathology

The tumor cells are characteristically medium to large, with pleomorphic nuclei that show convolutions or lobulations that may be pronounced (flower cells) (Fig. 15.1). In chronic and smoldering variants the cells may be predominantly small with round nuclei. The cytoplasm is basophilic. Giant cells may be seen. The skin shows dermal infiltration, frequently with extension of clusters of atypical cells into the epidermis. In chronic and smoldering cases the cutaneous infiltrate is usually subtle (Fig. 15.2). There may be associated hemophagocytosis, and in the bone marrow there may be associated osteoclastic activity.

In some cases large cells resembling the Reed–Sternberg cells of Hodgkin's lymphoma may be seen.

Table 15.2. Immunophenotype, Epstein–Barr virus status and genetic features of peripheral T-cell NHLs.

Neoplasm	CD3 S; C	CD5	CD7	CD4	CD8	CD25	CD30	CD52	TCR	EBV	Genetic abnormality	T-receptor genes
Adult T-cell leukemia/lymphoma	+	+	−	+	−	+	−/+	+	NA	−	Multiple	Rearranged
Peripheral T-cell lymphoma, unspecified	+/−	+/−	+/−	+/−	−/+	NA	−/+	−/+	αβ > γδ	−	Often complex	Rearranged
Angioimmunoblastic T-cell lymphoma	+	+	+	+/−	−/+	NA	−	−/+	αβ	Present in lymph nodes	Trisomy 3 and 5; additional X	Rearranged
Anaplastic large-cell lymphoma, T/null-cell, primary systemic type	+/−	+/−	NA	−/+	−/+	+	+	−	αβ	−	(see Table 15.3)	Rearranged
Subcutaneous panniculitis-like T-cell lymphoma	+	+	+	−	+	NA	−	NA	αβ	−	−	Rearranged
Cutaneous γδ T-cell lymphomas	+	−	+/−	−	−	NA	−/+	NA	γδ	−	−	Rearranged
Hepatosplenic gamma-delta T-cell lymphoma	+	−	+	−	−	NA	−	NA	γδ > αβ	−	i(7q) and trisomy 8	Rearranged
Extranodal NK/T-cell lymphoma, nasal type	−/+	−	−/+	−	−	NA	−	NA	−	+	del 6 and 13	−
Enteropathy-type T-cell lymphoma	+	+	+	−	+/−	NA	+/−	NA	αβ > γδ	−	LOH 9p21	Rearranged

S, surface; C, cytoplasmic; i, isochrome; del, deletion; LOH, loss of heterozygosity; +, >80%; −, >80%; +/−, >50% positive; −/+, >50% negative; NA, not available.

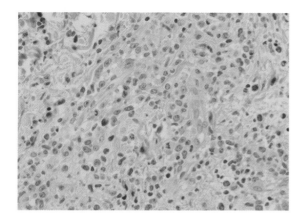

Figure 15.2. Adult T-cell leukemia/lymphoma (dermis of skin). A proliferation of large cells with convoluted nuclei that contain prominent nucleoli.

In most cases these are CD30-positive B cells that may also express CD15 and show evidence of EBV infection. These are likely to be reactive, and a reflection of the immunosuppression associated with the lymphoma.

Immunophenotypically the cells are mature T cells with no expression of TdT or CD1a. There is usually expression of CD2, CD3 and CD5, but lack of CD7 is common. Most cases are CD4+/CD8−, but CD4+/CD8+ and CD4−/CD8+ cases are occasionally seen. The cells are characteristically positive for CD25. Some cases may show expression of CD30, particularly in the large cells. Stains for TIA-1 and granzyme are usually negative.

Molecular pathology and cytogenetics

The prerequisite for the diagnosis is the demonstration of integrated HTLV-1 genomes in virtually all cases. TCR genes are clonally rearranged. Some recurring structural and numerical chromosome aberrations have been reported, among them trisomy for chromosomes 3p, 7q and 14q, and losses in 6q. These changes are predominantly encountered in aggressive variants.

Subtypes

ATLL is classified into four subtypes based on clinico-pathologic features and prognosis: acute, lymphoma, chronic and smoldering. In a recent study, patients with the acute type presented with hypercalcemia, leukemic manifestations and tumor lesions and had the worst prognosis, with a median survival of approximately six months. Lymphoma-type patients presented with low circulating abnormal lymphocytes ($< 1\%$) and nodal, liver, splenic, central nervous system, bone, and gastrointestinal disease, and had a median survival of 10 months. Chronic-type patients presented with $> 5\%$ abnormal circulating lymphocytes and had a median survival of 24 months, while the median survival of smoldering type had not yet been reached.

Treatment

ATLL is a difficult malignancy to treat. Patients may initially respond to combination chemotherapy, but overall survival is poor (median eight months). Response rates of 70–90% to combination interferon alpha (IFN-α) and zidovudine therapy have been demonstrated in ATLL, with associated median survival rates of 11–18 months. A clinical trial that investigated initial cytoreductive therapy with cyclophosphamide, doxorubicin, vincristine and prednisone (CHOP) followed by antinucleoside, IFN-α and oral etoposide therapy demonstrated encouraging results. A recent retrospective review of 44 patients diagnosed and treated for ATLL, however, found that patients who received infusional doxorubicin therapy had improvement in median overall survival as compared to patients who received the traditional CHOP-based treatment regimens. Furthermore, preliminary data from a Japanese phase III study show that patients treated with dose-intensified multi-agent chemotherapy VCAP (vincristine, cyclophosphamide, doxorubicin, prednisone), AMP (doxorubicin, ranimustine, prednisone) and VECP (vindesine, etoposide, carboplatin, prednisone) with intrathecal prophylaxis for aggressive ATLL had better overall survival than patients who received biweekly CHOP (overall survival at three years was 23.6% vs. 12.7%). Two reports have suggested a role for combination arsenic trioxide (As$_2$O$_3$) with IFN-α, which induces cell-cycle arrest and apoptosis both in HTLV-1 transformed cell lines and primary ATLL cells in culture. Proteasome inhibitors and all-trans retinoic acid (ATRA) have been shown to have an effect on ATLL cell-cycle progression as well, which may have implications for the clinical application of these agents in ATLL. Future research should include the investigation of recombinant toxins and monoclonal antibodies, such as denileukin diftitox (target CD25) and alemtuzumab (target CD52).

Peripheral T-cell lymphoma, unspecified (PTCL-u)

PTCL-u is predominantly a nodal lymphoma that represents the most common T-cell lymphoma subtype in Western countries, comprising approximately 50–60% of T-cell lymphomas and 5–7% of all NHL. PTCL-u usually affects male adults (male-to-female ratio 1.5), with a median age of 61 years (range 17–90) in a large study with 25% of patients presenting in stage I or II$_E$, 12% stage III and 63% stage IV. PTCL-u patients from this study commonly presented with unfavorable characteristics including B symptoms (40%), elevated LDH (66%), bulky tumor ≥ 10 cm (11%), non-ambulatory performance status (29%) and extranodal disease (56%), leading to the majority of patients (53%) falling into the unfavorable IPI category (score of 3–5). Other smaller studies of PTCL-u patients have corroborated male preponderance, B symptoms and extranodal disease (bone marrow > liver > skin > lung and bone).

Pathology

This is a polymorphous group of tumors that includes many subtypes previously identified as specific entities in the Kiel classification of lymphomas. The morphology is varied, but usually consists of a pleomorphic mix of medium and large cells that diffusely efface the lymph node architecture. Many of these cells have quite abundant clear cytoplasm. High endothelial venules are prominent and may have an arborising pattern. The background population includes a mixture of small lymphocytes, plasma cells, histiocytes and eosinophils.

In some cases the infiltrate is predominantly between lymphoid follicles, which may be hyperplastic (T-zone subtype) (Fig. 15.3). In these variants the cells are medium-sized with clear cytoplasm and little nuclear pleomorphism. Scattered large cells resembling Reed–Sternberg cells are often present. In the lymphoepithelioid variant (Lennert's lymphoma) the neoplastic cells are usually small. Clear cells are less frequent and there are clusters of epithelioid macrophages within the background infiltrate.

Immunophenotypically the cells are mature T cells that do not express TdT or CD1a but are positive for CD2, CD3, CD5 and CD7, although partial loss of T-cell antigen expression is frequent. The majority of cases are CD4-positive and negative for CD8, but

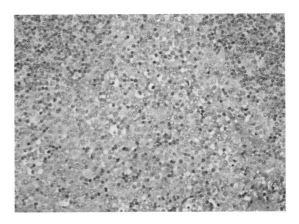

Figure 15.3. Peripheral T-cell lymphoma, unspecified (lymph node). A sheet of large cells with pleomorphic nuclei, which in this case lies between residual lymphoid follicles (T-zone pattern). Associated eosinophils are frequently present.

other combinations can be seen. In some cases the cells express CD30, and these must be distinguished from anaplastic large-cell lymphoma.

Molecular pathology and cytogenetics

The cytogenetic constitution of PTCL-u is still poorly defined and – in keeping with its variable morphologic features – no unifying cytogenetic aberration exists. Classical banding studies are rare, but have revealed recurring chromosomal aberrations. Recurring deletions have been described in the short arm of chromosome 1, the long arm of chromosome 6 and the short arm of chromosome 17. Gains are common in chromosomes 3, 7 and X. PTCL-u of the large-cell type is frequently characterized by a tetraploid karyotype. Only one recurring translocation, t(5;9)(q33;q22), has been identified so far, fusing *ITK* and *SYK* genes. Interestingly, this translocation may be indicative of a particular PTCL-u subtype morphologically characterized by a perifollicular and intrafollicular growth pattern. Studies using conventional comparative genomic hybridization (CGH) as a platform resulted in the revelation of a plethora of complex chromosomal alterations resulting in recurring imbalances, and in the definition of clearly nonrandom minimal overlapping target regions. Thus, the most frequent recurrent genetic losses in PTCL-u were encountered in 13q, 6q, 9p, 10q, 12q and 5q. Gains were observed in 7q, 17q, 16p, 8q, 9q and others. Some of these imbalances seem to occur simultaneously and may define particular PTCL-u subgroups.

Treatment

In many of the prognostic studies discussed above, most T-cell NHL patients were treated in the same manner as intermediate-grade B-cell patients, with anthracycline-based chemotherapy alone or with combinations including cisplatin and etoposide. Randomized trials comparing CHOP (cyclophospha-mide, doxorubicin, vincristine, prednisone) to other combination regimens confirmed CHOP as a stan-dard regimen for intermediate-grade B-cell NHL, but unfortunately these trials do not allow for subset analysis of T-cell patients. Rituximab should not be included in the treatment for PTCL-u (unless other conditions such as immune thrombocytopenic purpura exist), as CD20 is not expressed. Moreover, combined T-cell (from disease) and B-cell (from rituximab) suppression may result in prohibitive morbidity and mortality. Other therapeutic agents tested in T-cell NHL include purine and pyrimidine analogues, denileukin diftitox, and retinoic acid/ IFN-α combination. Nucleoside analogues such as 2'-deoxycoformin (dCF; pentostatin), fludarabine and 2-chlorodeoxyadenosine (2-CdA) have been tested mostly in patients with cutaneous NHL, although several anecdotal reports have reported activity in other T-cell NHL subtypes. Administered as an intravenous bolus daily over three days (at an initial dose of 5 mg/m^2 per day, repeated every 3–4 weeks), this has produced response rates to the ade-nosine deaminase (ADA) inhibitor, pentostatin, of 50% (7% complete response) in single-institution phase II studies, with median duration of responses of 4–6 months. One trial analyzed response according to CD26 (ADA binding protein) status, with five of nine CD26-negative patients responding to pentosta-tin. The pyrimidine antimetabolite, gemcitabine, has activity in relapsed/refractory T-cell NHL as a single agent, with reported response rates of 60% in small single-institution studies. Gemcitabine has also been studied in combination with cisplatin and methyl-prednisolone, with encouraging early results in relapsed Hodgkin's lymphoma and NHL.

Denileukin diftitox (DAB$_{389}$IL-2, Ontak) is a novel recombinant fusion protein consisting of peptide sequences for the enzymatically active, membrane-active and membrane-translocation domains of diphtheria toxin with recombinant interleukin 2 that has been studied mostly in cutaneous T-cell NHL, although clinical benefit has been reported in other T-cell NHL patients. Preliminary data from a phase II trial with single-agent denileukin diftitox showed a 40% overall response rate in relapsed/ refractory PTCL-u patients. A recent study reported on 17 patients with relapsed T-cell NHL using 13-cis-retinoic acid with IFN-α. A response rate of 31% was documented in four of six ALCL patients and one of seven PTCL-u, although median survival for the entire group of patients was 3.6 months. A recent European pilot study showed a 36% response rate with alemtuzumab in heavily pre-treated PTCL-u patients. Three of 14 patients had a complete response (CR) that lasted up to 12 months. However, there were significant hematological and infectious complications. Trials evaluating the efficacy of CHOP-alemtuzumab, dose-adjusted EPOCH-alemtuzumab (etoposide, vincristine, doxorubicin, bolus cyclo-phosphamide, oral prednisone) and CHOP-denileukin diftitox are currently under way.

Angioimmunoblastic T-cell lymphoma (AITL)

AITL, also known as angioimmunoblastic lymphade-nopathy with dysproteinemia, is one of the more common T-cell lymphomas, accounting for 15–20% of cases and 4–6% of all lymphomas. Mean age of presentation is 57 to 65 years, with a slight male pre-dominance, and the majority of patients present with stage III or IV disease. AITL is commonly a systemic disease with nodal involvement, with various asso-ciated disease features such as organomegaly, B symptoms (50–70%), skin rash, pruritis, pleural effu-sions, arthritis, eosinophilia and varied immunologic abnormalities (positive Coombs' test, cold agglutins, hemolytic anemia, antinuclear antibodies, rheuma-toid factors, cryoglobulins and polyclonal hyper-gammaglobulinemia).

Pathology

In established cases of AITL the lymph node is com-pletely effaced, but in early stages the neoplastic infiltrate is in the interfollicular area with residual lymphoid follicles which may be hyperplastic. In more advanced cases the follicles are atrophic and regressed. There is a polymorphous infiltrate of cells

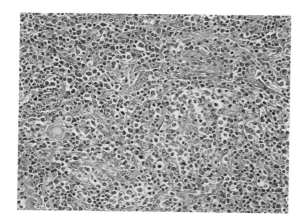

Figure 15.4. Angioimmunoblastic T-cell lymphoma. Many small vessels (high endothelial venules), histiocytes, scattered eosinophils and plasma cells are admixed with the tumor cells, which display clear cytoplasm. (From Rizvi *et al.* 2006. © American Society of Hematology.)

that include small, medium and large lymphoid cells, eosinophils, plasma cells and histiocytes (Fig. 15.4). A hallmark feature is the presence of abundant follicular dendritic cells (FDC). These are outside the confines of the germinal centers (whether reactive or atrophic) and form sheets around blood vessels in some of the more advanced cases. Where these sheets are pronounced, the clusters of FDCs can be seen on conventional (H&E) stained sections, but they may only be appreciated with immunocytochemical stains. In the background there is a pronounced vascular pattern with prominent high endothelial venules that show a markedly branched (arborising) pattern. The infiltrate frequently extends outside the lymph node across the capsule, but the peripheral sinus is usually preserved.

The neoplastic cells of AITL are mature T cells that do not express CD1a or TdT. They are positive for pan-T-cell antigens (CD2, CD3, CD5 and CD7) with rare antigen loss. The majority of cases express CD4 with no expression of CD8. A proportion of the neoplastic cells co-express CD10.

The background population contains a mixed population that includes many small CD8-positive T cells and plasma cells. The expanded proliferation of FDCs can be highlighted with antibodies against antigens expressed on these cells (CD21, CD23 and CD35). In most cases there is a residual small B-cell population that is usually compressed against the periphery of the node. Scattered large EBV-positive B cells are present in almost all cases.

Molecular pathology and cytogenetics

AITL represents an entity in which recurring chromosome abnormalities have been defined. TCR genes are rearranged in the majority of cases, but clonal rearrangements of IgH genes may be also detected in 20–30% of tumors. By *in-situ* hybridization, EBV early repeat (EBER) transcripts have been noted – in varying numbers of infected cells – in 60–95% of cases. Recurring chromosomal aberrations in AITL are trisomies 3 and 5 and, less frequently, an additional X chromosome. Some of these aberrations may be of prognostic importance.

Treatment

AITL typically follows an aggressive clinical course, although spontaneous regression occurs on rare occasions. Treatment with anthracycline-based combination chemotherapy results in CR rates of 50–70%, but only 10–30% of patients are long-term survivors. In one prospective, non-randomized multicenter study newly diagnosed "stable" AITL patients were treated with single-agent prednisone, and patients presenting with "life-threatening" disease or relapsed/refractory disease received combination chemotherapy. The CR rate was 29% with single-agent prednisone, while CR rates for relapsed/refractory patients and for patients treated initially with combination chemotherapy were 56% and 64%, respectively. With a median follow-up of 28 months, the OS and disease-free survival (DFS) were 40.5% and 32.3% respectively, although median OS was 15 months. There are anecdotal reports of relapsed AITL patients who have responded to immunosuppressive therapy, such as low-dose methotrexate/prednisone and cyclosporine, purine analogues and denileukin diftitox. Preliminary results from a study evaluating elderly AITL patients with CHOP plus rituximab were recently reported. Nine patients were treated, with eight achieving a CR after eight cycles of therapy. Two patients relapsed after 13 and 14 months, while one patient progressed after three cycles. All relapsed/refractory patients were salvaged with chemotherapy or alemtuzumab. All nine patients were alive, with eight of them having no evidence of disease, after a median follow-up of 12 months (7–53 months).

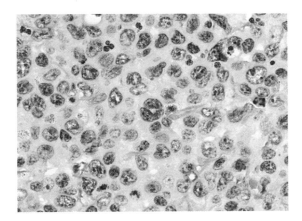

Figure 15.5. Anaplastic large-cell lymphoma. The infiltrate is composed of large transformed lymphocytes, including hallmark cells with kidney-shaped nuclei. (From Rizvi *et al*. 2006. © American Society of Hematology.)

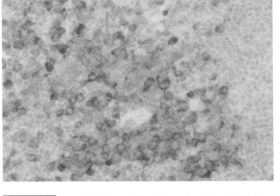

Figure 15.6. Anaplastic large cell lymphoma (lymph node). Staining for ALK1 gives a characteristic nuclear and cytoplasmic pattern associated with t(2;5).

Anaplastic large-cell lymphoma (ALCL), T/null-cell, primary systemic type

ALCL, primary systemic type, accounts for approximately 2–3% of all NHL. This disease mainly involves lymph nodes, although extranodal sites may be involved. ALCL may be divided in part based on the expression of the tyrosine kinase anaplastic lymphoma kinase (ALK). When heterogeneous patient populations are analyzed, the prevalence of ALK positivity in primary systemic ALCL cases is 50–60%. ALK-positive ALCL is typically diagnosed in men prior to age 35 (male-to-female ratio 3.0), with frequent systemic symptoms, extranodal disease and advanced-stage disease. ALK-negative patients are usually older (median age 61 years), with a male-to-female ratio of 0.9, and are less likely to present with extranodal disease.

Pathology

Although the mix of cells may be highly variable, all cases contain cells that have the characteristic appearance of abundant cytoplasm with large eccentric, horse-shoe or kidney-shaped nuclei, with a perinuclear area of eosinophilia in the cytoplasm (Fig. 15.5). Some cells show striking cytoplasmic nuclear pseudoinclusions (doughnut cells). The nuclei usually have clumped or dispersed chromatin with basophilic nucleoli. While infiltration of the lymph node may be diffuse in cases with partial infiltration of the node, the cells are frequently seen packing sinusoids mimicking metastatic tumor.

Several morphological variants have been described. A proportion of cases show mixed patterns and, in cases that relapse, the second lesion may be a different morphological variant from the first.

Common variant. This is the most frequent (70%). There are sheets of large cells as described above. A variant with sheets of more monotonous large cells, either as the sole finding or admixed with polymorphic areas, has also been described.

Lymphohistiocytic variant. In this variant (10%) the lymph node is effaced by a population of histiocytes with pale cytoplasm that may show erythrophagocytosis. There is usually an associated proliferation of small lymphocytes. The neoplastic cells may be scanty, and usually have a perivascular distribution. They may be larger than those of the common type and are best highlighted by staining for CD30.

Small-cell variant. In these cases (5–10%) the predominant cell is small to medium-sized and has irregular cerebriform nuclei. Large cells with a classical morphology are always present but may be scanty with a predominantly perivascular location.

Other morphological patterns. Several other morphological patterns of infiltration have been described, including lesions rich in giant cells and subtypes with sarcomatoid or signet-ring cells.

Immunophenotypically the neoplastic cells stain for CD30, with a membranous and perinuclear (golgi) pattern (Fig. 15.6). The small cells of the

Table 15.3. Characteristics of fusion proteins associated with ALK-positive ALCL.

Genetic aberration	Frequency	Fusion protein connected with TK domain of ALK 2p23	Size of fusion protein (kDa)	Staining pattern
t(2;5)(p23;q35)	73%	NPM	80	Cytoplasmic and nuclear
t(1;2)(q21;p23)	18%	TPM3	104	Cytoplasmic and nuclear
t(2;3)(p23;q21)	3%	TFG	97	Cytoplasmic
t(2;22)(p23;q11)	3%	CLTCL	250	Granular cytoplasmic
inv(2)(p23;q35)	3%	ATIC	96	Cytoplasmic

TK, tyrosine kinase; ALK, anaplastic lymphoma kinase; ALCL, anaplastic large-cell lymphoma; NPM, nucleophosmin gene; TPM3, non-muscle tropomyosin; TFG, tropomyosin receptor kinase-fused gene; CLTCL, clathrin heavy polypeptide-like gene; ATIC, 5-aminoimidazole-4-carboxamide ribonucleotide transformylase/inosine monophosphate cyclohydrolase. (From Rizvi *et al.* 2006. © American Society of Hematology.)

small-cell variant are frequently negative for CD30, but the scattered large cells express this antigen. The lymphoma cells characteristically show expression of one or more T-cell-related antigens, but loss of T-cell antigens may result in some cases showing an apparent "null" phenotype while showing T-cell lineage at the molecular level. Staining for CD3 is negative in up to 75%, and loss of CD5 and CD7 are also frequent. A higher proportion of cases are positive for CD2 and CD4, and CD43 is positive in about 75%. Staining for CD8 is usually negative. There is staining for cytotoxic granule-associated antigens (TIA-1, granzyme and perforin) in the majority of cases. Expression of CD45 is variable. Staining for EMA may be demonstrated in a proportion of cells in most cases. Expression of CD15 is very rare and if present is usually seen in only a small proportion of the neoplastic cells.

Staining for ALK is characteristic of this lymphoma, and is present in 60–85% of cases, mostly those occurring in children and young adults. The pattern of staining is variable and appears to be related to the underlying cytogenetic aberration, with the most common t(2;5) showing nuclear and cytoplasmic staining, while cytoplasmic staining alone is seen with t(1;2), t(2;3) and inv2. The t(2;17) is associated with granular cytoplasmic staining.

The determination of ALK positivity is important, as it denotes a significant favorable prognosis, with reported five-year overall survival rates of 79% versus 46% for ALK-negative ALCL cases. Moreover, the prognosis for ALK-positive and ALK-negative ALCL groups may be further divided based on CD56 positivity (neural cell-adhesion molecule), which portends a significantly worse outcome when it is expressed in either ALCL subgroup.

Molecular pathology and cytogenetics

Beginning in 1988, it was demonstrated that ALCL is associated with the chromosome translocation t(2;5). This non-random t(2;5) chromosome translocation has been cloned and is known to cause the fusion of the nucleophosmin (*NPM*) gene located at 5q35 to the gene at 2p23 encoding the receptor tyrosine kinase, ALK, resulting in the fusion protein NPM–ALK (Table 15.3). The transcription of the 80 kDa chimeric fusion protein NPM–ALK (also known as p80) results as a consequence of the *ALK* gene coming under the control of the NPM promoter. The presence of NPM–ALK may be detected by RT-PCR and FISH techniques. Polyclonal (ALK11) and monoclonal (ALK1 and ALKc) antibodies specific for the ALK portion of the molecule have been established that stain both the cytoplasm and nucleus in tissues containing the NPM–ALK translocation, which is documented in approximately 50–90% of primary systemic ALCL cases. When heterogeneous patient populations are analyzed, the prevalence of ALK positivity in primary systemic ALCL cases is 50–60%. Several series have documented that up to 30% of ALK-positive ALCL cases are found to be negative for the t(2;5) translocation, suggesting that other fusion proteins and chromosome translocations are involved with the 2q23 *ALK* gene other than NPM. Other fusion partners to the *ALK* gene include non-muscle tropomyosin (TPM3) forming t(1;2)(q21;23) and creating the chimeric protein TPM3–ALK, tropomyosin receptor kinase-fused gene (*TFG*) forming t(2;3)(p23;q21) and resulting in the TFG–ALK protein, clathrin heavy polypeptide-like gene (*CLTCL*) forming t(2;22) and resulting in the CLTCL–ALK protein, and 5-aminoimidazole-4-carboxamide-1-beta-D-ribonucleotide-transformylase/inosine-mono-phosphate-cyclohydrolase enzymatic activities (ATIC) caused by the inversion 2(p23;q35) and resulting in ATIC–ALK (Table 15.3). ALK-positive diffuse large B-cell lymphoma has been recently reported and is characterized by t(2;17)(p23;q23), which involves the *CLTC* gene at chromosome band 17q23 and the *ALK* gene at chromosome band 2p23.

The expression of the *ALK* gene is not confined to ALCL, thus decreasing the positive predictive value of this testing. Other disease entities that rarely express the *ALK* gene include neuroblastoma, rhabdomyo-sarcoma and inflammatory myofibroblastic tumors. There are also reports of the detection of *ALK* genes in non-neoplastic and "normal" peripheral blood cells. These data confirm that indiscriminate molecular testing should be avoided, but rather should be a complement to a detailed clinical and histologic work-up.

Other mechanisms of oncogenesis in ALCL include increased bcl-2, hypermethylation and *C-MYC* expression. Furthermore, the NPM–ALK fusion protein constitutively activates the phosphatidylinositol 3-kinase (PI3K)/Akt pathway, suggesting that this pathway may be involved in the molecular pathogenesis of ALCL.

Treatment

Therapy for pediatric ALCL is often based on prognostic risk factors, with treatment regimens modeled after high-grade B-cell NHL protocols. Following a brief cytoreductive pre-phase, short, intensified poly-agent chemotherapy is administered, with the number of cycles dependent on the stage of disease. Therapy for adult ALCL, systemic type, has commonly included anthracycline-based regimens. The response to therapy depends on ALK expression and prognostic factors such as the IPI score. Patients with IPI scores of 0 or 1 have survival rates above 90% while patients with unfavorable factors have

survival rates of 41%. The five-year OS for ALK-positive patients was 79% as compared to 46% for patients who were ALK-negative. Autologous stem-cell transplantation (ASCT) in first complete remission has been advocated by some groups, although this approach warrants prospective validation (see below). SGN-30, a chimeric monoclonal antibody directed against the CD30 antigen, is currently being evaluated in a phase II trial in patients with refractory or recurrent CD30-positive ALCL. Patients were heavily pre-treated with a median of three prior therapies (range 2–5). Eighteen of 20 patients were ALK-negative. One patient had a CR and remained in remission more than a year after therapy. Three patients had a partial response and three patients had stable disease while on treatment. The drug was well tolerated, with two possibly related grade 3/4 toxicities and only one definitely related grade 3/4 event.

Hepatosplenic T-cell lymphoma (HSTCL)

HSTCL is an uncommon T-cell lymphoma that is seen mainly in young males (median age 35). Patients present with B symptoms, prominent hepatosplenomegaly, anemia, neutropenia, thrombocytopenia (commonly severe), peripheral blood lymphocytosis and lymphadenopathy. It is often associated with an aggressive clinical course (median survival 16 months).

Pathology

HSTCL infiltrates the sinuses of the liver, bone marrow (two-thirds of patients) and splenic red pulp. HSTCL tumor cells are usually homogeneous, medium-sized lymphoid cells with round nuclei, moderately condensed chromatin and a pale cytoplasm. Erythrophagocytosis may be present in the spleen and bone marrow and circulating peripheral-blood tumor cells are seen in approximately 25–50% of patients (Fig. 15.7). TIA-1 is present in almost all cases, but commonly granzyme B and perforin are not present, indicating a non-activated cytotoxic T-cell phenotype. The tumor cells are usually CD4-, CD5- and CD8-negative, and CD3-, CD7- and CD56-positive.

Molecular pathology and cytogenetics

As with the other T-cell lymphomas already discussed, detection of clonal TCR gene rearrangements may prove essential in establishing a diagnosis of HSTCL, especially with complex histologic cases.

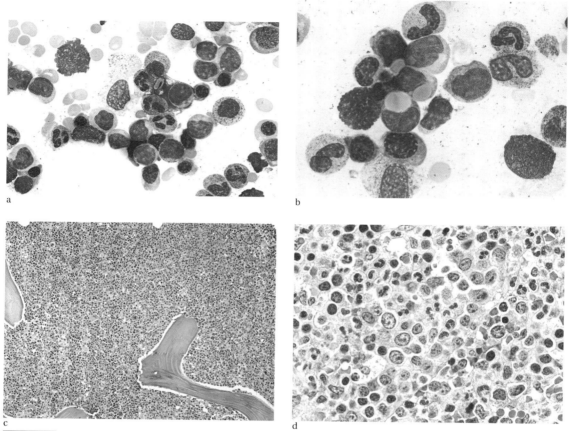

Figure 15.7. Hepatosplenic T-cell lymphoma involving the bone marrow. (a) The tumor cells in the bone marrow aspirate resemble blasts. They are medium-sized with dispersed chromatin and scant cytoplasm. (b) Two lymphoma cells display erythrophagocytosis. (c) Hypercellular bone marrow with almost all the normal hematopoietic cells replaced by lymphoma cells growing in sheets. (d) Lymphoma cells located within the lumen of a sinus. (From Rizvi *et al.* 2006. © American Society of Hematology.)

HSTCL likely arises from γδ T cells of the hepatic sinusoids and splenic red pulp, and most cases of HSTCL are demonstrated to have clonal TCR γ-gene or δ-gene rearrangements with a cytotoxic T-cell phenotype. Moreover, the Vγ1 or Vδ1 genes are preferentially expressed in this disease, reflecting in part the normal localization of γδ T lymphocytes that reside in the spleen, intestinal tissue and thymus. An αβ T-cell phenotype has been described with HSTCL. These infrequent αβ HSTCL cases interestingly occurred more commonly in women, but otherwise were characterized by clinicopathologic and cytogenetic features similar to γδ HSTCL. The primary recurrent chromosome abnormality in HSTCL demonstrated in many cases is isochromosome i(7q), although not

all series have documented i(7q) abnormalities in HSTCL. Furthermore, i(7q) is not specific for HSTCL, as this karyotype has been reported in acute leukemia, prolymphocytic leukemia and Wilms' tumor. Trisomy 8 has been frequently observed in HSTCL. Other chromosome aberrations less frequently detected in HSTCL include del(11q), t(1;14)(q21;q13), der(21)t(7;21) and complex karyotype.

Abnormal expression of *p21*, *p53* or other oncogenic gene pathways have not been identified in HSTCL. Reports of associated EBV have been conflicting, but some reports have documented strong EBER-1 expression in cases of HSTCL. A significant minority of HSTCL is recognized in post-transplant patients. Again, conflicting results regarding EBV positivity in

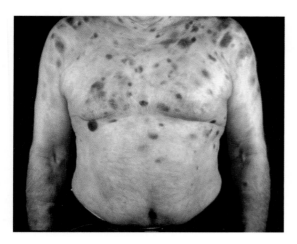

Figure 15.8. NK-cell lymphoma.

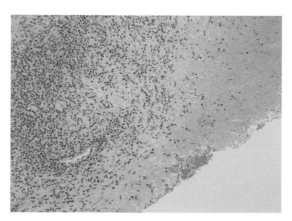

Figure 15.9. Extranodal NK-cell lymphoma, nasal type (nose). The surface mucosa is ulcerated and there is a sheet-like infiltrate of small to intermediate-sized cells focally surrounding small vessels.

this post-transplant T-cell lymphoma population have been reported, but the majority of cases have not had documented associated EBV or other viruses.

Treatment

The clinical course of HSTCL is commonly aggressive despite multi-agent chemotherapy. Anecdotal reports have described activity with the purine analogue pentostatin in relapsed patients. In a recent case report, a patient with αβ HSTCL was treated with alemtuzumab and subsequently went on to an unmatched, unrelated stem-cell transplant. The patient was alive with no evidence of disease after almost 21 months of follow-up.

Extranodal NK/T-cell lymphoma, nasal and nasal-type

Extranodal NK/T-cell lymphoma, nasal and nasal-type, formerly known as angiocentric lymphoma, is rare in Western countries and is more prevalent in Asia and South and Central America. The disease commonly presents in men at the median age of 43. It is associated with EBV and is typically characterized by extranodal presentation and localized stage I/II disease, but with angiodestructive proliferation and an aggressive clinical course. These tumors have a predilection for the nasal cavity and paranasal sinuses ("nasal"), although the "nasal type" designation encompasses other extranodal sites of NK/T-cell lymphomatous disease (skin, gastrointestinal, testis, kidney, upper respiratory tract and rarely orbit/eye) (Fig. 15.8).

Pathology

When there is surface mucosa there is usually extensive ulceration. In solid organs such as the testis there is necrosis. The lymphoma cells show a striking angiocentric, angioinvasive and angiodestructive pattern of infiltration. Cellular morphology is highly variable, with some cases showing monotonous small cells while other tumors are composed of cells that are medium, large or anaplastic. The cytoplasm is usually pale or clear and the nuclear chromatin is granular. Nucleoli are inconspicuous (Fig. 15.9).

In many cases there is an associated mixed inflammatory cell infiltrate which may mask the neoplastic population. In the nose/nasal cavity there may be striking hyperplasia of the surface squamous epithelium (pseudoepitheliomatous hyperplasia) mimicking well-differentiated squamous cell carcinoma.

Immunophenotypically the cells are positive for CD2 and CD56 (Fig. 15.10). There is cytoplasmic staining for CD3ε but no surface staining for CD3. There is expression of antigens associated with cytotoxic granules (TIA-1, granzyme and perforin). Occasional cases are positive for CD7, and CD30 can sometimes be seen. There is no staining for CD5, CD4, CD8, CD43 or CD45RO. Staining for CD16 and CD57 is also negative. The vast majority of cases show evidence of EBV infection. Cases negative for CD56 are only diagnosed if there is evidence of EBV infection together with presence of cytotoxic granules (Fig. 15.11).

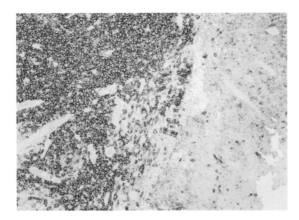

Figure 15.10. Extranodal NK-cell lymphoma, nasal type (nose). The neoplastic cells express CD56.

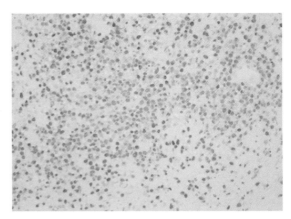

Figure 15.11. Extranodal NK-cell lymphoma, nasal type (nose). The neoplastic cells show evidence of infection by Epstein–Barr virus (*in-situ* hybridization for EBER).

Molecular pathology and cytogenetics

Most molecular studies of this disease have included small patient numbers, but many studies have been reported. The rearrangement of TCR genes has been inconsistently identified, being described anywhere from 0% to 60% in various studies. When present, γδ rearrangements are more common, while Ig rearrangements are germline. Studies have suggested that separation into distinct NK-cell and T-cell categories is feasible based on lineage-specific TCR rearrangements and immunophenotype. Cytogenetic abnormalities are common in extranodal NK/T-cell lymphoma, nasal type. Most reports have identified deletions of chromosome 6 (q21~25) to be the most frequent recurrent cytogenetic abnormality. Siu and colleagues demonstrated consistent patterns of allelic abnormalities, with loss of heterozygosity (LOH) at chromosome 6q in 91% of nasal lymphoma cases versus 50% of non-nasal NK lymphoma cases. Furthermore, they observed LOH at 13q in 33% of cases at presentation of disease, but in 100% of cases at relapse. A recent study by Ko and colleagues documented frequent losses at 1p, 17p and 12q, and gains at 2q, 13q and 10q, with infrequent chromosome 6q aberration. Other reported non-random chromosome abnormalities include isochromes 6p, 1q, 17q and 7q, 11q aberrations, $+$X and $+$8.

Identification of oncogenes related to extranodal NK/T-cell lymphoma has been difficult, in part because of insufficient recovery of viable, non-necrotic tissue for appropriate analyses. p53 has been shown to be overexpressed in many cases of extranodal NK/T-cell lymphomas, nasal type. However, p53 mutations are much more infrequently identified. Mutations of *k-ras* have been described in this lymphoma. Overexpression of p21 and p16 have been documented in NK/T-cell lymphoma, but the patterns of expression have been variable. It is not clear whether p21 overexpression is directly involved in the pathogenic process. EBV may play a role in the oncogenesis of extranodal NK/T-cell lymphoma, nasal type. EBER-1 RNA transcripts are detectable in the majority of cells in nearly all cases. Moreover, EBV-latent membrane protein (LMP-1) is expressed in most cases.

Treatment

Combined modality therapy incorporating doxorubicin-based chemotherapy (minimum six cycles for patients with stage III or IV disease), involved-field (IF) radiation (median dose 50 Gy, range 30–67 Gy) and intrathecal prophylaxis is recommended for extranodal NK/T-cell lymphoma (nasal) patients, although the benefit of the addition of chemotherapy to radiation has not been confirmed for limited-stage disease. Response rates for NK/T-cell lymphoma, nasal, have been reported to be near 85% (two-thirds CR) following radiation alone, although 50% of patients will experience local relapse and 25% systemic relapse with a predilection to extranodal sites such as testis, orbit, skin, gastrointestinal tract and central nervous system. In a recent report 77 patients with NK/T-cell sinonasal lymphoma (56 locoregional,

21 systemic disease) had a five-year OS rate of 36% (median follow-up 89 months).

The five-year DFS for patients with stage I/II disease is approximately 34–38% and the OS is between 57% and 65%, although systemic disease progression is often fatal. In patients with NK/T-cell sinonasal locoregional disease, a Taiwanese study found that combined chemotherapy/radiation or radiation alone resulted in better survival than chemotherapy alone (five-year survival rates 59%, 50% and 15%, respectively, $p < 0.01$). In addition, researchers from China retrospectively compared stage I_E patients who received IF radiation alone versus combined chemotherapy with radiotherapy. Of note, this group divided I_E patients into limited (confined to nasal cavity) and extensive (presenting with extension beyond the nasal cavity) stage I_E disease. Limited-stage I_E patients survived longer than extensive I_E patients overall (five-year OS 90% vs. 57%, $p < 0.001$). Moreover, comparing radiation alone with combined modality therapy, the five-year OS was not significantly different either for limited-stage I_E (89% and 92%, respectively) or for extensive I_E disease (54% and 58%). Korean researchers recently reported that patients with upper aerodigestive-tract involvement generally had better treatment outcomes than those with nasal involvement. Patients with systemic disease have poor long-term survival (five-year overall survival 20–25%), with high locoregional (> 50%) and systemic failure rates (> 70%). The traditional approach for stage III and IV extranodal NK/T-cell lymphoma (nasal) is combined modality therapy with doxorubicin-based chemotherapy and radiation therapy.

Enteropathy-type intestinal T-cell lymphoma (EITCL)

EITCL (also known as intestinal T-cell lymphoma) is a rare T-cell lymphoma of intra-epithelial lymphocytes that commonly presents with multiple circumferential jejunal ulcers in adults. Patients usually have a prior brief history of gluten-sensitive enteropathy. EITCL accounts for less than 1% of NHLs and has been recognized to have a poor prognosis, with reported five-year overall survival and disease-free survival rates of 20% and 3% respectively. This is in part related to many patients presenting with poor performance status.

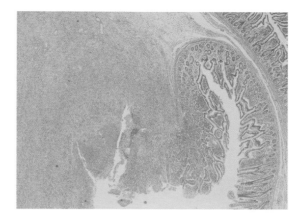

Figure 15.12. Enteropathy-type T-cell lymphoma (small intestine). An ulcerated tumor mass is present. The adjacent mucosa shows features of enteropathy including shortening of villous height.

EITCL may present without antecedent celiac disease history, but most patients have abdominal pain and weight loss. Evidence of serologic markers for celiac disease, such as positive anti-gliadin antibodies and/or HLA types (DQA1*0501/DQB1*0201/DRB1*0304) may be present at diagnosis. Moreover, these genotypes may represent patients with celiac disease at higher risk for development of EITCL. Small-bowel perforation or obstruction, gastrointestinal bleeding and enterocolic fistulae are recognized complications of this disease.

Pathology

Most commonly these tumors consist of a population of medium-to-large cells with little pleomorphism. In some cases there is more pleomorphism, and in some the cells have an anaplastic appearance. In a small number of cases the cells are monotonous and smaller with hyperchromatic nuclei and a thin rim of cytoplasm (Fig. 15.12). The tumor infiltrates the mucosa and usually extends through the entire bowel wall. Mucosal ulceration is very frequent and there may be mural perforation. The neoplastic cells may show infiltration of the epithelium (epitheliotropism). In early cases the neoplastic cells may be very scanty within an area of ulceration, with associated granulation tissue and inflammatory infiltrate (ulcerative jejunitis). There is frequently an eosinophil-rich infiltrate associated with the tumor (Fig. 15.13).

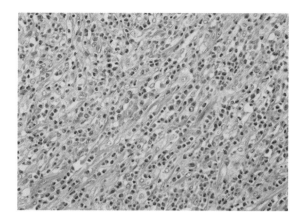

Figure 15.13. Enteropathy-type T-cell lymphoma (small intestine). The lymphoma is composed of a population of large cells with pleomorphic nuclei. In this case eosinophils are prominent.

The adjacent mucosa frequently shows morphological features of enteropathy with villous atrophy and increased numbers of intra-epithelial lymphocytes. In some cases the villous atrophy is lacking but the intra-epithelial lymphocytosis is retained.

Immunophenotypically the cells express the phenotype of mature T cells, with expression of CD3 and CD7. There is usually loss of CD5, and the tumor cells frequently lack both CD4 and CD8. The neoplastic cells characteristically express CD103, but antibodies against this antigen are at present not reactive in fixed, embedded material. CD30 may be expressed in some cases. Those cases with a small-cell morphology are often positive for CD56. In the majority of cases the cells contain cytotoxic granules.

The intra-epithelial T cells in the adjacent mucosa frequently show a similar phenotype to the neoplastic cells, with lack of CD4 and CD8.

Molecular pathology and cytogenetics

The TCR genes are rearranged in nearly all cases of EITCL (more commonly γ than β). Moreover, TCR gene rearrangements are often present in patients with EITCL who have evolved from celiac disease. In a recent study eight patients with overt EITCL were compared with 13 patients with celiac disease caused by a defined disorder, three patients with refractory celiac disease evolving into overt EITCL and two patients with ulcerative jejunitis. Clonal TCR-γ gene rearrangement was demonstrated with PCR in all resected jejunal specimens of the EITCL patients.

Furthermore, four of eight duodenal biopsy specimens from overt EITCL patients demonstrated positive clonality, compared to two of three with refractory celiac disease evolving into overt EITCL, two of two with ulcerative jejunitis (a disease associated with increased risk for development of EITCL), one of six with refractory celiac disease, and no patients with celiac disease caused by a defined disorder.

Chromosomal aberrations have rarely been reported with EITCL, though loss of heterozygosity at chromosome 9p21 is associated with the disease. One report documented that 22 of 23 EITCL tumors stained for p53, and 9 of 19 cases studied had collections of small lymphocytes in the affected bowel expressing p53. The role of p53 in the oncogenesis of EITCL is not known. Varied reports have documented EBV positivity (by PCR and FISH with EBER-1 analysis) in association with EITCL, including cases of EBV-related EITCL PTLD, suggesting a possible etiologic role of EBV in the pathogenesis of EITCL. Furthermore, analysis comparing the prevalence of EBV in Mexican and European patients with EITCL demonstrated that there are significant epidemiologic differences in EBV association (100% vs. 10%, respectively).

Treatment

Following diagnosis of EITCL, doxorubicin-based combination chemotherapy should be considered for each patient. Treatment is often complicated by the underlying malnutrition. Aggressive nutritional support with parenteral or enteral feeding is critical in the care of these patients. The majority of patients do not complete their planned chemotherapy courses due to complications such as perforation, gastrointestinal bleeding and fistula formation. It is imperative for patients with known celiac disease to adhere to a gluten-free diet.

STEM-CELL TRANSPLANTATION

The exact role of autologous or allogeneic stem-cell transplantation (SCT) in T-cell NHL has not been defined. Several case series have reported the outcome of patients with relapsed T-cell NHL following autologous, allogeneic and reduced-intensity SCT. PTCL-u and ALCL were the predominant subtypes in trials, and the three-year OS rates ranged from

36% to 58% following ASCT (median follow-up 36–43 months). High IPI (≥ 2) significantly predicted a worse outcome in one of these described trials, but not in another. Furthermore, ALCL (versus non-ALCL) predicted an improved outcome in the largest trial (three-year OS 79% vs. 44%, $p = 0.08$). Amongst ALCL patients, those who are ALK-positive have a better three-year overall survival than ALK-negative patients (100% vs. 75%), and the difference in EFS is much more pronounced (100% vs. 1%). Another study looked at ALK-negative ALCL patients only and found the OS to be 72 weeks.

Relapsed/refractory T-cell NHL patients were compared to diffuse large B-cell lymphoma (DLBCL) patients in the post-ASCT setting over a 12-year period. Thirty-six T-cell NHL patients with relapsed or primary refractory disease were compared to 97 patients with relapsed DLBCL. With a median follow-up of 42 months, T-cell NHL patients had a three-year OS rate of 48% compared to 53% for DLBCL patients. This study documented no significant outcome differences according to T-cell subtype, although PTCL-u patients had a trend for inferior three-year disease-free survival. There is some evidence that patients with T-cell NHL who do not achieve a CR after initial chemotherapy may experience long-term survival when salvaged with ASCT.

Stem-cell transplantation in first remission remains controversial. French and Italian investigators have documented long-term survival rates of approximately 90% for ALCL patients who received an ASCT in first CR. These results are encouraging, but patients with systemic ALCL (especially ALK-positive) have the best prognosis among those with T-cell NHL subtypes. The results of using ASCT as second-line therapy in relapsed/refractory mature T-cell or NK NHL were less encouraging. The cohort in this study included patients with PTCL-u ($n = 15$), ALCL ($n = 11$), AITL ($n = 5$), NK/T-cell lymphoma ($n = 4$), SPLTCL ($n = 2$) and one each with $\gamma\delta$ HSTCL and EITCL. The investigators concluded that only a few patients received a durable benefit from this approach. Prospective, randomized trials need to be performed to confirm these observations, especially in patients at higher risk. Small case series and anecdotal reports have described the feasibility and long-term survival for matched-sibling and unrelated allogeneic SCT for patients with chemotherapy-resistant T-cell NHL and patients with hemophagocytic syndrome.

RADIATION THERAPY

Due to the paucity of clinical trials, the integration of radiation therapy into the treatment plan of most T-cell NHL patients often models that of patients with B-cell NHL. Compared to DLBCL, those with T-cell NHL more commonly present with stage III/IV disease (48% and 74%, respectively) and T-cell patients frequently present with combined nodal and extra-nodal disease at diagnosis (especially PTCL-u, ALCL and AITL), thereby often obviating the need for the addition of radiation. Studies specifically addressing the benefits of radiation therapy to bulky sites for patients with advanced T-cell NHL have not been carried out.

EMERGING THERAPIES

Relevant proto-oncogenes and tumor suppressor genes involved in the pathogenesis of T-cell NHL represent potential candidates for molecular-based therapy. Gene therapy using adenoviral vector-mediated wild-type p53 gene transfer is being evaluated and may have application in certain T-cell lymphomas. In addition to denileukin diftitox, several other recombinant chimeric immunotoxins have been successfully produced, such as the anti-CD30 antibody combined with a mutant *Pseudomonas* exotoxin. A monoclonal antibody directed against CD2, CD4 and the human transferrin receptor (TfR) in HTLV-1-infected cells (mAb A24) is being evaluated. Protein kinase C modulating agents UCN-01 and bryostatin, pralatrexate, a novel antifolate, and nelarabine (506U78) are also being studied. Furthermore, histone deacetylase (HDAC) inhibitors (such as depsipeptide and SAHA) increase histone acetylation leading to cellular differentiation, decreased cell proliferation and induction of cell death, and are being examined in patients with T-cell NHL. The role of viral pathogenesis in T-cell NHL tumor development continues to be studied as a potential target of drug therapy.

Continuing research is needed, both to allow more accurate prediction of the course of the disease and to further elucidate the molecular oncogenesis of T-cell NHL. Prospective, multi-institution clinical trials remain critically important in order to determine the most effective treatment regimens that will continue to improve cure rates in these aggressive yet treatable, and often curable, diseases.

FURTHER READING

A clinical evaluation of the International Lymphoma Study Group classification of non-Hodgkin's lymphoma. The Non-Hodgkin's Lymphoma Classification Project. *Blood* **89** (1997), 3909–3918.

Ansell, S. M., Habermann, T. M., Kurtin, P. J. *et al*. Predictive capacity of the International Prognostic Factor Index in patients with peripheral T-cell lymphoma. *J. Clin. Oncol.* **15** (1997), 2296–2301.

Attygalle, A., Al-Jehani, R., Diss, T. C. *et al*. Neoplastic T cells in angioimmunoblastic T-cell lymphoma express CD10. *Blood* **99** (2002), 627–633.

Belhadj, K., Reyes, F., Farcet, J. P. *et al*. Hepatosplenic gammadelta T-cell lymphoma is a rare clinicopathologic entity with poor outcome: report on a series of 21 patients. *Blood* **102** (2003), 4261–4269.

Benharroch, D., Meguerian-bedoyan, Z., Lamant, L. *et al*. ALK-positive lymphoma: a single disease with a broad spectrum of morphology. *Blood* **91** (1998), 2076–2084.

Drexler, H. G., MacLeod, R. A., Borkhardt, A. and Janssen, J. W. Recurrent chromosomal translocations and fusion genes in leukemia–lymphoma cell lines. *Leukemia* **9** (1995), 480–500.

Falini, B., Pileri, S., Zinzani, P. L. *et al*. ALK+ lymphoma: clinico-pathological findings and outcome. *Blood* **93** (1999), 2697–2706.

Gallamini, A., Stelitano, C., Calvi, R. *et al*. Peripheral T-cell lymphoma unspecified (PTCL-U): a new prognostic model from a retrospective multicentric clinical study. *Blood* **103** (2004), 2474–2479.

Gascoyne, R. D., Aoun, P., Wu, D. *et al*. Prognostic significance of anaplastic lymphoma kinase (ALK) protein expression in adults with anaplastic large cell lymphoma. *Blood* **93** (1999), 3913–3921.

Gisselbrecht, C., Gaulard, P., Lepage, E. *et al*. Prognostic significance of T-cell phenotype in aggressive non-Hodgkin's lymphomas. Groupe d'Etudes des Lymphomes de l'Adulte (GELA). *Blood* **92** (1998), 76–82.

Harris, N. L., Jaffe, E. S., Diebold, J. *et al*. The World Health Organization classification of neoplastic diseases of the hemato-poietic and lymphoid tissues. Report of the Clinical Advisory Committee meeting, Airlie House, Virginia, November, 1997. *Ann. Oncol.* **10** (1999), 1419–1432.

Kanavaros, P., Lescs, M. C., Briere, J. *et al*. Nasal T-cell lymphoma: a clinicopathologic entity associated with peculiar phenotype and with Epstein–Barr virus. *Blood* **81** (1993), 2688–2695.

McArthur, H. L., Chhanabhai, M., Randy, G. D. *et al*. Evaluation of a New Prognostic Index for peripheral T-Cell lymphoma, unspecified (PTCL-US). *Blood* **106** (2005), 2812a.

Matutes, E., Brito-Babapulle, V., Swansbury, J. *et al*. Clinical and laboratory features of 78 cases of T-prolymphocytic leukemia. *Blood* **78** (1991), 3269–3274.

Melnyk, A., Rodriguez, A., Pugh, W. C. and Cabannillas, F. Evaluation of the Revised European–American Lymphoma classification confirms the clinical relevance of immunophenotype in 560 cases of aggressive non-Hodgkin's lymphoma. *Blood* **89** (1997), 4514–4520.

Morice, W. G., Kurtin, P. J., Tefferi, A. and Hanson, C. A. Distinct bone marrow findings in T-cell granular lymphocyte leukaemia revealed by paraffin section immunoperoxidase stains for CD8, TIA-1 and granzyme B. *Blood* **99** (2002), 268–274.

Osuji, N., Matutes, E., Catovsky, D., Lampert, I. A. and Wotherspoon, A. Histopathology of the spleen in T-cell large granular lymphocyte leukemia and T-cell prolymphocytic leukemia: a comparative review. *Am. J. Surg. Pathol.* **29** (2005), 935–941.

Pellatt, J., Sweetenham, J., Pickering, R. M., Brown, L. and Wilkins, B. A single-centre study of treatment outcomes and survival in 120 patients with peripheral T-cell non-Hodgkin's lymphoma. *Ann. Hematol.* **81** (2002), 267–272.

Rizvi, M. A., Evens, A. M., Tallman, M. S., Nelson, B. P. and Rosen, S. T. T-cell non-Hodgkin's lymphoma. *Blood* **107** (2006), 1255–1264.

Rudiger, T., Weisenburger, D. D., Anderson, J. R. *et al*. Peripheral T-cell lymphoma (excluding anaplastic large-cell lymphoma): results from the Non-Hodgkin's Lymphoma Classification Project. *Ann. Oncol.* **13** (2002), 140–149.

Salhany, K. E., Macon, W. R., Choi, J. K. *et al*. Subcutaneous panniculitis-like T-cell lymphoma: clinicopathologic, immunophenotypic, and genotypic analysis of alpha/beta and gamma/delta subtypes. *Am. J. Surg. Pathol.* **22** (1998), 881–893.

Savage, K. J., Chhanabhai, M., Voss, N. *et al*. Survival of limited stage peripheral T-cell lymphoma is similar to diffuse large B-cell lymphoma. *Blood* **106** (2005), 2817a.

16 CUTANEOUS LYMPHOMA

Julia Scarisbrick and Sean Whittaker

Pathology: Andrew Wotherspoon
Molecular cytogenetics: Andreas Rosenwald and German Ott

INTRODUCTION

The skin is the second most frequent extranodal site, after the gastrointestinal tract, for lymphoma. Cutaneous lymphomas have an annual incidence of 0.5–1.0 per 100 000, although recent Scandinavian studies have suggested an incidence of 4 per 100 000, possibly due to improved diagnosis and registration.

Primary cutaneous T-cell lymphoma (CTCL) comprises a heterogeneous group of non-Hodgkin's lymphomas, of which mycosis fungoides (MF) is the most common clinicopathologic subtype. Mycosis fungoides typically has an indolent course, but disease progression may occur in approximately 25% of patients. Sézary syndrome (SS), a leukemic form of CTCL, is very closely related to MF and has a poor prognosis, with a median survival of less than three years.

Primary cutaneous B-cell lymphomas (CBCL) are less common, comprising approximately 20% of all primary cutaneous lymphomas. They typically present with cutaneous papules, plaques or nodules and can be broadly divided into follicle center cell lymphoma, marginal zone lymphoma and large B-cell lymphoma.

The recent publication of the WHO EORTC classification system (Table 16.1) has clarified the classification of primary cutaneous lymphomas. The distinction of rare CTCL variants from MF/SS is critical, as the prognosis is poorer and treatment options are different.

PRIMARY CUTANEOUS T-CELL LYMPHOMAS (CTCL)

Mycosis fungoides

Mycosis fungoides (MF) is the commonest variant of primary CTCL, and it is generally associated with an indolent clinical course. The disease is characterized by cutaneous polymorphic atrophic erythematous patches and scaly plaques. Some patients progress from having limited patches and plaques to extensive thick plaques or tumors, and even erythroderma, and a minority will present with advanced disease. However, many patients do not develop disease progression.

Staging is based on cutaneous surface area involved and type of skin lesion: patches and plaques involving less than 10% of the body surface area (stage T1/IA; Fig. 16.1), more than 10% (stage T2/IB; Fig. 16.2), tumors (stage T3/IIB; Fig. 16.3) and erythrodermic disease (stage T4/III) (Fig 2). The prognosis of those with stage IA and 1B disease is excellent, with five-year survival rates of 100% and 96% respectively. The presence of cutaneous tumors is associated with a worse prognosis (five-year survival rates of 80%) (Table 16.2).

Histologic involvement of lymph nodes is a poor prognostic sign (stage IVA five-year survival 40%, median survival 13 months). Any systemic organ can be involved, and visceral disease is associated with rapid deterioration (stage IVB five-year survival 0%, median survival 13 months).

All patients with MF should have a full clinical examination and adequate diagnostic biopsies for histology, immunophenotypic and molecular studies, as patients with stage IA disease and a detectable T-cell clone have a poorer response to treatment.

Peripheral blood samples should be taken for routine hematology, biochemistry, serum LDH, Sézary cells, lymphocyte subsets, CD4:CD8 ratio, HTLV-I serology and TCR gene analysis. Any palpable bulky peripheral nodes should be biopsied. Staging CT scans of the chest, abdomen and pelvis are indicated

Lymphoma: Pathology, Diagnosis and Treatment, ed. Robert Marcus, John W. Sweetenham and Michael E. Williams. Published by Cambridge University Press. © Cambridge University Press 2007.

Table 16.1. WHO EORTC classification of cutaneous lymphomas with primary cutaneous manifestations.

Cutaneous T-cell and NK-cell lymphomas

Mycosis fungoides

MF variants and subtypes

   Folliculotropic MF

   Pagetoid reticulosis

   Granulomatous slack skin

Sézary syndrome

Adult T-cell leukemia/lymphoma

Primary cutaneous CD30+ lymphoproliferative disorders

   Primary cutaneous anaplastic large-cell lymphoma

   Lymphomatoid papulosis

Subcutaneous panniculitis-like T-cell lymphoma

Extranodal NK/T-cell lymphoma, nasal type

Primary cutaneous peripheral T-cell lymphoma, unspecified

Primary cutaneous aggressive epidermotropic CD8+
   T-cell lymphoma (provisional)

Cutaneous γ/δ T-cell lymphoma (provisional)

Primary cutaneous CD4+ small/medium-sized
   pleomorphic T-cell lymphoma (provisional)

Cutaneous B-cell lymphomas

Primary cutaneous marginal zone B-cell lymphoma

Primary cutaneous follicle center-cell lymphoma

Primary cutaneous large B-cell lymphoma, leg type

Primary cutaneous large B-cell lymphoma, other
   intravascular large B-cell lymphoma

Precursor hematologic neoplasm

CD4+/CD56+ hematodermic neoplasm (blastic NK-cell
   lymphoma)

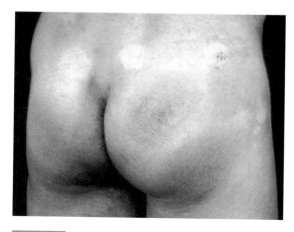

Figure 16.1. Mycosis fungoides, patch stage.

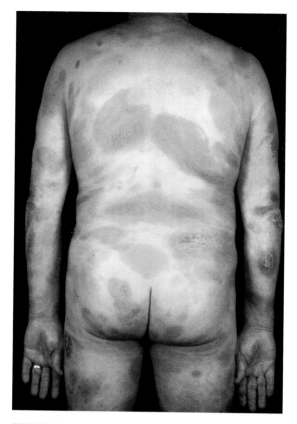

Figure 16.2. Mycosis fungoides, stage IB.

in all those patients with stage IIA–IV disease. Bone-marrow aspirate/trephine biopsies may be indicated in patients with stage IIB/III/IV MF and peripheral blood involvement, as indicated by Sézary cell counts representing >5% of the total leukocyte count, but they rarely yield useful clinical information.

Sézary syndrome

Sézary syndrome is defined by a clinical triad of erythroderma, peripheral lymphadenopathy and atypical mononuclear cells (Sézary cells) comprising 5% or more of peripheral blood leukocytes on a buffy coat smear (B1), or >20% of total lymphocyte count, or a total Sézary count of more than 1000×10^9/L (B2) (Figs. 16.4, 16.5). The presence of a peripheral-blood T-cell clone, as indicated by a CD4 : CD8 ratio > 10, by aberrant expression of pan-T-cell antigens, by cytogenetics or by TCR gene analysis, is now also required

Table 16.2. Prognosis in mycosis fungoides and Sézary syndrome according to disease stage.

Stage	IA	IB	IIA	IIB	III	IVA	IVB
Disease-specific 5-year survival (%)	100	96	68	80		40	0
Disease-specific 10-year survival (%)	98	83	68	42		20	0
Median survival	>32 yr	12.1–12.8 yr	10.0 yr	2.9 yr	3.6–4.6 yr	13 mo	13 mo
Overall disease progression	9%	20%	34%				
Free from relapse at 5 years	50%	36%	9%				
Free from relapse at 10 years		31%	3%				

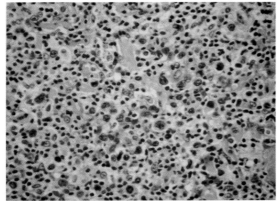

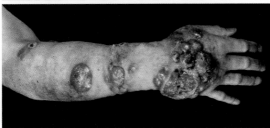

Figure 16.3. Mycosis fungoides, tumor stage.

to confirm a T-cell lymphoma/leukemia and distinguish from an inflammatory erythroderma.

Patients present with a generalized exfoliative erythroderma, ectropion, scalp alopecia, palmoplantar hyperkeratoses and nail dystrophy. Peripheral lymphadenopathy is often present. The distinction from erythrodermic MF (T4N0-4M0/stage III/IVA) is based on the degree of peripheral blood involvement

(>5 Sézary cells per 100 lymphocytes, T4N0-4M0 B1–2/stage III/IVA). The prognosis for patients with Sézary syndrome is poor, with a median survival of 35 months from diagnosis. The majority die of opportunistic infection. The prognosis is worse for those with histologic evidence of lymph-node involvement and a high blood tumor burden.

Pathology of mycosis fungoides and Sézary syndrome

In early stages MF is difficult to distinguish from dermatitis. Typical features such as the presence of intra-epidermal lymphocytes that are larger than normal lymphocytes with convoluted, cerebriform nuclei and a clear rim of cytoplasm (halo cells) or a linear pattern of infiltration along the dermo-epidermal junction are not specific. Pautrier microabscesses (clusters of atypical lymphoid cells in the epidermis) are found in only 10% of cases (Fig. 16.6). There is usually little spongiosis. Plasma cells and eosinophils are usually absent in early patch stages of MF.

In the more advanced thin-plaque stage the features are more established, with a dense infiltrate that includes cells with linear distribution in the basal layer of the epidermis and single-cell epidermotropism. The cells are often small with round or slightly irregular nuclei. In some cases halo cells predominate. There is a background of small lymphocytes, eosinophils, plasma cells and histiocytes (Fig. 16.7).

In the thick-plaque stage there is a dense band-like subepithelial infiltrate that includes a high number of

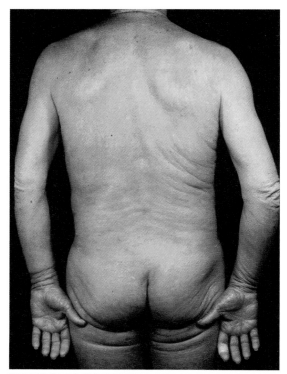

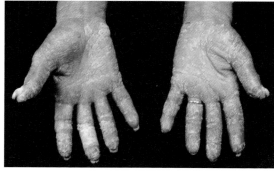

Figure 16.4. Sézary syndrome.

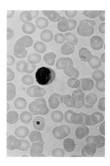 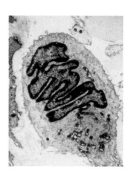

Figure 16.5. Sézary cell morphology.

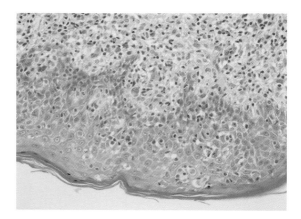

Figure 16.6. Mycosis fungoides (skin). A dense infiltrate of atypical lymphoid cells with convoluted nuclei focally extending into the epidermis.

atypical lymphoid cells with cerebriform nuclei. Small clusters of intra-epidermal lymphoid cells are frequent but Pautrier microabscesses are present in only 10%.

In tumor-stage lesions the infiltrate is more diffuse and epidermotropism may be absent. The cellular infiltrate is more polymorphic, with small, medium and large cells with cerebriform nuclei and occasional large transformed blastic cells that have prominent nucleoli.

In the folliculotropic subtype there is a dense infiltrate of small to medium-sized cells that infiltrate around and within the hair follicles with sparing of the intervening areas. The follicles show cystic dilation and plugging and there may be extracellular deposition of mucinous material.

In pagetoid reticulosis there is acanthotic epidermis that is infiltrated by halo cells either individually or in small clusters.

Granulomatous slack skin shows a band-like infiltrate in early stages but as the disease progresses there is infiltration of the dermis by small cells. In all cases there is an associated population of multinucleate giant histiocytic cells that often contain elastic fibres or lymphocytes within their cytoplasm.

In Sézary syndrome the features are similar to those of classical MF, with Pautrier microabscesses more frequently seen.

Lymph-node involvement by MF is characterized by dermatopathic-type changes in the early stages,

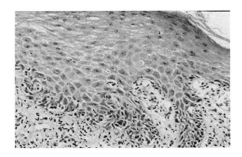

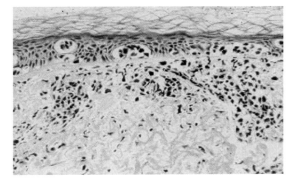

Figure 16.7. Mycosis fungoides pathology.

with atypical lymphocytes that are either scattered individually or present in small groups (category I involvement). With more advanced infiltration of the nodes there is partial involvement of the node by neoplastic cells, with a mainly paracortical distribution (category II) or massive, diffuse infiltration (category III).

The typical immunophenotype is that of a mature T cell, showing staining for CD2, CD3, CD5 and CD7. The cells are usually CD4-positive with lack of CD8, although an occasional CD8-positive case has been described. There is usually no staining for CD30. There is frequent loss of CD7, and as the disease progresses there may also be loss of CD2 and CD5, particularly in the intra-epidermal component. Expression of HECA antigen (associated with homing of lymphocytes to the skin) is present in the majority of cases. When transformation to a large-cell-predominant lesion occurs the cells often express CD30.

Molecular cytogenetics of mycosis fungoides and Sézary syndrome

Mycosis fungoides, the prototype of cutaneous T-cell lymphoma, initially presents in the skin and shows a characteristic stepwise clinical progression that probably reflects cumulative alterations of various genetic events involved in its pathogenesis. Monoclonal rearrangement of T-cell-receptor (TCR) gamma genes is a common finding in the tumor stage of MF, but is found in only half of early-stage cases. Molecular cytogenetic analysis has identified common genetic alterations in MF and Sézary syndrome, which represents the systemic form of the same disease. The most frequent chromosomal losses involve chromosomes 1p, 17p, 10/10q and 19, and chromosomal gains involve 4/4q, 18 and 17/17q. Numerical aberrations of chromosomes 6, 13, 15 and 17, and structural aberrations of chromosomes 3, 9 and 13, have been reported in MF, including early lesions. A pseudo-dicentric translocation (17;8)(p11.2;p11.2), identified by spectral karyotyping (SKY) analysis, may represent a recurrent structural aberration in these entities.

Recently, deletions or translocations affecting the human homologue of *unc-53*, the *NAV3* gene at chromosome 12q, were reported in MF and SS patients. The function of *NAV3* in human lymphoid cells is not known, but preliminary studies aiming at the silencing of *NAV3* with small interfering RNAs showed increased interleukin 2 (IL-2), but not CD25 expression, suggesting that *NAV3* may contribute to the growth, differentiation and apoptosis of the tumor cells as well as in skewing from a Th1 to Th2 phenotype during disease progression. In addition, one tumor sample was identified that harbored a *NAV3* deletion in one allele and a missense mutation of the other allele, supporting the hypothesis that *NAV3* may act as a classical tumor suppressor gene. Taken together, *NAV3* alterations were found in four of eight patients (50%) with early MF (stages IA–IIA) and 11 of 13 (85%) of patients with advanced MF and SS, suggesting that it may be the most frequent genetic lesion in cutaneous T-cell lymphoma. All patients with *NAV3* deletion or translocation suffered from frequent relapses or died from the disease.

In addition, the inactivation via deletions or promoter hypermethylation of several tumor suppressor genes including *SHP-1*, *p15*, *p16* and *hMLH1* has been reported. *SHP-1* is an important negative regulator involved in signaling through receptors for cytokines and growth factors, whose expression in often lost in MF and SS samples. Inactivation of p15 and p16 is reported in both early- and advanced-stage MF and SS by allelic loss or aberrant promoter methylation.

Recently, a genome-wide differential methylation hybridization analysis revealed a hypermethylated status of several additional putative tumor suppressor genes such as *BCL7a*, *PTPRG* and thrombospondin. Whether these events are causative or an epiphenomenon remains to be elucidated; nevertheless, these findings suggest the possible experimental use of demethylation agents in the therapy of these tumors.

Clonal rearrangement of TCR genes can be detected in most cases of granulomatous slack skin disease, which is referred to as a subtype of MF. Further molecular genetic data are not available because of the rarity of the disease; however, trisomy 8 was reported in two cases.

Characteristic cytogenetic abnormalities in Sézary syndrome include genomic losses at 1p, 10q, 14q and 15q that are obviously associated with clonal evolution of the tumor cells during disease progression. More recently, oligonucleotide array analysis provided interesting data based on the comparison between SS cells and CD4-positive T cells isolated from the peripheral blood of patients with atopic or chronic dermatitis and healthy volunteers. The SS samples displayed a relatively homogeneous gene expression pattern, with consistent upregulation of the two genes *Twist* and *EphrinA4* (*EphA4*). The *Twist* gene encodes a basic helix-loop-helix family transcriptional factor that is normally not expressed in lymphoid tissue and may inhibit apoptosis via antagonizing p53. EphA4 belongs to the Eph receptor subfamily of transmembrane protein tyrosine kinases and probably acts through an activation of the JAK/STAT pathway. A filter array analysis compared partially purified SS cells with in-vitro Th1- and Th1-skewed peripheral blood cells and found that the loss of STAT4 expression, together with the increased expression of *RhoB* and other genes, can discriminate SS patients from patients with inflammatory diseases. The discrepant data from both studies are probably due to the differences in study designs, patient sampling and data analysis.

Treatment of mycosis fungoides and Sézary syndrome

The choice of initial treatment for patients with MF and SS is dependent on the stage of the disease and the patients' performance status. The rationale for therapy in CTCL has been shaped by a randomized controlled trial in CTCL which compared palliative skin-directed therapy (topical mechlorethamine, superficial radiotherapy and phototherapy) with combined total-skin electron-beam and multi-agent chemotherapy in 103 patients. Response rates were higher in the chemotherapy group but morbidity was greater and there was no difference in disease-free or overall survival.

Skin-directed therapy includes topical treatments, phototherapy and radiotherapy. It is the first-line treatment for most patients with early-stage (IA–IIA) disease. Systemic treatments for advanced (IIB–IVB) or treatment-resistant early-stage disease should be given under the supervision of a multidisciplinary team, preferably as part of a randomized trial. The therapies for CTCL are listed below, and treatment options in the different stages of disease are shown in Table 16.3.

Skin-directed therapies
- topical corticosteroids
- topical chemotherapy
- other topical treatments
- phototherapy
- radiotherapy, including total-skin electron-beam therapy

Systemic therapies
- extracorporeal photopheresis
- immunotherapy
- monoclonal antibodies
- retinoids
- single- and multi-agent chemotherapy
- toxin therapies
- stem-cell transplantation
- experimental therapies

Skin-directed therapies
Topical corticosteroids

Emollients and topical corticosteroids are appropriate for patients with stage IA/B disease, to relieve symptoms of pruritus. Moderately potent topical corticosteroids may be used regularly for patches and thin plaques. Potent topical corticosteroids can produce a clinical response, although this is usually short-lived, and prolonged use can cause cutaneous atrophy.

Topical chemotherapy

Topical mechlorethamine (nitrogen mustard) 0.01% or 0.02% daily, either as an aqueous solution or in an

Table 16.3. Therapeutic options in primary CTCL and CBCL.

Stage/disease entity	First line	Second line	Novel/developing therapies
IA	No therapy or SDT	No therapy or SDT	Bexarotene gel
IB	SDT	PUVA + IFN-2α, TSEB, oral bexarotene	Denileukin diftitox, HDACI
IIA	SDT	PUVA + IFN-2α, TSEB, oral bexarotene	Denileukin diftitox, HDACI
IIB	Radiotherapy/TSEB, chemotherapy (liposomal doxorubicin)	IFN-2α, denileukin diftitox, oral bexarotene, multiagent chemotherapy (reduced-dose CHOP)	HDACI, ASCT, RISTs
III	PUVA ± IFN-2α, ECP ± IFN-2α, methotrexate, oral bexarotene	TSEB, denileukin diftitox, single agent chemotherapy (chlorambucil or deoxycoformycin), antibody therapy (alemtuzumab)	HDACI, ASCT, RISTs
IVA	Radiotherapy/TSEB, single-agent chemotherapy (gemcitabine/ liposomal doxorubicin)	IFN-2α, denileukin diftitox, multi-agent chemotherapy (reduced dose CHOP), antibody therapy (alemtuzumab)	HDACI, ASCT, RISTs
IVB	Palliative radiotherapy/ chemotherapy	—	ASCT, RISTs
Lymphomatoid papulosis	UVB or PUVA, radiotherapy, methotrexate	—	—
Primary cutaneous ALCL	Primary excision, radiotherapy	Chemotherapy for extracutaneous disease	—
Subcutaneous panniculitis-like TCL	Liposomal doxorubicin, radiotherapy, corticosteroids	Multiagent chemotherapy (eg. CHOP)	ASCT, RISTs
Primary cutaneous epidermotropic CD8+ TCL	Liposomal doxorubicin, TSEB	Multiagent chemotherapy (eg. CHOP)	ASCT, RISTs
Primary cutaneous small/medium pleomorphic TCL	Primary excision, radiotherapy	Chemotherapy (cyclophosphamide) IFN-2α	—
Primary cutaneous MZL	No treatment, primary excision, radiotherapy	Chlorambucil, IFN-2α (sc or intralesional), multi-agent chemotherapy with rituximab for nodal disease (CHOP-R)	Intralesional rituximab
Primary cutaneous FCCL	Radiotherapy	Liposomal doxorubicin, multi-agent chemotherapy with rituximab (CHOP-R)	Intralesional rituximab
Primary cutaneous LBCL	Radiotherapy	Multi-agent chemotherapy with rituximab (CHOP-R)	Intralesional rituximab

ointment base, is effective for early-stage disease, with response rates of 51–80% for IA, 26–68% for IB and 61% for IIA disease. Nitrogen mustard can cause an irritant or allergic contact dermatitis (35–58%). It must not be used in pregnancy and it is carcinogenic, with rare reports of non-melanoma skin cancer in patients treated with topical mechlorethamine.

Topical carmustine (BCNU) is an alternative topical chemotherapeutic agent in CTCL with similar efficacy to nitrogen mustard. Alternate or daily treatment with 10 mg of BCNU dissolved in 60 ml of 95% alcohol, or 20–40% BCNU ointment, may be used. Hypersensitivity reactions are less frequent than with nitrogen mustard, occurring in 5–10% of patients. All patients receiving treatment with carmustine (unlike nitrogen mustard) should have regular monitoring of their full blood counts, and treatment is normally given for limited periods (e.g. 2–4 weeks) to avoid myelosuppression.

Other topical treatments

Recently a novel retinoid, 1% Targretin (bexarotene) gel, has been approved by the FDA for topical therapy in stage I MF for patients who are resistant or intolerant of other topical therapies. It is a retinoid X receptor agonist (RXR) and may be useful for patients resistant to other skin-directed therapies. It has a response rate of 63% in IA/B disease, with complete responses (CR) in 21% and a median duration of two years.

Other topical treatments which have been used in small numbers of patients with some efficacy include imiquimod and a topical form of methotrexate, but formal studies are lacking at present.

Phototherapy and photochemotherapy

PUVA, broad-band UVB, narrow-band UVB and high-dose UVA-1 phototherapy have all been used in MF with considerable success, but there have been no adequate comparative studies of different phototherapy regimens in CTCL. UVB may be associated with a lower risk of cutaneous carcinogenesis than PUVA, but is less effective in patients with dark skin and thick plaques. Narrow-band UVB produces less irritation and erythema than broad-band UVB. A retrospective study of 56 patients with early-stage MF (1A and 1B) suggested that narrow-band UVB is at least as effective as PUVA in terms of both response and relapse-free interval, but most clinical experience has involved PUVA therapy.

The clinical benefit of PUVA (photochemotherapy) in patch/plaque-stage MF was noted three decades ago, and CR rates of 79–88% in stage IA and 52–59% in stage IB disease have been reported. PUVA remains one of the most effective therapies for patients with stage 1B/IIA disease. Treatment schedules have varied but normally involve treatment two or three times a week with oral 8-methoxypsoralen and UVA in regular dosage increments until maximum tolerated dose is reached. Treatment is continued until complete or best partial response has been achieved. Flexural sites ("sanctuary sites") often fail to respond completely, and the duration of response varies. UVA will not penetrate deeply enough to effectively treat folliculotropic MF or tumor-stage disease, and it is rarely tolerated in erythrodermic (stage III) disease.

One study has shown that 56% of stage IA and 39% of stage IB complete PUVA responders had no recurrence of disease after 44 months follow-up without maintenance therapy. However, relapse following PUVA therapy is commonly reported, and patients often require repeated courses over many years. Between 30% and 50% of patients may remain disease-free for 10 years, but late relapses still occur, and survival is not affected by relapse status. Many patients will inevitably have a high total cumulative UVA dose, and the risks of non-melanoma and melanoma skin cancer are consequently increased for these patients. Maintenance therapy is rarely effective at preventing relapse and therefore should if possible be avoided, particularly as this group of patients may go on to receive other carcinogenic therapies, increasing their risk of secondary malignancies.

Effort should be made to restrict the total PUVA dose to less than 200 treatment sessions or a total cumulative dose of $1200 \, J/cm^2$. However, in exceptional circumstances patients may receive a greater total dose if it is clinically justified and has the consent of the patient.

Radiotherapy and total-skin electron-beam therapy

MF and other CTCL variants are extremely radiosensitive. Individual thick plaques, eroded plaques or tumors can be treated successfully with relatively low-dose superficial orthovoltage radiotherapy (2 or 3 fractions of 400 cGy at 80–120 kV). Large tumors may require a higher energy. Closely adjacent and overlapping fields can often be retreated because of the low doses used.

Electron-beam therapy is also used to treat local disease, and the energy used depends on the depth of disease. Whole-body total-skin electron-beam (TSEB) therapy has also been extensively used to treat resistant widespread cutaneous disease.

A meta-analysis of open uncontrolled and mostly retrospective studies of TSEB as monotherapy in 952 patients with CTCL established that responses are stage-dependent, with complete responses of 96% in stage IA–IIA disease, but relapse rates are high, indicating that this approach is not curative in early-stage disease. In stage IIB disease complete responses are less common (36%), but erythrodermic (stage III) disease shows complete responses of 60%. Greater skin-surface dose fractionation (32–36 Gy) and higher energy (4–6 MeV electrons) are associated with a higher rate of complete response, and five-year relapse-free survivals of 10–23% were noted. A comparative retrospective study of TSEB versus topical mechlorethamine in early-stage MF showed similar response rates and duration of response, suggesting that TSEB therapy should be reserved for those who fail first- and second-line therapies.

Adverse effects of TSEB include temporary alopecia, telangiectasia and skin malignancies, and treatment is only available in a limited number of centers. Although TSEB is usually given only once in a lifetime, several reports have documented patients who have received two or three courses, although the total dose tolerated and duration of response have been lower with subsequent courses.

Systemic therapies
Extracorporeal photopheresis

Extracorporeal photopheresis (ECP) involves administration of oral psoralen, followed by ex-vivo collection of an enriched buffy coat preparation using a cell separator. These leukocytes are then exposed to UVA before being returned to the patient. This regimen is repeated on two successive days and the two-day cycle repeated monthly or at two-weekly intervals. In-vitro evidence suggests that a proportion of the UVA-exposed leukocytes, including some tumor lymphocytes, undergo apoptosis, and that dendritic cells are activated during the ex-vivo circulation, with induction of a host anti-tumor immune response after the treated cells are returned to the patient. Recent evidence has also shown activation of dendritic cells during an expanded period of ex-vivo incubation overnight (transimmunization).

ECP is licensed by the FDA for the treatment of CTCL, but there are no randomized studies to clarify whether ECP has an impact on overall survival. The original open study of ECP in 29 patients with erythrodermic CTCL (stage III/IVA) reported a response rate of 73%, but response rates in patients with earlier stages of MF were much lower (38%). Subsequently a median survival of 62 months was reported in the original cohort of 29 erythrodermic patients, which compares favorably with historical controls (30 months). A study of 33 patients with SS treated with ECP reported a median survival of 39 months, which was similar to historical controls from the same institution. A systematic review of response rates in erythrodermic disease (stage III/IVA) treated with ECP has shown overall response rates of 35–71%, with CR rates of 14–26%. ECP has not been found to be of benefit in stage IB patients who have molecular evidence of a peripheral-blood clone. There have been claims that the CD8 count is critical in predicting whether patients will respond to ECP, although others have provided evidence that the total baseline Sézary count is the best predictor of response.

Preliminary non-randomized cohort studies suggest that the combination of interferon alpha and ECP is more effective than ECP alone. There are also isolated case reports of combined ECP and interferon gamma inducing complete clinical and molecular responses.

Immunotherapy

Immunotherapy may enhance the anti-tumor host immune responses by promoting the generation of cytotoxic T cells and Th1 cytokine responses. Interferon alpha has been used most frequently, with overall response rates of 45–74% and CR rates of 10–27%. Various dosage schedules have been employed (3 MU × 3/wk – 36 MU/d), and it appears that response rates are higher for larger doses (overall response of 78% vs. 37% for the lower-dose schedule), but dose-limiting toxicities include fever, chills, malaise, leukopenia, thrombocytopenia and liver dysfunction. Overall response rates are also higher in early (IB–IIA, 88%) compared to late (III–IV, 63%) stages of disease.

Combined interferon α and RAR retinoids produce similar response rates to interferon alone and are not recommended. A randomized controlled study comparing PUVA and interferon α with interferon α and acitretin in early-stage disease showed complete response rates of 70% and 38%, respectively, but there are no data on duration of response. Uncontrolled studies of combined PUVA and interferon α (maximum tolerated dose 12 MU/m^2 × 3/wk) have shown overall responses rates of 100% and complete response rates of 62%. This combination may also be useful in patients with resistant early-stage disease, such as those with thick plaques and folliculotropic disease.

Small pilot studies have shown that interferon γ can produce clinical responses in CTCL, but the therapeutic value remains to be established. Interleukin 12 has also been shown to produce a clinical response, and the benefit of IL-12 appears to be due to potent stimulation of interferon gamma.

Monoclonal antibody therapy

Humanized chimeric anti-CD4 monoclonal antibody has shown response rates of 50–75%. Patients with a clinical response develop an eczema-like reaction, and CD4 depletion may be prolonged for up to one year. Recent phase II studies using a fully humanized anti-CD4 antibody (HuMaxCD4) have shown similar response rates. A radiolabeled anti-CD5 antibody has also been used in MF with some objective results and Campath (anti-CD52/alemtuzimab) has also been administered to patients with advanced stages of disease, with demonstrable but short-lived clinical responses. This approach is associated with a high rate of cytomegalovirus (CMV) reactivation and prolonged immunosuppression.

Retinoids

Retinoids are vitamin-A derivatives which have been shown to be of clinical benefit for CTCL. Both acitretin and isotretinoin have been shown to have similar but low rates of response in CTCL. Side effects include teratogenicity, dryness of the mucous membranes and hyperlipidemia.

Bexarotene (Targretin) is the only retinoid that selectively binds and activates the RXR receptor and has been shown to promote apoptosis and inhibit cell proliferation. It is relatively selective and therefore should have little effect on the RAR receptor involved in cell differentiation. In phase II and III studies of 152 patients with CTCL, response rates of 20–67% have

been reported. The most effective tolerated oral dose is 300 mg/m^2 per day, although responses improve with higher doses. It is teratogenic, and most patients develop hyperlipidemia, requiring treatment with lipid-lowering agents, and central hypothyroidism.

Open studies comparing PUVA with combined PUVA and acitretin have shown a similar CR rate (73% vs. 72%), although the cumulative dose to best response was lower in patients receiving the combination therapy.

Systemic chemotherapy

MF and SS are relatively chemoresistant malignancies, probably due to the low proliferative rate of tumor cells and high prevalence of p53 mutations. Complete responses are seen in about 33% but are frequently short-lived. Chemotherapy is not suitable or clinically effective for patch/plaque-stage disease (IA–IIA). In addition, individual tumors (IIB) and effaced lymph nodes (IVA) will respond to local radiotherapy, but chemotherapy can be given for those with good performance status who have extensive nodal or visceral disease. CHOP has been the most frequently used multi-agent regimen, and may produce a CR of 38% in stage IIB–IVB with a median duration of only 5–41 months. However, multi-agent regimens are highly immunosuppressive; bone-marrow suppression may be severe and overall duration of response is usually very short-lived. In such patients, infection or septicemia are frequently preterminal.

Single-agent chemotherapies that have been shown to produce a clinical response in stage IIB–IVB disease include oral chlorambucil, methotrexate and etoposide, and intravenous 2-deoxycoformycin, 2-chlorodeoxyadenosine and fludarabine. Open studies of 2-deoxycoformycin in MF and SS have reported response rates of 35–71%, with CR rates of 10–33%. Methotrexate (single weekly doses of 5–125 mg) has been reported to produce a CR rate of 41% in 29 patients with erythrodermic (stage III/T4) disease, with a median survival of 8.4 years, but this study was uncontrolled. Deoxycoformycin and methotrexate are the preferred second-line therapies for stage III disease. In a recent trial, pegylated liposomal doxorubicin was found to be effective and safe in patients with recurrent or recalcitrant MF (stage IIB–IVA), and resulted in a response rate of 88%. Doxorubicin is the preferred treatment for patients with extensive cutaneous tumors, but responses are short-lived. Recently gemcitabine has been used in CTCL with some success.

Toxin therapies

Denileukin diftitox, a DAB_{389}-IL-2 fusion toxin (Ontak) has received FDA approval for the treatment of resistant or recurrent CTCL. It is a recombinant fusion protein which inhibits protein synthesis in tumor cells expressing high levels of the IL-2 receptor (CD25+ cells) resulting in apoptosis. Phase III studies of 71 heavily pre-treated patients with stage IB–IVA disease and more than 20% CD25+ lymphocytes showed an overall response rate of 30% including 10% with complete responses lasting at least six weeks. The median duration of response was 6.9 months (range 2.7–46.1 months).

The optimally tolerated intravenous dose is 18 μg/kg per day for five days, repeated every 21 days for 4–8 cycles. Adverse effects include fever, chills, myalgia, nausea and vomiting and a mild increase in trans-aminase levels. Acute hypersensitivity reactions occur in 60% of patients, invariably within 24 hours of the initial infusion. A vascular leak syndrome characterized by hypotension, hypoalbuminemia and edema occurs in 25% of patients. Myelosuppression is rare. 5% of adverse effects are severe or life-threatening. The duration of clinical response has not yet been established.

Stem-cell transplantation

Recent pilot studies assessing the use of TSEB and/or total-body irradiation combined with high-dose conditioning chemotherapy prior to autologous stem-cell transplantation (ASCT) in patients with stage IIB/IVA disease have shown good clinical responses, but high relapse rates. There are no data available at present to indicate if this approach affects disease-free or overall survival. Allogeneic stem-cell transplantation (allo-SCT) has only been used in a few patients, with encouraging results, but the associated mortality suggests that this approach is difficult to justify. However a graft-versus-lymphoma effect may be therapeutically important and non-myeloablative allo-SCT may have a role for selected younger CTCL patients with advanced stages of disease. A recent study of eight patients with advanced CTCL who underwent either a full or reduced-intensity conditioning regimen and allo-SCT showed

that all achieved a complete clinical remission and resolution of molecular and cytogenetic markers of disease within 30–60 days after SCT. Two patients died from transplantation-related complications, but after a median follow-up of 56 months the other six patients remained alive without evidence of lymphoma.

Emerging novel therapies

Suberoyleranilide hydroxamic acid (SAHA) is an oral histone deacetylase (HDAC) inhibitor. In a phase II open-label study with oral SAHA eight of 33 patients with advanced, refractory CTCL experienced partial responses. The most common side effects seen in the study were fatigue, diarrhea, nausea, change in taste, dry mouth, decreased appetite and thrombocytopenia.

Depsipeptide (FK228) is an intravenous HDAC inhibitor. In a phase I trial of depsipeptide, three patients with CTCL had a partial response, and one patient with a peripheral T-cell lymphoma had a complete response. Sézary cells isolated from patients after treatment showed increased histone acetylation. Side effects include electrocardiogram changes, fatigue, nausea, vomiting, anorexia, transient leukopenia and thrombocytopenia.

Mycosis fungoides clinicopathologic variants

Pagetoid reticulosis

Pagetoid reticulosis is a localized solitary variant of CTCL characterized clinically by an isolated, persistent scaly plaque, commonly involving an acral site, and histologically by intense epidermotropism. It was first described in 1939; it is rare but appears to affect younger adults. A more generalized variant with multiple plaques at other sites has also been described (Ketron–Goodman), but it is likely that this represents the more recently described CD8-positive epidermotropic CTCL variant. The natural history of pagetoid reticulosis is of very slow local extension with an excellent prognosis. Successful remission and cure has been reported with both surgical excision and low-dose superficial radiotherapy.

Folliculotropic and syringotropic MF

Folliculotropic and syringotropic variants of MF may occur. Clinically these present as multiple small

Table 16.4. Prognosis in different cutaneous T-cell lymphomas.

Lymphoma	Disease-specific 5-year survival (%)	Median survival
Lymphomatoid papulosis	100	–
Primary cutaneous CD30+ anaplastic large-cell lymphoma	90–95	–
Subcutaneous panniculitis-like T-cell lymphoma	82	–
Primary cutaneous peripheral T-cell lymphoma, unspecified	16	–
Primary cutaneous epidermotropic CD8+ T-cell lymphoma	18	–
Primary cutaneous CD4+ small/medium-sized pleomorphic T-cell lymphoma	60–80	–
Extranodal NK/T-cell lymphoma, nasal type	–	15 months

(1–3 mm) red macules and papules clustered around hair follicles and frequently associated with alopecia. Histologically atypical lymphocytes show tropism for hair-follicle or sweat-gland epithelium and rarely demonstrate epidermotropism.

Recent studies suggest that the prognosis of folliculotropic variants of MF are worse. Follicular mucinosis may occur in association with MF or as a separate entity. Clinically there is follicular plugging and hair loss, and boggy erythematous plaques may be present with complete alopecia. Histologically, mucinous degeneration can be seen deposited throughout the follicular epithelium. If the hair follicles have been destroyed, scarring alopecia may occur.

Because of the perifollicular localization of the dermal infiltrates, folliculotropic MF is often less responsive to skin-targeted therapies, such as PUVA and topical nitrogen mustard, than classical plaque-stage MF. In such cases total-skin electron-beam irradiation is an effective treatment, but sustained complete remissions are rarely achieved. PUVA combined with retinoids or interferon alpha may be considered, and persistent tumors can be treated with radiotherapy.

Granulomatous variants of MF

Granulomatous slack skin presents with redundant erythematous folds typically in flexural sites. The histology is granulomatous, often with extensive areas of elastolysis, and the atypical lymphocytic infiltrate may be sparse and may not show epidermotropism. The condition must be distinguished from other forms of cutis laxa. Granulomatous infiltration has

also been described in clinical MF without the typical features of slack skin.

Granulomatous slack skin may be treated with radiotherapy with some efficacy.

CD30-POSITIVE T-CELL LYMPHOPROLIFERATIVE DISORDERS OF THE SKIN

Primary cutaneous CD30-positive lymphoproliferative disorders represent a spectrum of disorders consisting of lymphomatoid papulosis and primary cutaneous CD30-positive large-cell anaplastic lymphoma. Critically, primary cutaneous CD30-positive large-cell lymphomas are associated with a good prognosis, in contrast to histological transformation of mycosis fungoides with tumor-cell CD30-positive expression, and systemic nodal CD30-positive lymphomas.

Lymphomatoid papulosis

The term lymphomatoid papulosis was first coined in 1968 by Macaulay to describe a "self-healing rhythmical paradoxical papular eruption, histologically malignant but clinically benign." Recurrent crops of papular/nodular lesions predominantly affect the limbs, although any body site may be involved and regional localized variants may occur. These lesions may grow rapidly over a few days and develop ulcerated necrotic centres. Healing occurs slowly, with fine atrophic or varioliform scars. Recurrent lesions are common but the prognosis is excellent (Table 16.4). Patients are at risk of developing CD30-positive large-cell anaplastic T-cell lymphoma, MF and Hodgkin's lymphoma (< 5% of cases). Patients with MF may also develop lymphomatoid papulosis, which is reported to be a favorable prognostic feature in MF.

Pathology

Three histological patterns of lymphomatoid papulosis have been described. Type A lesions contain scattered large cells that resemble Reed–Sternberg cells within a dense background infiltrate that includes neutrophils, eosinophils, histiocytes and a few plasma cells (Fig 16.8). Type B lesions are more reminiscent of MF, with a band-like infiltrate of cerebriform-type cells that show epidermotropism. Type C lesions contain prominent clusters/cohesive sheets of atypical large cells.

Immunophenotypically the cells are mature T cells with expression of CD3. In most cases there is expression of CD2 and/or CD5, but both may be lost. Staining for CD7 is often absent. The cells are usually CD4-positive with lack of CD8, and there is expression of CD25 and HLA-DR. In type A and C lesions the large cells are positive for CD30 and negative for CD15. The small cerebriform cells of type B lesions are CD30-negative. There is expression of TIA-1 and granzyme in the majority of cases.

Treatment

There is no current treatment which alters the clinical course of lymphomatoid papulosis. Lesions are extremely radiosensitive but as they resolve spontaneously this is only necessary for larger necrotic lesions. Topical or intralesional steroids and topical nitrogen mustard applied to developing lesions may accelerate clearance, but have little effect on well-developed lesions. Narrow-band UVB therapy or PUVA may be preventative while patients are on treatment. Low-dose oral methotrexate is effective and may reduce or prevent the frequency and severity of new lesions. There is no evidence that intensive combination chemotherapy is effective for lymphomatoid papulosis, and chemotherapy is contraindicated. Therapeutic options are shown in Table 16.3.

Primary cutaneous CD30-positive anaplastic large-cell lymphoma

Primary cutaneous CD30-positive anaplastic large-cell lymphoma (ALCL) is a cutaneous T-cell lymphoma variant confined to the skin. These lymphomas are usually seen in adults and present as large solitary nodules which may ulcerate, most often on the trunk. Multiple lesions may occur but there are no associated patches or plaques of MF. In contrast to lymphomatoid papulosis, the histology shows an extensive infiltrate of CD30-positive atypical large anaplastic cells. Individual lesions may partially or totally regress spontaneously, and disease may remain localized to a limb (Fig 16.9). Progression to extracutaneous sites is rare but has been reported in 10%. The prognosis for

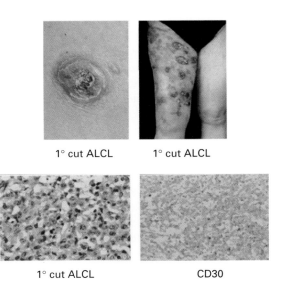

1° cut ALCL   1° cut ALCL

1° cut ALCL   CD30

Figure 16.9. Primary cutaneous CD30-positive ALCL.

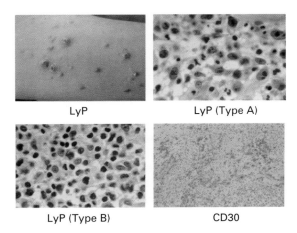

LyP   LyP (Type A)

LyP (Type B)   CD30

Figure 16.8. Lymphomatoid papulosis.

patients with primary cutaneous disease is excellent (five-year survival rates of 90–95%, Table 16.4). However, staging consisting of bone-marrow and CT scans is required in all patients to exclude secondary cutaneous involvement in primary nodal CD30+ ALK+ lymphomas.

Pathology

Morphologically these lesions are characterised by a dense dermal infiltrate of large cells with immunoblastic, pleomorphic or anaplastic morphology. Epidermotropism may be seen. Large bizarre cells with irregular nuclei and abundant pale cytoplasm are present, and some of these may have multiple nucleoli. There may be an associated infiltrate of small lymphocytes, but eosinophils and plasma cells are not prominent.

Immunophenotypically CD30 is present in over 75% of large cells. These cells also express CD2, CD3, CD5 and CD25, although variable loss of CD2, CD3 and CD5 is common. The cells are positive for cytotoxic granules (TIA-1 and granzyme) but do not express epithelial membrane antigen (EMA), and they are negative for ALK in the vast majority of cases. Expression of HECA is seen in about 50% of cases.

Treatment

Both excision and localized radiotherapy are acceptable methods of treating isolated lesions. Nodal involvement may also respond to radiotherapy. Oral methotrexate is also effective. Multi-agent chemotherapy including CHOP can be effective but is not recommended unless extracutaneous sites are involved because of the excellent prognosis and high recurrence rate with short duration of benefit. Therapeutic options are shown in Table 16.3.

Molecular cytogenetics of CD30-positive T-cell lymphoproliferative disorders of the skin

TCR genes are clonally rearranged in the vast majority of cases. NPM–ALK fusion transcripts generated from the translocation t(2;5)(p23;q35), characteristic of systemic ALCL, have infrequently been reported in occasional cutaneous ALCL and lymphomatoid papulosis samples. These cases, however, may represent a cutaneous manifestation of primary systemic disease. Comparative genomic hybridization (CGH)

studies have revealed genomic gains at chromosomes 1/1p, 5, 6, 7, 8/8p and 19. Recently, microarray-based CGH analysis was performed in a series of cutaneous ALCL that demonstrated copy number gains of *FGFR1* (8p11), *NRAS* (1p13.2), *MYCN* (2p24.1), *RAF1* (3p35), *CTSB* (8p22), *FES* (15q26.1) and *CBFA2* (21q22.3) oncogenes. In the same series, amplifications of *CTSB*, *RAF1*, *REL* (2p13), *JUNB* (19p13.2), *MYCN* and *YES1* (18p11.3) were found.

SUBCUTANEOUS PANNICULITIS-LIKE T-CELL LYMPHOMA

Subcutaneous panniculitis-like T-cell lymphoma (SPTCL) is a lymphoproliferative disease originating and presenting in the subcutaneous tissue and predominantly affecting adults. It is characterized clinically by solitary or multiple subcutaneous nodules and plaques, which mainly involve the legs. There are two subsets, namely those derived from gamma/delta T cells, which have a poor prognosis and are usually CD56-positive with histologic evidence of epidermotropic, dermal and subcutaneous involvement, and a more indolent group derived from alpha/beta T cells, which are CD8-positive and show histologic involvement of only the subcutis. A hemophagocytic syndrome is a frequent complication of gamma/delta SPTCL in which patients present with fever, pancytopenia and hepatosplenomegaly. It usually indicates a fulminant downhill clinical course. However, if therapy for the underlying lymphoma is instituted and successful, the hemophagocytic syndrome may remit. Dissemination to lymph nodes and other organs is uncommon, and usually occurs late in the clinical course.

Pathology

The infiltrate is characteristically subcutaneous, with involvement of the lobules of the subcutaneous fat resembling lobular panniculitis. There is prominent apoptosis, and fat necrosis is frequently present. Characteristically there is rimming of the lobular adipocytes by atypical lymphoid cells. The neoplastic cell morphology is variable, ranging from small cells with round nuclei and inconspicuous nucleoli to larger cells with dense chromatin. Plasma cells and reactive lymphoid follicles are usually absent (Fig. 16.10).

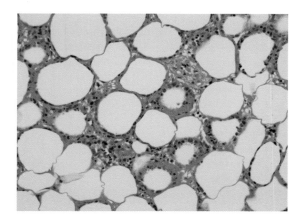

Figure 16.10. Subcutaneous panniculitis-like T-cell lymphoma (skin). The subcutaneous fat is infiltrated by atypical lymphoid cells that surround adipocytes. Apoptotic debris is prominent.

Immunophenotypically the cells express a mature T-cell phenotype and stain for CD2, CD3 and CD5. The cells are characteristically positive for CD8 with lack of CD4, and there is expression of cytotoxic granule-related proteins TIA-1, granzyme and perforin. Staining for CD30 is usually negative. The cells express TCRαβ in the majority of cases (about 75%), while the remainder are positive for TCRγδ. The cases expressing TCRγδ are usually negative for CD4 and CD8 and may express CD56. There is no evidence of EBV.

Treatment

Patients are generally treated with doxorubicin-based chemotherapy and local radiation therapy. However, recent studies suggest that many patients with indolent disease can be successfully treated with systemic corticosteroids. In aggressive disease preconditioning chemotherapy followed by an autologous or allogeneic SCT may be the only therapeutic option for improving survival. Therapeutic options are shown in Table 16.3.

PRIMARY CUTANEOUS PERIPHERAL T-CELL LYMPHOMA, UNSPECIFIED

This category encompasses all primary CTCLs which are not currently well defined on the basis of clinicopathologic criteria outlined for other CTCL variants above. It includes primary cutaneous aggressive epidermotropic CD8-positive T-cell lymphoma, cutaneous gamma/delta-positive T-cell lymphoma, which has been discussed above in the context of SPTCL, and primary cutaneous CD4-positive small/medium-sized pleomorphic T-cell lymphoma.

Primary cutaneous aggressive epidermotropic CD8-positive T-cell lymphoma

Primary cutaneous aggressive CD8-positive TCL typically presents with widespread papules, plaques, nodules and/or tumors which may show erosions, ulceration and necrosis. Mucosal involvement may occur. Characteristically there are no typical polymorphic scaly or atrophic patches/plaques of MF. These lymphomas express CD8 and cytotoxic proteins with a striking epidermotropic infiltrate. Although there are currently few reports of this entity, the distinctive pathological and immunophenotypic features and poor prognosis (five-year survival 18%, Table 16.4) suggest that it represents a distinct subtype of CTCL. CNS involvement can occur and nodal dissemination is uncommon.

There is a poor response to radiotherapy and chemotherapy. Patients are generally treated with doxorubicin-based multi-agent chemotherapy, and younger patients may be eligible for autologous or allogeneic SCT. Therapeutic options are shown in Table 16.3.

Primary cutaneous CD4-positive small/medium-sized pleomorphic T-cell lymphoma

This CTCL variant presents with non-specific erythematous nodules on the face, neck or upper trunk. Multiple lesions may occur, but with no clinical evidence of MF. In most cases there is a favorable clinical course and systemic involvement is unusual (five-year survival 75%, Table 16.4).

Histologically there are nodular and diffuse infiltrates of small to medium-sized pleomorphic T cells, which may infiltrate into the subcutis. Epidermotropism may be present.

In view of the excellent prognosis, patients with solitary localized skin lesions may be treated with surgical excision or radiotherapy. Cyclophosphamide as single-agent therapy and interferon alpha are effective in patients with more generalized skin disease. Therapeutic options are shown in Table 16.3.

PRIMARY CUTANEOUS B-CELL LYMPHOMAS (CBCL)

Primary CBCLs constitute approximately one-quarter of all primary cutaneous lymphomas. Full staging investigations are essential for all patients with a CBCL to exclude a primary nodal lymphoma with secondary cutaneous involvement. The prognoses associated with the various diagnostic entities are shown in Table 16.5.

Molecular analysis of primary cutaneous B-cell lymphoma demonstrates clonally rearranged immunoglobulin receptor genes in the majority of cases. Few data are available concerning the immunoglobulin receptor configuration; however, preferential usage of the IgV_H family member 2-70, ongoing mutations, and low rates of replacement mutations in framework regions have been reported. These findings suggest a negative antigen selection pressure and indicate that local antigens could modulate the growth of primary cutaneous B-cell lymphoma.

Primary cutaneous marginal zone B-cell lymphoma/immunocytoma

Primary cutaneous marginal zone B-cell lymphomas (PCMZL) are indolent lymphomas which present as asymptomatic solitary or multiple dermal papules, plaques or nodules on any body site, although the trunk is most often involved. Benign monoclonal paraproteinaemia may be present. There is a slight male predominance. The estimated five-year survival is excellent (98–100%, Table 16.5). Nodal involvement is very rare.

Pathology
PCMZLs are derived from post-germinal-center cells and are characterized by a proliferation of small lymphocytes, lymphoplasmacytoid cells and plasma cells with monotypic cytoplasmic immunoglobulin.

Molecular cytogenetics
The translocation t(11;18)(q21;q21), representing the most common translocation in extranodal marginal zone B-cell lymphoma, has not been demonstrated in PCMZL. The translocation t(14;18)(q32;q21),

Table 16.5. Prognosis in different cutaneous B-cell lymphomas.

Disease entity	Disease-specific 5-year survival (%)
Primary cutaneous marginal zone lymphoma	99
Primary cutaneous follicle center-cell lymphoma	95
Primary cutaneous large B-cell lymphoma	50–55

involving the IgH locus and the *MALT1* gene, is reported frequently and according to some studies can be demonstrated in one-third of cases. The recently described t(3;14)(p13;q32), which results in the deregulation of the *FOXP1* gene, has also been detected in PCMZL; however, its overall frequency is not established. Similar to the *API2–MALT1* fusion, aberrations involving the *BCL-10* gene have not been identified in cutaneous MZBL. Recent studies provide data linking primary cutaneous B-cell lymphoma with *Borrelia burgdorferi* infection, providing a rationale for systemic antibiotic treatment.

Treatment
Patients with solitary or few cutaneous lesions can be treated with radiotherapy or surgical excision, or an expectant lesion may be followed. In patients with associated *B. burgdorferi* infection, systemic antibiotics should be tried first. For patients presenting with multifocal skin lesions, chlorambucil or intralesional/subcutaneous administration of interferon alpha may produce complete responses in approximately 50% of patients. Excellent results have also been obtained with systemic and intralesional anti-CD20 antibody (rituximab). Patients with secondary nodal involvement may require more aggressive chemotherapy treatment. Therapeutic options are shown in Table 16.3.

Primary cutaneous follicle center-cell lymphoma

Primary cutaneous follicle center-cell lymphoma (PCFCCL), previously known as Crosti's lymphoma, is an indolent lymphoma. Patients present with

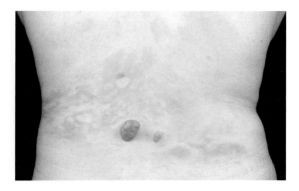

Figure 16.11. Primary cutaneous follicle center cell lymphoma.

clinically solitary or grouped purple papules, plaques or nodules, most commonly on the head, neck or trunk, although any body site may be involved (Fig. 16.11). Lesions increase slowly over time without treatment and new nodules may develop over a period of years. The estimated five-year survival of PCFCCL is 94–97% (Table 16.5).

Pathology

The growth pattern of these lesions may be follicular, follicular and diffuse, or purely diffuse. The infiltrate is within the dermis and may extend into the subcutaneous tissue. In most cases there is a Grenz zone between the infiltrate and the overlying epidermis. There is a variable mixture of centrocyte and centroblast cells which, in the follicular type, gives a monotonous appearance to the follicle centers without the characteristic zoning of reactive germinal centers. Macrophages with tangible bodies are scanty. In contrast to nodal follicular lymphoma, grading of these lymphomas is not performed as this has not been shown to be prognostically useful.

Immunophenotypically the cells are positive for CD20 and CD79a and lack CD5. Expression of CD23 may be seen in some cases. Staining for CD10 is variable, but most cases are positive for bcl-6. The cells lack bcl-2 protein expression in most cases. There is no expression for MUM1/IRF4. Where a follicular growth pattern is present, underlying follicular dendritic cell meshworks can be highlighted by CD21, CD23 or CD35.

Molecular cytogenetics

In contrast to nodal follicular lymphoma, the cutaneous FL variants lack the translocation t(14;18)(q32;q21) that results in the deregulated expression of *BCL-2*. In

PCFCCL, inactivation of $p15^{INK4b}$ and $p16^{INK4a}$ tumor suppressor genes is frequently reported, most often as a result of promoter hypermethylation.

Treatment

In patients with localized or few scattered skin lesions, radiotherapy is the preferred mode of treatment. Cutaneous relapses can be treated with further radiotherapy. Anthracycline-based chemotherapy (such as doxorubicin) is required only in patients with very extensive cutaneous disease and patients developing extracutaneous disease. Systemic or intralesional anti-CD20 antibody (rituximab) therapy has been effective in small numbers of patients. Therapeutic options are shown in Table 16.3.

Primary cutaneous large B-cell lymphoma

Primary cutaneous large B-cell lymphomas (PCLBCL) typically present as large dermal nodules or tumors which are either solitary or multifocal and characterized by a diffuse proliferation of large B cells consisting of centroblasts and immunoblasts. These lymphomas tend to develop on the lower limbs (Fig. 16.12). This has led to the classification of these lymphomas as LBCL of the leg type, although PCLBCL can also occur less commonly at other sites. It affects an elderly population with a female predominance. The prognosis of primary cutaneous large B-cell lymphoma is poor, with a five-year survival of 50–55% (Table 16.5).

Pathology

There is a diffuse dermal infiltrate of large lymphoid cells, with destruction of the adnexal structures. Extension into the subcutaneous tissue may be present. There is usually a subepidermal Grenz zone. The cells resemble centroblasts with vesicular nuclei containing multiple nucleoli that are often attached to the nuclear membrane. Some cases have significant numbers of immunoblast-like cells.

Immunophenotypically the cells express CD20 and CD79a and lack CD5 and CD10. Expression of bcl-6 is variable but is usually positive. There is strong staining for MUM1/IRF4 but CD138 is not expressed. There is strong staining for bcl-2 protein.

Molecular cytogenetics

Cases of primary cutaneous LBCL lack translocations commonly encountered in nodal DLBCL. Recent

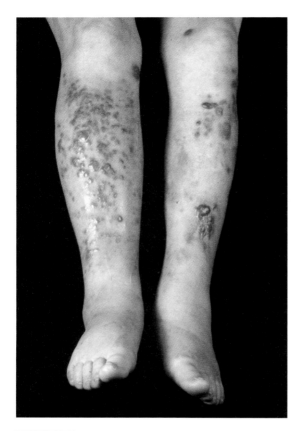

Figure 16.12. Large B-cell lymphoma involving the leg.

array-based CGH studies have demonstrated different genomic imbalances in both PCFCCL and PCLBCL leg-type. The most frequent alterations in PCFCCL were high-level amplifications of *c-REL* at 2p16, and deletions at chromosomal band 14q32, while PCLBCL harbored amplifications at 18q21, including both *BCL-2* and *MALT1* genes, and deletions of a small region at 9p21 containing the *CDKN2A, CDKN2B* and *NSG-x* genes. Gene expression profiling of cutaneous B-cell lymphomas has demonstrated increased expression of several genes associated with proliferation (*Pim1, Pim2, MYC, MUM1/IRF4* and *Oct2*) in PCLBCL leg-type and an activated B-cell (ABC)-like signature, while PCFCCL is characterized by a germinal-center B-cell (GCB)-like expression pattern and overexpression of the *SPINK2* gene.

Treatment

In elderly patients with solitary tumors radiotherapy may be appropriate but multi-agent chemotherapy is usually required for multifocal disease. The role of rituximab in primary cutaneous disease has yet to be determined but this has proved effective in relapsed nodal DLBCL in combination with CHOP chemotherapy. Intralesional rituximab may be effective. Therapeutic options are shown in Table 16.3.

FURTHER READING

Bekkenk, M. W., Geelen, F. A. M. J., van Voorst Vader, P. C. *et al.* Primary and secondary cutaneous CD30 positive lymphoproliferative disorders. *Blood* **95** (2000), 3653–3661.

Bekkenk, M. W., Vermeer, M. H., Geerts, M. L. *et al.* Treatment of multifocal primary cutaneous B-cell lymphoma: a clinical follow-up study of 29 patients. *J. Clin. Oncol.* **17** (1999), 2471–2478.

Bunn, P. A., Jr. and Lamberg, S. I. Report of the Committee on Staging and Classification of Cutaneous T-Cell Lymphomas. *Cancer Treat. Rep.* **63** (1979), 725–728.

Grange, F., Bekkenk, M., Wechsler, J. *et al.* Prognostic factors in primary cutaneous large B-cell lymphomas: a European multicenter study. *J. Clin. Oncol.* **19** (2001), 3602–3610.

Hoefnagel, J. J., Vermeer, M. H., Jansen, P. M. *et al.* Primary cutaneous marginal zone B-cell lymphoma: clinical and therapeutic features in 50 cases. *Arch. Dermatol.* **141** (2005), 1139–1145.

Jones, G. W., Kacinski, B. M., Wilson, L. D. *et al.* Total skin electron radiation in the management of mycosis fungoides: consensus of the European Organisation for Research and Treatment of Cancer (EORTC) Cutaneous Lymphoma Project Group. *J. Am. Acad. Dermatol.* **47** (2002), 364–370.

Kaye, F. J., Bunn, P. A. Jr., Steinberg, S. M. *et al.* A randomized trial comparing combination electron beam radiation and chemotherapy with topical therapy in the initial treatment of mycosis fungoides. *N. Engl. J. Med.* **321** (1989), 1784–1790.

Kim, Y. H., Liu, H. L., Mraz-Gernhard, S., Varghese, A. and Hoppe, R. T. Long-term outcome of 525 patients with mycosis fungoides and Sézary syndrome: clinical prognostic factors and risk for disease progression. *Arch. Dermatol.* **139** (2003), 857–866.

Mehregan, D. A., Su, W. P. and Kurtin, P. J. Subcutaneous T-cell lymphoma: a clinical, histopathologic, and immunohistochemical study of six cases. *J. Cutan. Pathol.* **21** (1994), 110–117.

Santucci, M., Biggeri, A., Feller, A. C., Massi, D. and Burg, G. Efficacy of histologic criteria for diagnosing early mycosis fungoides: an EORTC cutaneous lymphoma study group investigation. European Organization for Research and Treatment of Cancer. *Am. J. Surg. Pathol.* **24** (2000), 40–50.

Scarisbrick, J. J., Whittaker, S., Evans, A. V. *et al.* Prognostic significance of tumor burden in the blood of patients with erythrodermic primary cutaneous T-cell lymphoma. *Blood* **97** (2001), 624–630.

Smoller, B. R., Bishop, K., Glusac, E., Kim, Y. H. and Hendrickson, M. Reassessment of histologic parameters in the diagnosis of mycosis fungoides. *Am. J. Surg. Pathol.* **19** (1995), 1423–1430.

van Doorn, R., Van Haselen, C. W., van Voorst Vader, P. C. *et al.* Mycosis fungoides: disease evolution and prognosis of 309 Dutch patients. *Arch. Dermatol.* **136** (2000), 504–510.

van Doorn, R., Scheffer, E. and Willemze, R. Follicular mycosis fungoides, a distinct disease entity with or without associated follicular mucinosis: a clinicopathologic and follow-up study of 51 patients. *Arch. Dermatol.* **138** (2002), 191–198.

Vonderheid, E. C., Bernengo, M. G., Burg, G. *et al.* Update on erythrodermic cutaneous T-cell lymphoma: report of the International Society for Cutaneous Lymphomas. *J. Am. Acad. Dermatol.* **46** (2002), 95–106.

Whittaker, S. J., Marsden, J. R., Spittle, M., and Russell Jones, R. Joint British Association of Dermatologists and U.K. Cutaneous Lymphoma Group guidelines for the management of primary cutaneous T-cell lymphomas. *Br. J. Dermatol.* **149** (2003), 1095–1107.

Willemze, R., Meyer, C. J., Van Vloten, W. A. and Scheffer, E. The clinical and histological spectrum of lymphomatoid papulosis. *Br. J. Dermatol.* **107** (1982), 131–144.

Willemze, R., Jaffe, E. S., Burg G. WHO-EORTC classification for cutaneous lymphomas. *Blood* **105** (2005), 3768–3785.

Zackheim, H. S., Amin, S., Kashani-Sabet, M. and McMillan, A. Prognosis in cutaneous T-cell lymphoma by skin stage: long-term survival in 489 patients. *J. Am. Acad. Dermatol.* **40** (1999), 418–425.

Michele Spina, Robert Marcus and Umberto Tirelli

Pathology: Andrew Wotherspoon
Molecular cytogenetics: Andreas Rosenwald and German Ott

INTRODUCTION

Immunodepleted patients are at higher risk for developing lymphoproliferative disorders (LPD), above all non-Hodgkin's lymphomas (NHL). Even though the association between primary immunodeficiency diseases (e.g. X-linked lymphoproliferative syndrome, common variable immunodeficiency, ataxia telangiectasia and Wiskott–Aldrich syndrome) and LPDs, on the one hand, and between LPDs and autoimmune diseases, on the other, is well known, the leading causes of immunosuppression are considered at present to be organ transplantation and HIV infection. Generally, lymphomas in immunocompromised hosts differ from lymphomas in the general population in histopathological findings, increased extranodal involvement, a more aggressive clinical course, poorer response to conventional therapies and poorer outcome.

In patients who undergo solid-organ transplantation, the risk for lymphoma is strongly influenced by the type of organ transplanted: during the first year after kidney or heart transplantation it is 20 and 120 times higher, respectively, than in the general population. The majority of lymphomas develop within the first three months after transplantation, even if some cases are reported after prolonged immunodepression. Overall the risk of cancer in organ-transplant recipients is well known: the frequency of cancer after renal transplantation was reported to be 6% in the United States and 8.3% in the Nordic countries, that is 4.5–6.3 times higher than in the general population. In a large series of 1844 renal-transplant recipients in Italy a significantly increased incidence of Kaposi's sarcoma, cancers of the lip, liver and kidney, and NHL was observed.

The incidence of HIV-related NHLs (HIV-NHL) has increased since 1981. Primary brain lymphoma has recently been included in the CDC AIDS case definition, while systemic intermediate- to high-grade NHLs have been regarded as AIDS-defining illnesses since 1986. Since the onset of the HIV pandemic NHL is the second most frequent cancer – after Kaposi's sarcoma – in AIDS patients, with a homogeneous distribution among all HIV risk groups. The introduction of highly active antiretroviral therapy (HAART) into clinical practice has had a dramatic effect on the epidemiology of HIV-related tumors and also of NHLs. When pre- and post-HAART cancer incidence rates in HIV-positive individuals were compared, a considerable decrease in the incidence of Kaposi's sarcoma and also of primary central nervous system NHL was reported. In the case of systemic NHLs, most longitudinal studies in patients with HIV infection show reduced incidence rates after 1997, that is since HAART has become available. However, recent findings demonstrate a slight increase in systemic NHLs as an initial AIDS-defining diagnosis, which may be due to a sharp decline in the incidence of opportunistic infections and also to a remarkably improved survival of HIV-infected patients, although their immunodeficiency is a risk factor for lymphoma.

NHLs differ greatly in pathology and clinical features, but some common characteristics can indeed

Lymphoma: Pathology, Diagnosis and Treatment, ed. Robert Marcus, John W. Sweetenham and Michael E. Williams. Published by Cambridge University Press. © Cambridge University Press 2007.

be observed, including B-cell origin, high-grade histology and aggressive clinical behavior. Based on their pathology and clinical features, HIV-NHLs can be differentiated into systemic NHLs, primary brain lymphomas (PBLs) and primary effusion lymphomas (PELs).

According to the WHO classification, HIV-NHLs and post-transplant LPDs (PTLD) are clinically and pathologically independent entities, as against LPDs occurring in immunocompetent hosts. HIV-NHLs are usually B-cell origin with high-grade malignity, including small non-cleaved-cell lymphoma (SNCCL, 40%) and diffuse large B-cell lymphoma (DLBCL, 60%). SNCCL includes Burkitt's and Burkitt-like lymphoma; DLBCL incorporates large non-cleaved-cell lymphoma (LNCCL, 25%), immunoblastic lymphoma plasmocytoid (IBL-P, 25%) and CD30 (Ki-1)-positive B-cell anaplastic large-cell lymphoma (ALCL, 10%).

PATHOLOGY

Post-transplant lymphoproliferative disorders (PTLD)

Early lesions (plasmacytic hyperplasia, infectious mononucleosis-like)

There is partial or incomplete effacement of the lymph node or tonsil architecture and there may be reactive lymphoid follicles. In the plasmacytic hyperplasia cases the infiltrate consists predominantly of plasma cells with scanty immunoblasts, while the infectious mononucleosis cases have a polymorphous infiltrate, seen in primary Epstein–Barr virus (EBV) infections, with numerous immunoblasts in a background of T cells and plasma cells. Immunophenotypically the cells show a typical antigen expression for their cell types. The immunoblasts are typically positive for EBV LMP-1.

Polymorphic PTLD

There is effacement of the tissue by a polymorphic infiltrate including immunoblasts and plasma cells. These are differentiated from the early lesions by the presence of architectural effacement, but in contrast to typical lymphomas there is a mixture of cell types. In some cases these may resemble the "polymorphic immunocytoma" lesions previously described in earlier lymphoma classifications. There may be immunoblasts

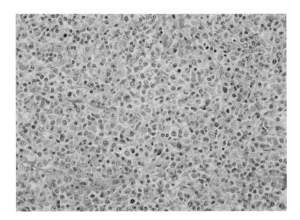

Figure 17.1. Post-transplant lymphoproliferative disorder. There is a sheet of lymphoid cells, all of which are large cells, although there is some pleomorphism consistent with a monomorphous post-transplant lymphoproliferative disorder resembling diffuse large B-cell lymphoma.

with markedly atypical, bizarre morphology, and necrosis is frequently present. Immunophenotypically the cells express appropriate antigens. The B cells may be either polytypic or monotypic for immunoglobulin. EBV LMP-1 is present in the immunoblasts in the majority of cases.

Monomorphic PTLD

These lesions are morphologically recognizable as lymphomas. They are usually B-cell and should be classified using terminology associated with the non-transplant setting. The majority of cases are DLBCL. Many of these are immunoblastic type, but a significant number show plasmablastic differentiation. Some cases are anaplastic, and a minority show features of Burkitt's lymphoma. Immunophenotypically the cells express CD20 and CD79a, and there is monotypic immunoglobulin expression in 50% of cases. The majority show EBV infection, with staining for LMP-1. Staining for CD43 and CD45RO is common. (Fig. 17.1).

Rarely the lesions have the appearance of plasmacytoma, and some post-transplant patients develop myeloma. These may or may not be associated with EBV infection.

Cases of T-cell lymphoma-like lesions are occasionally seen, and these show the morphology and immunophenotype of equivalent lesions in non-transplant patients. EBV detection is variable.

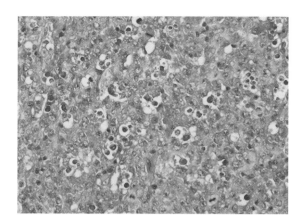

Figure 17.2. Lymphoma in HIV-positive patient. In this case the morphology is of diffuse large B-cell lymphoma. The cells have a high proliferation, and scattered macrophages with apoptotic debris give a "starry sky" appearance.

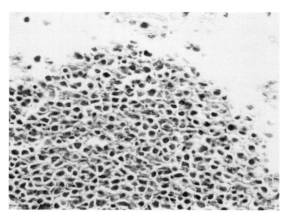

Figure 17.3. Primary effusion lymphoma (pleural effusion). A cluster of large cells within effusion fluid showing degenerative changes.

Hodgkin's-like PTLDs are also recognized, and these are classified as for those seen in non-transplant patients. The Reed–Sternberg cells are more commonly associated with B-cell antigen expression than in classical Hodgkin's lymphoma, and EBV is almost always seen.

Methotrexate-associated lymphoproliferative disorders

The morphology of these lesions is variable but the majority are DLBCL, lymphoplasmacytic lymphoma or Hodgkin's lymphoma. Less frequently they are follicular, while Burkitt's and T-cell lymphomas are rare. The immunophenotype is similar to that seen for the lymphoma types seen in the immunocompetent patient, but EBV is present in about 50% of cases.

HIV-associated lymphomas

Morphologically the lymphomas share features that are similar to those seen in the immunocompetent patient (Fig. 17.2). About 30% of cases have features similar to those seen in classical Burkitt's lymphoma, and of these about 30% will be associated with EBV. Burkitt's lymphoma with plasmablastic differentiation appears to be almost confined to the AIDS setting, and is characterized by cells with more abundant cytoplasm and an eccentric nucleus that contains a central nucleolus. EBV can be demonstrated in 50–75% of these cases. A proportion of cases will have the appearance of diffuse large B-cell lymphomas, composed of centroblasts with a variable number of immunoblasts. These lymphomas account for about 25% of HIV-associated lymphomas and are associated with EBV in almost a third of cases. Immunoblastic lymphomas are rarer (10% of HIV-associated lymphoma) but are more frequently associated with EBV (90%) and account for most of the primary CNS lymphomas in this setting. Other lymphomas that are seen more specifically in the HIV patient include primary effusion lymphoma (Fig. 17.3) and plasmablastic lymphoma of the oral cavity.

MOLECULAR PATHOLOGY AND CYTOGENETICS

Lymphoproliferative disorders in patients who are immunosuppressed for various reasons represent a spectrum of diseases different from that of sporadic lymphomas. Genetic studies aiming at the identification of a clonal lymphoproliferation and the presence of chromosomal/molecular alterations may be crucial in determining both prognosis and treatment.

Primary immune disorders (PID)

Lymphoproliferations occurring in primary immune disorders are variable both morphologically and with respect to biology. This variability reflects the pathogenetic heterogeneity of the disorders. With

Table 17.1. Molecular genetic features in PTLD.

Category	IgH clonality	EBV status	Oncogene/tumor suppressor gene alterations
Early lesion PTLD	Polyclonal	Absent Polyclonal Clonal	Absent
Polymorphic PTLD	Monoclonal Oligoclonal	Clonal	Present
Monomorphic PTLD	Monoclonal	Clonal	Present

the notable exception of ataxia telangiectasia (AT), lymphoproliferative disorders arising in the setting of PID are usually of B-cell lineage, and DLBCL is the most common form of PID-LPD. These tumors are frequently associated with Epstein–Barr virus (EBV) infection owing to impaired immune surveillance. Monoclonal IgH rearrangements are found in cases morphologically corresponding to malignant lymphoma.

Post-transplant lymphoproliferative disorders (PTLD)

In early lesions of infectious mononucleosis-like PTLD or plasmacytic hyperplasia that occur early after organ transplantation (3–4 months), an EBV infection can be demonstrated in many instances, especially in infectious mononucleosis-like lesions. Tandem repeat analyses have revealed polyclonal, oligoclonal or monoclonal virus populations. Usually, no distinctly monoclonal rearrangements of IgH genes can be detected, and chromosomal alterations are notably absent.

Polymorphic PTLD is associated with EBV in most cases, with the viral antigen expression profile usually suggesting EBV latency types 2 or 3. In polymorphic PTLD, clonality analyses usually reveal monoclonal or (rarely) oligoclonal tumor-cell populations. Interestingly enough, the investigation of multiple tumor nodules within one organ (e.g. gastrointestinal tract) may show different clones in each lesion.

Monomorphic PTLD is morphologically identical to sporadic aggressive lymphomas. EBV infection is usually present and, as in polymorphic PTLD, monoclonal EBV episomes are the rule. Cases with latency type 1 may occur. Monomorphic PTLD usually harbor monoclonal tumor-cell populations (Table 17.1).

The analysis of genetic alterations may be of major biological and clinical importance in PTLD. Early lesions characteristically lack genetic alterations, as has been shown for *BCL-1*, *BCL-2*, *MYC*, *RAS*, *TP53* and other genes. In contrast, polymorphic PTLD in part and monomorphic PTLD as a rule are characterized by structural alterations in several of these genes, indicating the evolution of genetically altered, autonomous cell clones. The analysis of the configuration of *BCL-6* suggests that structural alterations of this gene in the process of somatic hypermutation are an important step in the progression of PTLD. The presence of *BCL-6* mutations has been shown to strongly predict for shorter survival and refractoriness to reduced immunosuppression and/or surgical excision of tumors. More recently, CGH analysis has also suggested the occurrence of non-random chromosomal imbalances in hotspot regions such as 8q24, 3q27 and others. Moreover, CGH alterations detected in monomorphic PTLD were similar to those known from sporadic lymphomas in immunocompetent patients.

Methotrexate-associated lymphoproliferative disorders

The most characteristic clinical setting for the occurrence of these disorders is represented by methotrexate (MTX) treatment in rheumatoid disorders like rheumatoid arthritis or polymyositis. The majority of the cases are associated with EBV, and MTX treatment may, besides inducing immunosuppression, also facilitate EBV reactivation.

Apart from the genetic features discussed above pertaining to both immunodeficiency-related and sporadic lymphomas, lymphoproliferations occurring in immunologically compromised patients may also display some genetic alterations not, or only rarely, encountered in sporadic tumors in immuno-competent hosts. Thus, the mutator phenotype eli-cited by mutations/inactivations of DNA mismatch repair genes has been exclusively demonstrated in HIV-associated NHL and PTLD, but not in a large cohort of sporadic lymphomas.

HIV-associated lymphomas

Lymphomas occurring in the setting of infection with HIV are aggressive neoplasms in most instances. IgH genes are rearranged in the vast majority of tumors, and EBV association is variable, depending on the histological subtype and the site of origin. IgV$_H$ ana-lysis has shown somatically mutated genes in most cases.

HIV-associated Burkitt's lymphoma (BL) generally harbors, like its sporadic counterpart, translocations involving *MYC*, and point mutations of the gene have also been detected. HIV-related DLBCLs, frequently of immunoblastic/plasmablastic type, also harbor *MYC* alterations in a proportion (20%) of cases. In contrast to BL, they often show deregulation of *BCL-6*, either via translocations or by mutations of the 5′ noncoding region of the gene. *RAS* mutations may be a character-istic feature in HIV-associated DLBCL. *TP53* muta-tions/deletions have been demonstrated in both BL and DLBCL arising in the setting of HIV-associated immunodeficiency. A number of proto-oncogenes involved in signal transduction or transcription (*PIM1*, *PAX5*, *MYC* and *RhoH/TTF*) are targeted by aberrant somatic hypermutation in HIV-related lym-phoid neoplasms, thus possibly deregulating their transcription.

CLINICAL PRESENTATION AND INVESTIGATIONS

Clinical features and natural history of NHLs in immunosuppressed patients differ greatly from those observed in the general population. In most patients lymphomas are clinically advanced, with fre-quent – sometimes unusual – extranodal involve-ment: central nervous system, bone marrow, colon and rectum, skin, heart and ureter. Exact causes for this clinical presentation are unknown, but they could be ascribed to defects in the various adhesion molecules. In the general population over 60% of

NHLs are confined to the lymph nodes, but it is rare to find an NHL in an immunosuppressed patient that does not have evidence of extranodal involvement. At onset, NHLs in immunosuppressed hosts fall within Ann Arbor stages III and IV in over 70% of the cases, with extranodal involvement in 70–98%. The most common extranodal sites are the gastrointestinal tract, the bone marrow and the central nervous sys-tem. The most common symptoms – besides site-specific features – are fever, night sweats and marked weight loss at the time of diagnosis (75%). Typically, NHLs are bulky (nodal masses > 10 cm in diameter) with a rapid growth rate, and serum lactate dehydro-genase (LDH) levels are well above the normal range. Staging must include CT scans of the chest, abdomen, pelvis and brain, and bone-marrow biopsy. Further investigations should be carried out only if clinically indicated. Moreover, a lumbar puncture must be per-formed to exclude meningeal involvement, which is reported – most often asymptomatically – in almost 20% of the patients.

POST-TRANSPLANT LYMPHOPROLIFERATIVE DISORDERS

Post-transplant lymphoproliferative disorders are a well-recognized and potentially life-threatening com-plication after solid-organ transplantation. PTLD is a relatively common malignancy after transplantation and is seen in up to 10% of all solid-organ transplant recipients. It is the most common form of post-transplant malignancy in children, and in adults it is the second most common malignancy after skin can-cer. In both children and adults it is the most common cause of cancer-related mortality after solid-organ transplantation, and the reported overall mortality for PTLD often exceeds 50%. Up to 85% of PTLDs are of B-cell lineage and most of these (over 80%) are associated with EBV infection. Around 10–15% of PTLDs are of T-cell lineage, around 30% of which are associated with EBV.

Etiology and presentation

According to WHO classification, PLTD can be divided into three groups: (a) diffuse B-cell hyper-plasia, characterized by differentiated plasma cells and preservation of the normal lymphoid archi-tecture; (b) polymorphic PTLD, characterized by nuclear atypia, tumor necrosis and destruction of the underlying lymphoid architecture; (c) mono-morphic PTLD, including high-grade invasive lymphoma of B- or T-lymphocyte centroblasts. Monomorphic B-cell PTLD can be further divided into diffuse large-cell lymphomas and Burkitt's or Burkitt's-like lymphomas that display characteristic chromosomal translocations. Monomorphic T-cell PTLD can be further divided according to whether it is large-cell, anaplastic or unspecified in type. EBV is closely involved in the pathogenesis of PTLD, and the majority of cases of PTLD arise in response to primary infection with EBV or reactivation of pre-viously acquired EBV. The incidence of PTLD after solid-organ transplantation is markedly different in children and adults, and also varies according to the type of organ transplant. In adult recipients, PTLD has been reported to occur in 1.0–2.3% of kidney transplants, 1.0–2.8% of liver transplants, 1.0–6.3% of heart transplants, 2.4–5.8% of heart–lung trans-plants, 4.2–10% of lung transplants and up to 20% of small-bowel transplants. The incidence of PTLD is significantly higher in pediatric recipients, and has been reported in 1.2–10.1% of kidney transplants, 4–15% of liver transplants and 6.4–19.5% of lung, heart and heart-lung transplants.

Although PTLD may occur at any time after trans-plantation, the risk of developing PTLD is greater within the first year and declines over time thereafter. A report by the Transplant Collaborative Study showed the incidence of PTLD to be 224/100 000 in the first year, 54/100 000 in the second year and 31/ 100 000 in the sixth year following transplantation. PTLD arises, in large part, as a consequence of the potent immunosuppressive agents necessary to pre-vent allograft rejection. The risk following adminis-tration of specific immunosuppressive agents is still a matter of controversy. The incidence of lymphomas was found to increase after the introduction of cyclo-sporine but it turned out that this was due to the influence of other risk co-factors. In other large series, treatment with cyclosporine did not enhance the risk for lymphoma compared to azathioprine therapy. However, a number of small retrospective studies have suggested that the routine introduction of cyclosporine as an immunosuppressive agent in the 1980s was associated with an increased incidence of PTLD. Experiences with FK506-based immunosup-pression and tacrolimus are limited, although an increased incidence of lymphomas has been reported in both adults and children. It has been speculated that the intensity of the immunosuppression, rather than an individual agent, plays a key role in the devel-opment of lymphoma, which is supported by the higher incidence of lymphoma in non-renal trans-plant recipients receiving higher doses of immuno-suppression. Moreover, patients who have weakened immune systems prior to transplantation, such as the elderly or those with pre-existing cytomegalovirus (CMV) infection, may be particularly vulnerable to over-immunosuppression and hence PTLD.

Therapy

The management of PTLD poses a major therapeutic challenge, and although there is reasonable agree-ment about the overall principles of treatment, there is still considerable controversy about the optimal treatment of individual patients.

Surgical resection and/or local radiotherapy should be considered in patients with suitable loca-lized disease. The initial treatment in all patients with PTLD is to reduce immunosuppression in the hope that this will increase anti-tumor activity. The approach to reducing immunosuppressive therapy needs to be carefully individualized and will depend on the nature and extent of disease and the type of transplant recipient, i.e. whether they have a life-supporting graft (e.g. heart) or non-life-supporting graft (e.g. kidney). Cyclosporine or tacrolimus dosage are typically reduced, over 4–6 weeks, to give whole-blood trough levels of around 25–50% of normal therapeutic level, depending on the extent of disease and type of graft. Anti-proliferative drugs such as azathioprine or mycophenolate mofetil should be reduced or stopped. A response to reduc-tion in immunosuppression is usually seen within 2–4 weeks, with a long-term remission of around 50–60%. Generally, polyclonal PTLD developing dur-ing the first year after transplantation (early disease) responds well to reduced immunosuppression, whereas monoclonal tumors are unresponsive to a reduction in immunosuppression and have a very high mortality.

Chemotherapy is commonly used in the treatment of PTLD when reduction in immunosuppression fails to control the disease. It is also often used in combi-nation with reduced immunosuppression as initial

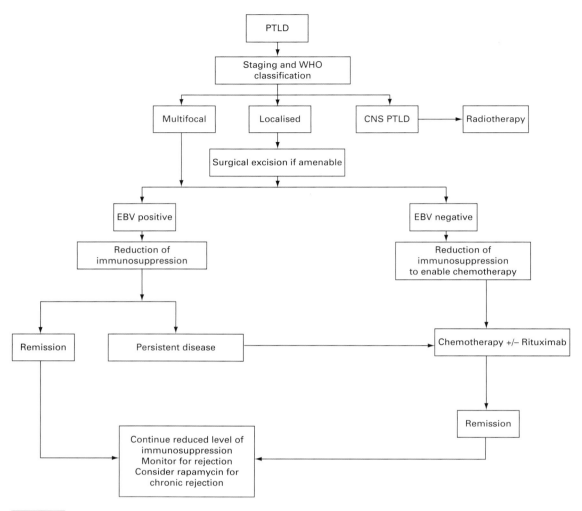

Figure 17.4. Treatment algorithm for post-transplant lymphoproliferative disorders.

therapy for the more aggressive monoclonal types of PTLD seen in late disease. With the use of standard chemotherapy regimens (CHOP, VACOP-B, VAPEC-B) the complete response (CR) rate was 40–60%, with a high mortality from treatment-related toxicity. Considering the high toxicity rate of chemotherapy and the short duration of CR, other approaches have been tested. Since PTLD is usually due to neoplastic proliferation of B cells, the use of monoclonal antibodies to deplete B cells is a logical therapeutic approach, and rituximab has been recently used in the treatment of patients with PTLD after solid-organ transplantation as an adjunct to reduction of immunosuppression or chemotherapy. From the analysis

of small published series, rituximab appears to improve the remission rate of PTLD when used in combination with other therapies, even if it does not restore the cytotoxic T-lymphocyte (CTL) function essential for long-term EBV control, and relapse may therefore be a problem. Interferon α and anti-IL-6 have been tried as adjuvants along with reduction, but at present there is insufficient evidence to recommend their routine use. Adoptive T-cell therapy using EBV-specific CTL lines has generated considerable recent interest as a treatment for PTLD. This approach has been used with success as prophylaxis and treatment of PTLD after stem-cell transplantation using CTL lines derived from the donor and specific for EBV gene products. However, further clinical trials focusing on the safety of this approach are needed to confirm these promising preliminary results.

A treatment algorithm for PTLD is shown in Figure 17.4.

HIV-ASSOCIATED LYMPHOMAS

Non-Hodgkin's lymphomas

Since the introduction of HAART into clinical practice, the outcome for patients with HIV-related tumors has improved. In recent years a huge amount of published data has demonstrated the beneficial effect of HAART on the clinical presentation of NHLs in HIV-positive patients. A comparison between the clinical features of the disease in HAART-treated and HAART-naive patients has shown that the patients who develop NHLs while taking HAART are older and present with a minor degree of extranodal involvement, especially of bone marrow and meninges. Unfortunately, patients with post-HAART HIV-NHL still have a significantly worse outlook than HIV-negative individuals with aggressive NHLs. Burkitt's lymphoma is more frequent in HIV-infected patients, and they present with more advanced disease, more extensive extranodal involvement (most commonly gastrointestinally), higher IPI score and frequently higher LDH levels. HAART has a positive impact on outcome for patients receiving antiretroviral therapy, with survival and disease-free progression significantly better than in HAART-naive patients; above all, a significantly improved disease-free survival rate (possibly a result of the improved immune deficit) has been reported. But when the outcome of patients with HIV-NHL is compared to that of HIV-negative patients with NHL, overall survival is shorter in the first group, maybe because of the lower CR rates, even if response-adjusted overall survival is similar in both groups. However, it has to be recognized that in the HAART era a curative care takes priority over a palliative approach in all patients, regardless of their HIV status.

Therapy

There is still much controversy regarding treatment of HIV-NHLs. Based on the pathology and clinical features, aggressive chemotherapy treatment would be required, but this is often incompatible with the complications related to the underlying HIV infection. Chemotherapy-induced anemia may actually further compromise the immune cell function of patients with HIV infection, which would in turn induce the occurrence of opportunistic infections and/or the progression of the infection. Last but not least, leukopenia, which is frequently observed because of HIV-related myelodysplastic alterations of the bone marrow in this population, makes the use of conventional chemotherapy regimens very difficult. The reduced chemotherapy-related hematological tolerance reduces the dose intensity of antiproliferative agents but also increases morbidity due to opportunistic infections occurring during the treatment. Because of the role of the immune deficit as a prognostic factor, and also because of the virological and clinical effects of antiretroviral therapy, it is recommended to combine HAART with antiproliferative agents even if the combined treatment may induce crossed myelotoxicity, which requires the administration of hematopoietic growth factors, and in particular of G-CSF, a cytokine that causes no increases in HIV replication.

The prospective studies on the treatment of HIV-NHLs that were performed in the pre-HAART era, or that were started before the introduction of the new antiretroviral agents, belong to three major research lines. The first, followed by American investigators, involves low-dose chemotherapy protocols that are administered indiscriminately to all patients; the second research approach, supported by European investigators, consists of different dose-intensity treatment protocols stratified by risk group (good, intermediate and poor prognosis); the third research line, another American approach, includes the administration by continuous-infusion chemotherapy to patients who have not been stratified by risk group. Low-dose m-BACOD (methotrexate, bleomycin, doxorubicin, cyclophosphamide, vincristine, dexamethasone) is associated with CR rates (46–56%) and median survival (6.5–8 months) that are comparable with those achieved with standard doses (CR > 50%, median survival 7–8 months), but severe toxicity (G3–G4 according to WHO) is significantly lower with the administration of lower doses (51% vs. 70%, $p < 0.008$).

In May 1993, the European Intergroup NHL-HIV Study started the first randomized study on the effectiveness of different dose-intensity chemotherapy regimens in the treatment of NHL, with patients stratified by presence/absence of certain prognostic factors ($CD4 < 100/\mu L$, prior AIDS diagnosis, performance status ≥ 2). A total of 485 patients were enrolled, but the study results refer only to patients that were followed up for at least one year. In the low-risk group (no unfavorable prognostic factors) patients were randomized between the intensive ACVBP (doxorubicin, cyclophosphamide, vindesine, bleomycin, prednisone) regimen and the less aggressive CHOP (cyclophosphamide, doxorubicin, vincristine, prednisone) therapy with G-CSF support. In the intermediate-risk group (only one unfavorable prognostic factor) randomization was between CHOP and low-dose CHOP (reduced by 50%). In the high-risk group (two or three unfavorable prognostic factors) patients were randomized between low-dose CHOP and palliative vincristine plus prednisone. In the low-risk group both ACVBP and CHOP arms reached similar CR (66% vs. 60%) and five-year survival rates (51% vs. 47%). In the intermediate-risk group, the CR rate was significantly higher after standard CHOP than with low-dose CHOP (49% vs. 32%, $p < 0.05$), even though five-year overall survival rates were similar (28% vs. 24%).

In the high-risk group the CR rate was much higher in the low-dose CHOP arm than in the group that had received vincristine plus prednisone (20% vs. 5%). The five-year overall survival rates were similar (11% for low-dose CHOP vs. 3% for vincristine plus prednisone). The only factors influencing survival rates were the administration of HAART, HIV score and the IPI score. Investigators concluded that the study, which was terminated before monoclonal antibodies became available, showed that CHOP was the standard chemotherapy regimen for HIV-related NHLs, as for NHLs in the general population, and that increasing the treatment dose-intensity in patients with good prognosis had no effect on outcome.

Continuous infusional CDE (cyclophosphamide, doxorubicin, etoposide) for four days is the first study protocol within the third research line concerning treatment of HIV-related NHLs. The rationale for this study was provided by preclinical evidence suggesting that continuous infusional administration of antiproliferative agents is more effective than administration in bolus. With the CDE regimen CR was 45%, two-year overall was survival 43% and two-year

failure-free survival was 36%. The prevalence of severe opportunistic infections during chemotherapy and follow-up was 14%, and once again HAART had a positive impact on the patients' outcome, with improved survival and lower toxicity rates. The new continuous infusional "dose-modified" EPOCH (etoposide, prednisone, vincristine, cyclophosphamide, doxorubicin) regimen, in which cyclophosphamide dose adjustment was based on CD4-positive cell count (cycle 1) and then on myelotoxicity (cycles 2–6), has been used so far to treat good-prognosis patients (median $CD4 > 200/\mu L$). Preliminary results are very satisfactory in terms of CR (74%), progression-free (92%) and overall survival rates (60%) at 53 months.

Monoclonal antibodies

In recent years, the introduction of rituximab has significantly improved the survival of NHL patients in the general population, compared with patients receiving CHOP alone. Based on these data, several authors have explored the feasibility and effectiveness of rituximab in combination with chemotherapy in patients with HIV-related NHL. The Italian Cooperative Group on AIDS and Tumors (GICAT) examined the administration of rituximab (375 mg/m^2 on day 1) plus infusional CDE (cyclophosphamide 187.5 mg/m^2 per day, doxorubicin 12.5 mg/m^2 per day, etoposide 60 mg/m^2 per day, administered by continuous intravenous infusion for four days) every four weeks for a total of six cycles, with concomitant HAART and G-CSF support. In all, 74 patients were enrolled and 75% of them responded to treatment, with 70% reaching CR and 5% partial response (PR). Treatment-related toxicity was acceptable in this patient setting except for infectious events: 19 non-opportunistic infections developed in 23% of the patients during neutropenia, and 14% of the patients were diagnosed with AIDS-defining opportunistic infections during chemotherapy or in the first three months after conclusion of the treatment plan. After a median follow-up of 16 months (range 1–57 months), median survival had not been reached, with a two-year overall survival rate of 62%, disease-free survival 89% and progression-free survival 86%. Univariate analysis identified Burkitt histotype, homosexual lifestyle and positive viremia at the end of chemotherapy as negative prognostic factors, whereas multivariate analysis showed that only Burkitt histotype and

Swinnen, L. J. Organ transplant-related lymphoma. *Curr. Treat. Options Oncol.* **2** (2001), 301–308.

Taylor, A. R., Marcus, R. and Bradley, J. A. Post-transplant lymphoproliferative disorders (PTLD) after solid organ transplantation. *Crit. Rev. Oncol. Hematol.* **56** (2005), 155–167.

Vaccher, E., Spina, M., di Gennaro, G. *et al.* Concomitant cyclophosphamide, doxorubicin, vincristine, and prednisone chemotherapy plus highly active antiretroviral therapy in patients with human immunodeficiency virus-related, non-Hodgkin lymphoma. *Cancer* **91** (2001), 155–163.

Vaccher, E., Tirelli, U., Spina, M. *et al.* Age and serum LDH level are independent prognostic factors in HIV related non-Hodgkin's lymphoma: a single institution study of 96 patients. *J. Clin. Oncol.* **14** (1996), 2217–2223.

INDEX